# Native American Health

*Then and Now*

By

**Sue Johnson**

Native American Health: Then and Now

By Sue Johnson

This book first published 2024

Ethics International Press Ltd, UK

British Library Cataloguing in Publication Data

A catalogue record for this book is available from the British Library

Print Book ISBN: 978-1-80441-385-2

eBook ISBN: 978-1-80441-386-9

# Dedication

This book would not have been possible without the support and mentoring of two valued colleagues: Pamela Dickerson, PhD, RN, NPDA-BC®, FAAN and Eric Wurzbacher, BA.

Their input and advice was invaluable and enabled me to explore Indigenous perspectives on health and healing then and now.

I second John Lowe's sentiments in the Preface, that this study "serve as a catalyst for dialogue, reflection, and ultimately, positive change". Our Indigenous people deserve no less.

# Table of Contents

# Index of tribes covered in this book

# Preface

Before the Pilgrims landed and the Virginia colony began, what is now the United States was populated by multiple indigenous tribes. Each tribal society practiced its own customs to promote health—physical, social, emotional, spiritual, and intellectual. This is the story of those health and healing practices and how interactions with settlers and explorers affected their health—then and now.

Native tribes are in multiple locations throughout the United States and many of them were relocated (voluntarily or involuntarily) to different geographic regions. To help the reader understand health & healing and impact of health on interaction with White culture, each tribe's entries will begin where the tribe originated and progress to their current location(s).

# Foreword

As we embark on this compelling journey through the pages of "Native American Health—Then & Now," we are invited to explore the rich tapestry of Indigenous tribes that inhabited what is now the United States. As a Native American, I appreciate this exploration as not merely a historical chronicle but an essential understanding of the intricate relationship between these tribes and their holistic approach to health – physical, social, emotional, spiritual, and intellectual.

The author, drawing from a deeply personal connection to the subject matter, takes us back to their roots in Bradford, Pennsylvania, near the Seneca Reservation at Onoville, New York. This proximity unveils an intimate perspective on the impacts of historical events like the construction of the Kinzua Dam a project that reshaped landscapes and, more importantly, disrupted the lives and traditions of the Seneca Nation.

The narrative unfolds with a poignant reflection on the consequences of the dam's construction, highlighting the forced relocation of communities, loss of homes, and the erosion of cultural practices. Through the lens of the Seneca Nation's struggle against the backdrop of the Flood Control Act of 1936, we witness the tragic collision of promises made and promises broken, as the United States Supreme Court ruled against the tribe, relying on racist ideologies.

The author's exploration of this historical injustice serves as a microcosm of the broader narrative woven throughout this book. From the New England Tribes to Native Hawaiians, each chapter unearths the unique health and healing practices of Indigenous peoples while shedding light on the enduring impact of colonial encounters. These encounters, often marked by displacement, violence, and cultural suppression, have left indelible marks on the physical, social, emotional, spiritual, and intellectual well-being of Native American communities.

As we delve into the chapters that traverse the diverse regions of the United States, we are confronted with the stark realities faced by

Indigenous tribes – the Carlisle Indian Industrial School's assimilation efforts, the harrowing Trail of Tears during the Southern Tribes' Removal Period, and the complex dynamics of Tribal Gaming in the Midwest. Additionally, we examine the pervasive issue of violence against Native women among the Great Plains Tribes, the intricacies of tribal government and recognition in the Rocky Mountain Tribes, and the challenges posed by the Bureau of Indian Affairs and reservations in the Southwest.

The author's narrative prowess guides us through the intricate tapestry of Indigenous experiences, weaving together stories of resilience, cultural reclamation, and the ongoing pursuit of holistic health. It is a poignant reminder that the history of Native American tribes is not confined to the past; it reverberates through time, impacting generations and shaping the present reality.

This book stands as a testament to the resilience of Indigenous peoples, urging readers to reflect on the importance of understanding and respecting the diverse health and healing practices that have sustained these communities for centuries. As we turn each page, let us be mindful of the collective responsibility to acknowledge the profound contributions of the First Americans and strive for a future marked by mutual respect, understanding, and healing.

May this exploration into Indigenous perspectives on health and healing serve as a catalyst for dialogue, reflection, and, ultimately, positive change.

John Lowe, RN, PhD, FAAN


Joseph Blades Centennial Memorial Professor in Nursing
Director: Indigenous Nursing Research Enhancement (INRE) Post-Doc
Fellowship Program
Faculty Affiliate Native American and Indigenous Studies
The University of Texas, Austin, Texas

# Introduction

This is my seventh book, and it is truly special to me. I was born and raised in Bradford, Pennsylvania 15 miles from the Seneca Reservation at Onoville, New York. In 1960 when I was a high school freshman, the U.S. Army Corps of Engineers began construction of what would become the Kinzua Dam to protect Pittsburgh from flooding and pollution. I didn't understand the legal or tribal issues. I just remembered that the great Seneca chief Cornplanter was buried in a cemetery on reservation land that would be flooded. Supposedly, he was reinterred on higher land and his marker was removed to reflect this. I went to the new site a few years later overlooking the new Kinzua Dam to see his marker.

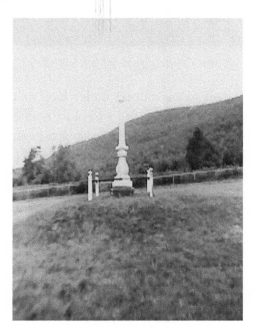

*Cornplanter Memorial 1970*

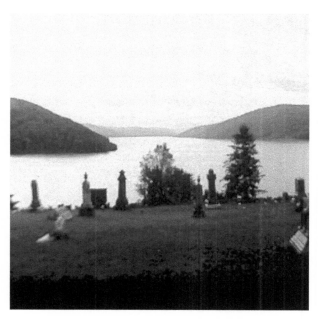

*Cornplanter Cemetery overlooking Kinzua Bay 1970*

I knew the Seneca had towns buried under tons of water, but didn't understand how it all happened until I was older and studied the history of the area. When Pittsburgh flooded in 1936, Congress passed the Flood Control Act of 1936. After World War II and Korea, Congress and the Corps of Engineers moved forward with construction of a dam that would eventually cost the Seneca nine communities and 10,000 acres of their Allegany Territory. 600 people lost their homes when residents were forcibly relocated and their towns burned. The Seneca tried to legally challenge the Dam based on the Treaty of Canandaigua of 1794. The treaty established Seneca territory as all of Western New York. According to the treaty negotiated with George Washington's consent, "the United States will never claim the same, nor disturb the Seneka Nation ... in the free use and enjoyment thereof: but it shall remain theirs, until they choose to sell the same to the people of the United States, who have the right to purchase." (Diaz-Gonzalez, 2020).

The Seneca Nation believed in Washington's promises and the treaty and fought the case to the Supreme Court. In ruling against the tribe, the Court relied on racist ideas to defend their decision. Allowing the federal government to displace the Seneca Citizens, they used a passage from an earlier case *Beecher v. Weatherby* that the government would "be governed by such considerations of justice as would control a Christian people in their treatment of an ignorant and dependent race" (Diaz-Gonzalez, 2020).

The tribe hired a civil engineer who believed the Kinzua Dam was not an optimal flooding solution. He developed and presented the Conewango-Cattaraugus Plan for a diversion dam near Coldspring, New York. The plan had several advantages, including having Lake Erie as an outlet with much greater water storage. Flood protection would increase, there would be more opportunities for hydropower exploration, and the lake at Conewango didn't have the seasonal fluctuations of Allegany Reservoir. He and the Seneca Nation delayed the project for three years with support from celebrities like Eleanor Roosevelt and Johnny Cash. However, in 1957 the Corps hired an engineering firm to evaluate all plans. The Corps was the firm's largest client and they stated that the Conewango-Cattaraugus plan would cost too much.

Groundbreaking began in 1960 and losses were not just physical. The New York State public education system had pushed assimilation for Native children for many years. The Seneca language could not be spoken in school and the loss of homes affected traditional Seneca life, including use of the language at home. According to Stephen Gordon, a Seneca elder, "They wanted us to become a part of the melting pot. And in order to do that, it was important that the education system drill it into us that you have to learn English, you have to learn mathematics, you have to learn history. And that your history doesn't matter" (Diaz-Gonzalez, 2020).

Since its completion in 1965, the Kinzua Dam operates by the Corps varying the amount of water in the 27-mile-long Allegany Reservoir-holding it during heavy precipitation and releasing it in dry spells. Most of the sediment is near the reservoir's northern border in the Seneca Allegany Territory. Climate change and water-resistant structures and roads in the floodplain are causing flooding upstream to communities that never experienced flooding before (Diaz-Gonzalez, 2020).

The Seneca Nation has worked successfully to reclaim its culture, language, and ceremonies so its young people can integrate these into their lives. They continue to love their remaining land and care for it as their ancestors did.

What happened to the Seneca also happened and still happens to other Native American tribes. Their painful history is not unique, but Whites like me must understand what these indigenous people brought to the land we know as the United States and how interaction with White culture has impacted their physical, social, emotional, spiritual, and intellectual health.

They deserve our respect as the First Americans!

Sue Johnson

# Chapter 1
# New England Tribes

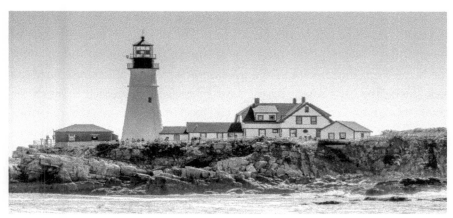

Several tribes lived in the New England area prior to and after the arrival of White settlers. They were the Abenaki, Micmac, Pennacook, Pequot, Mohegan, Narragansett, Nipmuc, Woronoco, and Wampanoag tribes.

## *Abenaki*

Abenaki means People of the Eastern Dawn and the tribe lived in Vermont, New Hampshire and parts of Massachusetts and Maine as well as in eastern Canada. Currently, there are four state recognized Abenaki tribes in Vermont and other Abenaki tribes that are not state or federally recognized. Each of the four state recognized tribes has its own website: the Elnu Abenaki Tribe of Southern Vermont; the Koasek Traditional Band of the Koas Abenaki Nation in Central Vermont; the Abenaki Nation of Missisquoi St Francis/Sokoki Band; and the Nulhegan Band of the Coosuk Tribe Abenaki Nation (Abenaki Arts & Education Center, 2018).

**Note:** State and Federal recognition will be discussed in a later chapter.

## Health & Healing Then

The Abenaki word for medicine is Nebizun. Its root word Nebi is Abenaki for water, which was important for its healing powers, highways for travel and maintaining the plants, fish, birds, animals, and other wildlife essential to the Abenaki way of life (Longtoe Sheehan, 2022). Healers or shamans, mostly male, routinely went alone into the woods for fasts of several days where they received a sacred prayer, ritual or healing medicine from the Creator. They used a variety of treatments to cure the sick including sweating, herbs, and plant-based medicines such as laxatives, salves, and teas. They also believed in special, magical remedies using dance and symbols. When the person was near death, food was withheld, a practice that occurs in modern society where dying individuals may refuse food and fluids (encyclopedia.com, 2018).

## Health & Healing Now

Today a female spiritual elder uses traditional Abenaki medicine to help people dealing with homelessness, divorce, addiction, abuse, sexual violence, or suicidal ideation. She spent many years learning the prayers, sacred rituals, and ceremonies she uses to voluntarily provide spiritual guidance. She believes that services like hers should be free and does refer individuals in active withdrawal or psychiatric crisis to agencies that can provide intensive support and treatment. Suicide prevention is especially important because Abenaki believe the spirit of a person who has committed suicide is trapped between two worlds and must seek the Creator's forgiveness before moving on. This healer willingly shares her knowledge with all who ask and supports Abenaki who don't know about their native traditions. This may include officiating at a baby naming ceremony or praying at the bedside of a dying relative. Besides keeping the Abenaki health traditions alive today, the healer has acceptance by Abenaki people who distrust mainstream White culture (Picard, 2019).

## Impact on Health of Interaction with White Culture Then

Other history texts will relate the impact of wars and colonization on indigenous tribes. Since the focus of this manuscript is on health practices then and now, the story of eugenics and the Abenaki people is applicable here. In the early 1900s public and private agencies were created in Vermont to help needy children. Between 1925-1928 the Eugenics Survey of Vermont conducted research and identified families the surveyors considered degenerate. The Vermont Commission on Country Life was created in the following three years to promote positive eugenics and "normal" families. After 1931 Vermonters were educated about eugenics and how to solve the problem of the "unfit" in the state with sterilization as an option. Since some Abenaki had intermarried with French Canadians, the Abenaki were considered to have "bad heredity" making them targets for sterilization until 1957 (uvm.edu, 2013). Young women were sterilized at 15 without knowledge about what the procedure meant for their future. Being listed in the eugenics survey resulted in denying Abenaki heritage (Hardy, 2021).

This tragic period of ethnocide (killing of culture) included a mental intent to destroy as well as physical sterilization to prevent procreation.

## Impact on Health of Interaction with White Culture Now

Vermont has acknowledged and apologized for state-sanctioned eugenics and the Abenaki Alliance is willing to work with the newly appointed Truth and Reconciliation Commission by sharing their cultural and lived experiences to create more positive, beneficial, and compassionate relationships. They are using physical, social, emotional, spiritual, and intellectual health to help create a more inclusive future for the tribe and other Vermonters (Abenaki.edu.org, 2023).

## *Micmac*

The Micmac (Mi'kmaq) Nation is located in Presque Isle, Maine. Twenty-seven other bands live in Canada. Micmac means "my kin-friends". The tribe was federally recognized in 1991. They continue to make a variety of traditional baskets and work on economic opportunities (Micmac-nsn.gov, 2023).

## Health & Healing Then

Medicine to the Micmac tribe was a spiritual way to heal illnesses of body, mind and spirit. Sacred plant medicines were given to villages with sick people by strangers who were plant persons in human form. After the villagers helped the stranger, he showed them his true identity and showed them how to prepare medicinal plants by putting them in teas. Some of these plants were strawberry, teaberry, sweet flag, yellow birch and pine. If the illness was severe, the afflicted person was concerned about an evil eye or bewitchment. Shamans called 'puoins' were called to share their spiritual knowledge to cure the sick person. The puoin would ask the sick person about dreams and activities to determine the cause of the illness and what medicines to use. The puoin also sang special songs and dances to help draw out the illness. When this happened, he would put the illness into an object so the sick person could destroy the object to aid in recovery (Mic-nsn.gov, 2023).

The Micmac also used medicine bags or pouches worn around the neck. These bags contained medicine to fight off illness. Contents included herbs to drink in tea and symbols for strength and power, such as a bear claw. The puoin selected the contents of the medicine bag. Along with stones, bones, and rattles made from declawed animals, the bags contained birchbark figures to represent spirits. The rattles and singing by the puoin were integral in returning the sick person to health (Mic-nsn.gov, 2023).

## Health & Healing Now

Today the Micmac (Mi'kmaq) Nation has a health clinic that includes grief counseling, chronic disease management, community health services that include health maintenance (diabetes, heart health, elder health, youth health), home and workplace safety, assistance in accessing health care services, and referrals and tracking outreach services (Mic-nsn.gov, 2023).

The behavioral health program respects each person's path to recovery and well-being while honoring the cultural beliefs of the community. Behavioral health providers offer several services in the office and refer community members for outside resources, including mental health counseling, substance use disorder counseling for the person and affected others, tobacco cessation treatment services, and adult case management (Mic-nsn.org).

## Impact on Health of Interaction with White Culture Then

The Micmac tribe was the largest indigenous population in New England and Eastern Canada in 1600 with about 26,000 members. Since 27 of the 28 Micmac bands lived in Nova Scotia, the Canadian Anthropology Society studied their population decline in the centuries since then due to dietary changes, alcohol, reduced resistance to endemic diseases, destruction of game and lands for hunting and gathering, and deliberate starvation and exposure. By 1843 the Micmac population there was reduced to 1,300 from these causes. As Micmac moved from a diet of mainly meat and fish to European dried foods, hardtack, and brandy their resistance to endemic diseases was reduced. The English also served poisoned food to the Micmac on occasion and infected them with smallpox due to "poisoned" woolen goods in trading. French soldiers also inadvertently contracted typhus at sea and transmitted this disease to the Micmac on arrival resulting in the deaths of 1/3rd of the tribe or about 4,000 people Outbreaks of smallpox, whooping cough, measles, typhus, typhoid fever and infectious hepatitis occurred in multiple years. When the Canadian government offered vaccination for smallpox, many Micmac were suspicious and refused to take the vaccine. The English also embarked on a genocide campaign by burning large tracts of forest lands that destroyed the natives' settlements and the game they relied on for food, clothing and trade items. During cold Nova Scotia winters, the Micmac faced malnutrition, starvation and exposure without clothing or blankets. New diseases followed these poor living conditions, including tuberculosis, rheumatism, and bronchitis. In 1867 the Canadian government assumed responsibility for the indigenous population resulting in 2,048 Micmac in the 1921 Census of Canada (Miller, 1982).

## Impact on Health of Interaction with White Culture Now

The Mi'kmaq Nation in Maine with 1,489 members has a Health Department with clinic appointments offered five days a week except for Federal and Tribal holidays. The clinic's purpose is to educate and provide "services that encourage and promote responsibility for personal, family, and tribal wellness" (Mic-nsn.gov, 2023).

## Pennacook

The Pennacook tribe is extinct today. Originally, the Pennacook were a large Confederacy of about 12,000 living in 30 villages in New Hampshire, Vermont, and Massachusetts. Their name is from "penakuk" meaning "at the bottom of the hill.

### Health & Healing Then

The Pennacook lifestyle was identical to the Abenaki. Their leader was a sachem who used supernatural powers to mediate between tribal members and spirits (Wikipedia, 2023).

### Impact on Health of Interaction with White Culture Then

The Pennacook were adversely affected by epidemics of smallpox, typhus, measles, influenza, and diphtheria contracted from direct contact with European and English settlers. As their population dwindled, the Pennacook participation in conflicts between the French and English resulted in dispersal into the Abenaki tribe and into Canada. Today, many of their descendants are among the Abenaki tribe in New Hampshire, Vermont, Massachusetts, Maine, and Canada ((Weiser-Alexander, 2021).

## Pequot

The Pequot people live in Connecticut which was their original homeland. Many historians believe their name means "destroyer", but the Pequot call themselves the "fox people" (mptn-nsn.gov, 2023). There are two Pequot bands today: the Eastern Pequot Tribal Nation in New London (state, but not federally recognized) and the Mashantucket (Western) Pequot Tribal Nation in Mashantucket (federally recognized). Today, the tribe owns a successful casino on one of the oldest, continuously occupied reservations in North America (mptn-nsn.gov, 2023).

## Health & Healing Then

The Pequot used herbs for medicinal purposes. Fresh white pine needles were steeped to make a tea to treat colds. Infusion of the inner bark and that of the sugar maple were cough remedies (mptn-nsn.gov, 2023).

## Health & Healing Now

Today Pequot Health Care manages health care and prescription plans for Native tribes and other commercial enterprises (mtpn-nsn.gov, 2023).

## Impact on Health of Interaction with White Culture Then

Many of their traditions along with their language were destroyed in the Pequot War of 1634-1638 with English colonists where many tribal members were killed, enslaved or dispersed (Wikipedia, 2023). The Pequot War decimated the tribe and over the next 200 years, the Pequots fought to keep their remaining land. The Eastern Pequot Tribal Nation was granted their current reservation of 224 acres in 1683 (originally 500 acres or more) and continue to live there growing crops, basket weaving, hunting, and holding traditional gatherings (easternpequottribal-nation.org, 2021). By 1856 the reservation of the (Western) Pequot Tribal Nation was only 213 acres due to illegal land sales.

## Impact on Health of Interaction with White Culture Now

By the 1970s the tribe began developing economic self-sufficiency and revitalizing their culture. The Pequot have worked to become self-sustaining, by seeking additional tools, material, and equipment to achieve that goal They also created a community garden to educate and sustain those in need and engage in selling cord wood, maple syrup, and garden vegetables as well as a swine project and opening a hydroponic greenhouse (easternpequottribalnation.org, 2021). They have placed in trust 1,250 acres by successfully suing to reclaim their land (mptn-nsn.gov, 2023).

## *Mohegan*

The Mohegan tribe, known as the "Wolf People", lives in Connecticut and is federally recognized. The tribe has followed the Mohegan Way—living and working cooperatively within the tribe and in the non-native community—since Sachem Uncas who left the Pequot tribe in the 1600s and allied his Mohegans with the English. This decision preserved enough of the tribe's autonomy to maintain its identity and achieve ultimate success. Today, the Mohegan Tribe owns and operates six casinos and hotels, the Connecticut Sun women's basketball team, and plans to open a resort in South Korea in 2023 (The Mohegan Tribe, 2023).

### Health & Healing Then

Corn was a source of spiritual and physical nourishment. Parched corn was ground as yokeag by women for the annual Corn Festival to thank the Creator for this gift (the Mohegan Tribe, 2023).

### Health & Healing Now

Corn is celebrated today by the Mohegan at the Wigwam Festival. Wigwam means "welcome" or "come in the house" and it includes crafts, food items, storytelling, and traditional dance. The Tribe donates over $1 million annually to support community organizations. Their Uncasville Medical Center provides primary and specialty care for the tribe and the community. The Mohegan Tribal Fire Department provides basic and advanced life support, with fire and hazmat support 24/7 to the region (The Mohegan Tribe, 2023).

### Impact on Health of Interaction with White Culture Then

Alliance with the English kept the Mohegans from many of the illnesses and depredations that plagued other tribes. The Mohegan Way helped the tribe maintain its traditions while maintaining beneficial relationships with their non-native neighbors and educating them about Mohegan culture.

## Impact on Health of Interaction with White Culture Now

When their land claims case was resolved in 1995, the Tribe negotiated an agreement with Connecticut to permit Class III gaming and opened a casino that is a major economic success for the tribe and the entire region by investing in education, housing, and paying tribute to Mohegan cultural tradition (Burgess & Spilde, 2004).

## *Narragansett*

The Narragansett (a federally recognized tribe) live in Rhode Island. Their name comes from "people of the small point", a reference to their homelands. They were farmers who grew corn, squash, and beans, hunters, and fishermen (Alchin, 2017). Today, their Department of Community Planning and Natural Resources works to develop a sound economic base leading to job creation and expansion of existing businesses while protecting the natural environment (Narragansett Indian Tribe, 2022).

## Health & Healing Then

The Green Corn Ceremony was a sacred ceremony where corn was presented to the Creator or Great Spirit (Alchin, 2017) Medicine men and women influenced the tribe by preserving historic and cultural traditions in the past and today (Santiago, 2019).

## Health & Healing Now

Today, the tribe has health care programs about: dental services; smoking cessation; mental health counseling; financial assistance; education about other healthcare services in the state; Medicare savings programs; nutrition and yoga classes; heat wave education; and pandemic education. Wellness bags are distributed at the Annual August Powwow (Narragansett Indian Tribe, 2022).

## Impact on Health of Interaction with White Culture Then

The Narragansett were not affected by the infectious diseases brought by White colonists in the 1600s. However, in 1675 they joined King Phillip of the Wampanoag tribe in an effort to drive the colonists out of Massachusetts and many of their women, children, and old men were massacred in their winter camp in the Great Swamp. After that, the tribe dispersed. Some were killed and others sold into slavery. Hunting and farming areas were depleted, and the colonists introduced hogs to the coastal area which destroyed clam beds (a traditional food source for the Narragansett). As reservation lands were sold for debt, the Narragansett fought to keep their remaining land and traditional ways. The State of Rhode Island illegally "detribalized" them in the 1880s. The tribal council continued to function, and the Narragansett Tribe of Indians was finally recognized and  incorporated in December 1934. They reclaimed 1,800 acres of tribal land in a lawsuit in 1978 (Narragansett Indian Tribe, 2022).

### Impact of Health on Interaction with White Culture Now

The Tribe is involved with federally-funded programs through The Department of Indian Health Services and the Bureau of Indian Affairs to provide services to members for their physical and mental health (Narragansett Indian Tribe, 2022).

## Nipmuc

The Nipmuc Nation of about 600 people resides on the 3.5-acre Hassanamisco Reservation in Massachusetts. They are known as "the people of the freshwater pond" because of their location along rivers and streams, but called themselves the "Beaver Tail Hill People" (Pakachoag or place where the river turns). They lived by hunting, gathering, planting and harvesting crops and were good stewards of the land. They even took corn to starving colonists in Boston. They are currently a state recognized tribe which focuses on preserving the land, self-sufficiency, and the heritage of their ancestors (nipmucnation.org, 2021 & Oleson, 2014).

### Health & Healing Then

The Nipmuc had a complex social structure and their own religion. Their farming and medicine skills were superior to the White culture in the 1600s. They used digitalis to treat heart conditions and buried fish heads as fertilizer for crops.

## Health & Healing Now

The Nipmuc Indian Development Corporation (NIDC) has a grant to conduct a food assessment of tribal members. It is designed to help members understand the dangers of processed foods and assess conditions affected by food intake, such as diabetes, obesity, heart disease, and asthma triggered by allergies (NIDC, n.d.).

## Impact on Health of Interaction with White Culture Then

The first interaction with White culture was positive by welcoming the English colonists. However, settlers and farmers subsequently built towns and displaced the Nipmuc. The beaver they depended on were gone, healers could not practice their skills, and many Nipmuc died of smallpox and other infectious diseases contracted from the colonists (Oleson, 2014).

## Impact of Health on Interaction with White Culture Now

Today the Nipmuc use traditional planting techniques to help feed their community. They study and create native medicine using local plants and support herbalists, artists, and tribal entrepreneurs as they blend tradition with today's environment (nippi.org, 2023).

## *Woronoco*

The Woronoco tribe no longer exists. It was located in Massachusetts and many members expired in 1617 due to endemic illness. The remainder died in 1633 in a smallpox epidemic, except for a few who assimilated into other tribes (Bruchac, 2005 & Deerfield History Museum, 2020).

## Health & Healing Then

No information is available about health practices of this tribe.

## Impact on Health of Interaction with White Culture Then

No information is available about the interaction of this tribe with White culture.

## *Wampanoag*

There are two federally recognized Wampanoag tribes: the Wampanoag Tribe of Gay Head (Aquinnah) in Martha's Vineyard and the Mashpee Wampanoag Tribe in Mashpee on Cape Cod, Massachusetts. Known as the "People of the First Light" each reservation has its own tribal council, medicine man, clan mothers, and government structures. Both focus on protecting the land and preserving water quality (Wampanoagtribe-nsn.gov & Mashpeewampanoagtribe-nsn.gov).

### Health & Healing Then

Women elders exercised significant power and served as spiritual leaders. Women provided the crops of corn, bean and squash and followed conservation practices long before these were common while men were hunters and fishermen. Tea from the bark of winged or dwarf sumac was used to clean blisters and tea from its root was used to treat dysentery. Parts of the sassafras tree had medicinal uses. Hazelnut bark tea treated hives and fevers and a poultice of this was used to close cuts and wounds. Shamans conducted religious ceremonies called Powwows and women practiced natural holistic healing that combined ceremonial prayers and cleansing practices such as sweat lodges to use the earth's energies to achieve harmony of body, mind, and soul (Simaratana, 2011).

### Health & Healing Now

The Mashpee annual Powwow is a traditional celebration of tribal culture with drumming, dancing, games, songs, contests, and a traditional clambake. The Aquinnah Wampanoag Tribe celebrates Cranberry Day annually after the cranberry harvest to thank the Creator for the harvest with dancing and singing (Wampanoagtribe-nsn.gov & Mashpeewam-panoagtribe-nsn.gov).

### Impact on Health of Interaction with White Culture Then

In 1616 European traders brought yellow fever to their first contact with the Wampanoag Nation and nearly two-thirds of the population died, especially small children and Elders. After helping the pilgrims in the early years of that century, the Wampanoag continued to see the land they depended on for survival reduced as White settlers appropriated the land for themselves. King Phillip's War resulted in the deaths of 40% of the Wampanoag population and enslaving of many healthy men. Emphasis on assimilation by White culture resulted in children being sent to the Carlisle Indian School from 1904-1916 (Wampanoagtribe-nsn.gov & Mashpeewampanoagtribe-nsn.gov).

## Impact on Health of Interaction with White Culture Now

The Mashpee Wampanoag Tribe has been adversely impacted by the opioid epidemic and has launched a marketing program to educate the community about opioid use and how to fight addiction and overdoses (Mashpeewampanoagtribe-nsn.gov). The Wampanoag Health Service has a registered nurse for urgent care services and to answer health-related questions. A doctor is available in a clinic on the fourth Monday each month and during General Membership meetings (Wampanoagtribe-nsn.gov)

## The Carlisle Indian Industrial School       1879-1918

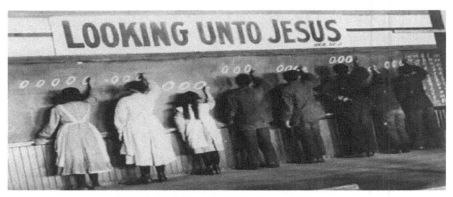

*"Kill the Indian, Save the Man" --Lt. Col. Richard Henry Pratt [proponent of Carlisle Indian Industrial School] (Carlisle Indian School Project, 2020).*

The Carlisle Indian Industrial School and other Native Boarding Schools affected many tribes and impacted the physical, emotional, and mental health of their students throughout their lives. These will be referenced under each indigenous tribe that was impacted, but will be analyzed in depth here.

In 1879 the first government-run boarding school opened for Native Americans at the site of a former military post in Carlisle, Pennsylvania. The goal of the school was forced assimilation into White culture by Native children. Children of many tribes were removed from their families and displaced in Carlisle in a strange, forbidding environment. Some were as young as four-years old and all were required to cease wearing Native clothing, speaking their Native languages, wearing long hair, and practicing their culture and customs. They were required to adopt Christianity and endured discipline that included corporal punishment and solitary confinement. Carlisle and the church-operated schools that followed wanted the children to fully assimilate into White culture and punished those who refused (Carlisle Indian School Project), 2020).

Today there are 186 graves on the site of children who died at the Carlisle School and eventually the lives of children in over 140 tribes across the United States were impacted in these schools. The physical scars may have healed, but the emotional scars remain today. According to the Carlisle Indian School Project website:

"Students lost their language, their cultural traditions, and their connection to their tribes and families. Parents lost children. Tribes lost members of their community and tribal traditions" (Carlisle Indian School Project, 2020).

On June 22, 2022, Deb Haaland, the first Native American Secretary of the Interior, testified before the Senate Committee on Indian Affairs about a bill to establish the Truth and Healing Commission on Indian Boarding School Policies. She shared that her grandparents were removed from their families and placed in Federal Indian boarding schools at eight-years of age and did not return until age thirteen. She led the first departmental investigation into this system with the following reported findings:

- "The federal Indian boarding school system consisted of 408 federal Indian boarding schools across 37 states or then-territories, including 21 schools in Alaska and 7 schools in Hawaii";
- "Approximately 50 percent of federal Indian boarding schools may have received support or involvement from a religious institution or organization, including funding, infrastructure, and personnel";
- 'The federal government at times paid religious institutions and organizations for Native children to enter federal Indian boarding schools that these institutions and organizations operated"; and
- "Approximately 53 different schools contain marked or unmarked burial sites" (Carlisle Indian School Project, 2020).

As this investigation continues, the Department of the Interior plans to focus on expanding Tribal access to mental health resources. Policies must reflect revitalization of Native health care, education, languages, and cultural practices as well as the "Road to Healing" to hear from survivors and descendants about their experiences and to connect them with mental health support. A permanent collection of their oral histories will be essential to learn from this tragic history. According to Secretary Haaland, "While we cannot change that history, I believe that our nation will benefit from a full understanding of the truth of what took place and a focus on healing the wounds of the past" (Carlisle Indian School Project, 2020).

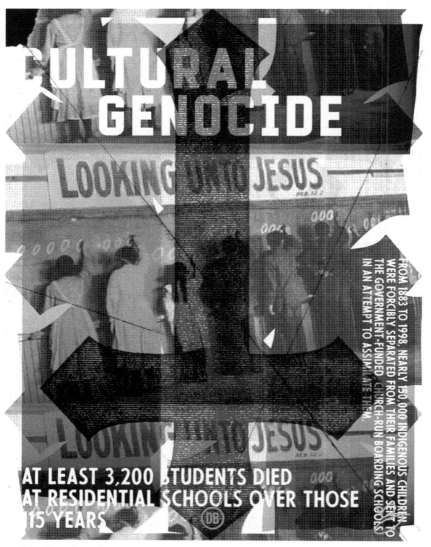

# Chapter 2
# Mid-Atlantic Tribes

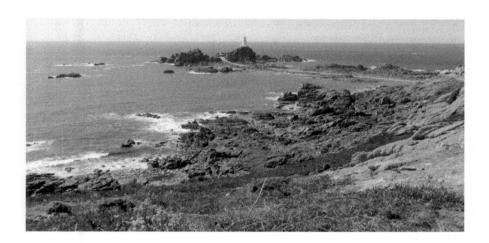

Tribes in the Mid-Atlantic region were Accohannock, Cayuga, Delaware, Erie, Honniasont, Lenni Lenape, Mohawk, Mingo, Nanticoke, Oneida, Onondaga, Piscataway, Seneca, Shawnee, Susquehannock, and Tuscarora.

## *Accohannock*

The Accohannock Tribe is recognized by the State of Maryland. The original tribe intermarried with colonists and African Americans and assimilated into Black culture. (Maryland Archives, 2022) Many other tribes and researchers believe that the current Accohannock is a reincarnation of the original tribe and does not qualify as a Native nation (Tkacik, 2018).

### Health & Healing Then

The original tribe-Accomac-was known is "the other side of water place" (Wikipedia.org, 2023). They were fishermen, trappers, hunters, and farmers on Chesapeake Bay. They grew corn, squash, and other foods. A peaceful people, the clan mothers prayed and received a vision to marry with the colonists until the tribe could be reborn (AAANativeArts.com, 1999-2023).

## Health & Healing Now

Poverty is a challenge facing the Tribe, including unemployment, lack of education and job skills, substance use, family violence, health and medical issues. The Administration for Native Americans awarded the tribe a grant in 2008-2010 to develop Bending Water Park and provide economic opportunities for tribal members. Six small park businesses generated some needed income. By the project's conclusion, attendance and revenues did not meet expectations and there was no funding for permanent facilities or a welcome center (Administration for Native Americans, 2010). Today, the Tribe still has the Bending Water Park and advertises it as Water Trails for kayaking or canoeing. The Park is listed as a rustic camping site (Somerset County, 2023).

## Impact on Health of Interaction with White Culture Then

The original tribe was decimated by smallpox and other diseases as well as attacks from the colonists Assimilation and intermarriage occurred in the original tribe over 300 years (AAANativeArts.com, 1999-2023).

## Impact on Health of Interaction with White Culture Now

Today they host an annual Native American Heritage Festival and Powwow, and most are not able to continue the traditional occupations of their ancestors (AAANativeArts.com, 1999-2023).

# Cayuga

The Cayuga Nation is called "The People of the Great Swamp" and are located in the Finger Lakes region of New York State. They are federally recognized and involved in multiple enterprises for their community, including a casino in Union Springs and a new gaming facility in Seneca Falls (cayuganation-nsn.gov).

## Health & Healing Then

The Cayuga believed that  a tribe of underworld humanlike demons caused disease and misfortune. They cured disease by appealing to the demons in a friendly manner. Cayuga medicine societies prescribed herbs and used powerfully haunting masks to treat the underlying causes of illness (Speck, 1950).

## Health & Healing Now

As a matrilineal society, the Cayuga have five clans led by a Clan Mother. The clans are represented by birds and animals in the elements of air, water, and land. Their ceremonies throughout the year express thanks to the creator, the spirit world, the natural world, and the people. These ceremonies include prayer, storytelling, songs, and dances using instruments like gourd rattles and water drums. (cayuganation-nsn.gov). The Cayuga also grow produce which they distribute weekly to over 100 Nation households along with distributing dried and canned goods at season's end (cayuganation-nsn.gov).

## Impact on Health of Interaction with White Culture Then

The Cayuga avoided the epidemics that plagued tribes in New England and had a stable government by Clan Mothers until the Revolutionary War. The Cayuga were loyal to their families and their land and found themselves on both sides of the War. Despite attempts at neutrality, their villages were burned, and orchards destroyed by American forces in 1777. They were forced from their land, and it was given to American soldiers. Although a treaty in 1794 re-established the current reservation, New York State ignored the treaty and took 250 years to successfully achieve the intent of the original Treaty of Canandaigua (cayuganation-nsn.gov).

## Impact on Health of Interaction with White Culture Now

Today the Cayuga reservation is 64,015 acres (cayuganation-nsn.gov), Divisions within the Nation between traditionalists and the tribal government today are avoided by New York State authorities so the tribal members can settle their own disputes. In late 2022, the Cayuga Nation donated $70,000 to the Union Springs Fire Department to purchase a new Medical Rescue vehicle and protect the community (cayuganation-nsn.gov).

## Delaware/Lenni Lenape

The Delaware or Lenni Lenape tribe lived in New Jersey, New York, and Pennsylvania. The Lenape were considered the parent tribe with Lenni (original) and Lenape (Indian).The Delaware were called "grandfather". Today, they are located in Oklahoma and Kansas as part of the Cherokee Nation following removal to Indian Territory. Today, the Delaware Nation (Anadarko, OK) and the Delaware Tribe of Indians (Bartlesville, OK) are federally recognized (delawarenation-nsn.gov & delaware-tribe.org). Three Lenape tribes in Delaware and New Jersey are state recognized (Legends of America, 2023; lenapeindiantribeofdelaware.com, 2010 and delawaretribe.org, 2023).

### Health & Healing Then

The Delaware/Lenape used natural remedies to cure diseases and wounds. Both men and women were healers who collected plants, roots, and barks in the proper seasons and cured or dried them to preserve them for future use. Bark from different trees had multiple uses-to reduce fever, stop vomiting, relieve constipation, cure chest colds, relieve hoarseness, and cure toothache. Blackberry roots were used to cure diarrhea and dysentery. Dried leaves in a tea were used for spider bites and sore throats. They addressed the Creator when gathering medicinal herbs as well as the spirit of the plants gathered (McCartlin & Rementer, 1986).

### Health & Healing Now

In 2022 the Delaware Nation assisted 774 tribal members with clothing, food, utility bills, vision, dental, and prescription needs (delawarenation-nsn.gov). The Delaware Tribe of Indians has a health and wellness center open Monday-Friday, but without medical personnel. They also have an Elder Nutrition Program which provides lunches to Native Americans 55 years or older (delawaretribe.org).

## Impact on Health of Interaction with White Culture Then

The Delaware/Lenape were also devastated by epidemics of European diseases in the 1600s. They were continually pushed west as more settlers arrived, especially after 90 peaceful Delaware were slaughtered at the mission village of Gnadenhutten, Ohio in 1782 (Legends of America, 2023 & delawaretribe.org, 2023).

## Impact on Health of Interaction with White Culture Now

The Delaware Nation has programs for families in crisis, including Indian Child Welfare (provides counseling service for abusive, neglectful parents to keep children in the home), Promoting Safe & Stable Families (provides protective and preventive services), and Children & Family Services (protects rights of children and families under the Child Welfare Act) (delawarenation-nsn.gov).

## *Erie*

The Erie people no longer exist as an indigenous tribe. They were known as the Cat Nation and lived on the Southern shore of Lake Erie. After war with the Iroquois Confederacy, the remaining survivors joined the Huron-Wyandot or Seneca tribes. (World Atlas, 2017).

## Health & Healing Then

The Erie hunted, fished, and grew corn, beans, and squash. Erie burial customs included "crying ceremonies" that lasted five days. These included dancing and singing with the dead placed on tall scaffolds. Every 10-12 years, the Erie held another large ceremony where the remaining bones were buried (World Atlas, 2017).

## Impact on Health of Interaction with White Culture Then

The Erie had little interaction with White Culture prior to their demise as a tribe.

## *Honniasont*

The Honniasont is no longer in existence. The name means "wearing something around the neck" and the tribe was reported destroyed by the Susquehanna and Seneca. The few survivors settled among the Seneca.

### Health & Healing Then

No information is available about their health practices.

### Impact on Health of Interaction with White Culture Then

There is no indication of interaction with White Culture.

## *Mohawk*

The St. Regis Mohawk Tribe's reservation is in both New York State and the Ontario and Quebec provinces in Canada. The Mohawk name is "People of the Flint" and they historically are "Keepers of the Eastern Door" of the Iroquois Confederacy. The Mohawk are divided into three clans-Turtle, Bear, and Wolf (Seaver, 2023). Today, the Saint Regis Mohawk Tribe is federally recognized and "administers its own environmental, social, policing, economic, health and educational programs, policies, laws and regulations" (srmt-nsn.gov). The tribe also has a Tribal Gaming Commission to regulate and oversee the Akwesasne Mohawk Casino Resort and the Mohawk Bingo Palace" (srmt-nsn.org).

### Health & Healing Then

Mohawk longhouses were common areas for entertainment, education, religious ceremonies and daily activities. Their spiritual system was based on the ongoing conflict between good and evil and they believed that interpreting dreams could give direction to the waking world and deliver messages. Many of their religious leaders devoted time to interpret dreams of community members and help them achieve spiritual balance or successfully complete quests to them by dream givers or traditionally divine spirits. The Two Row Wampum Belt symbolized respect and peace among nations through the River of Life which each nation navigated (Seaver, 2023). Healers used plants to treat wounds sore throats, fevers, scurvy, head lice, and even hypertension and childbirth complications (srmt-nsn.gov).

## Health & Healing Now

Spiritual ceremonies celebrate appreciation, such as the Strawberry Ceremony or Maple Ceremony. Tobacco burning ceremonies are used for a number of purposes and tobacco is considered sacred. (srmt-nsn.gov).

## Impact on Health of Interaction with White Culture Then

In the 1600s European settlers brought smallpox and other diseases that resulted in numerous deaths. Many other Mohawk succumbed to war with the settlers and starvation from loss of tribal land (Seaver, 2023).

## Impact on Health of Interaction with White Culture Now

Today the Saint Regis Mohawk Health Services  ensures that Mohawk patients receive professional care with courtesy and respect. Their Mission is "Body, Mind & Spirit in Harmony with our Environment". Their Community and Family Services Division has child support, family support, homeowners' assistance, tribal vocational rehabilitation, and community advocacy programs. Their community advocacy programs address domestic violence, victim and family issues, and safe home shelter services (srmt-nsn.gov).

## *Mingo*

The Mingo are no longer a separate tribe. They migrated to Ohio in the 1850s, joined other Cayuga and Seneca bands and eventually migrated to Oklahoma. In 1937, the combined tribe became the Seneca-Cayuga Tribe of Oklahoma (revwartalk.com, 2014). They will be discussed in that regional group.

## *Nanticoke*

The Nanticoke Nation today live in Delaware and are a state recognized tribe. Their name means "tidewater people". Today, they use the

Nanticoke Indian Museum to share their culture and heritage by educating the public (nanticokeindians.org, 2011).

## Health & Healing Then

The Nanticoke had an excellent lifestyle. They were proficient farmers with abundant crops of beans, squash, corn, pumpkins, tobacco, and sunflowers. They ate luscious seafood and hunting was successful. They used every part of sea creatures and animals without waste. They used (and still do) powwows to preserve traditions, sing to the Creator, and dance in celebration of their heritage (nanticokeindians.org, 2011). Plants, barks, roots and herbs had medicinal uses. Many have been discussed earlier, but tobacco deserves recognition as an offering to the Creator and its uses to cure earache, toothache, and indigestion ((nanticoke-lenapemuseum.org, 2017).

## Health & Healing Now

Today's powwows serve traditional foods, such as succotash and fry bread as well as hot dogs and hamburgers. Tribal spokesmen share stories about the regalia for each dance. The regalia keep the Nanticoke culture alive and are integral to the powwow heritage celebration (nanticokeindians.org, 2011).

## Impact on Health of Interaction with White Culture Then

In the 1600s the Nanticoke initially befriended the colonists. By the end of the century White settlers depleted the game and farmlands the Nanticoke needed to survive. Treaties took more Nanticoke lands. Alcohol sales also adversely impacted the Nanticoke who lost land and valuable furs to unscrupulous traders (nanticokeindians.org, 2011). Perhaps, the most difficult aspect of interaction with White Culture was the biracially segregated system in Delaware where census-takers were told not to classify the Nanticoke as Native American. They were to be classified as anything but White and usually as Mulatto or Black. Although the Nanticoke had founded their own school in the 1800s, they were teased and taunted. If they went to the White school, they and the Blacks had to sit upstairs. Only Nanticoke who were light-skinned were able to pass and sit downstairs. They weren't allowed on the rides at the amusement park and couldn't swim at the White beach. Although this has changed over the years, the pain remains, and today's Nanticoke share their heritage and educate others  to ensure it doesn't happen again (Delaware Public Media, 2015).

## Impact on Health of Interaction with White Culture Now

The Nanticoke Indian Museum is designated as a National Historic Landmark and today's Nanticoke people make jewelry and craft items for sale there to tourists visiting the displays. The Tribe also offers special tours for community groups and schools to share how Native arts are created. This income source also is an opportunity to showcase Nanticoke culture (nanticokeindians.org, 2011).

## *Oneida*

The Oneida Indian Nation lives in Central New York and is federally recognized. The Oneida Nation of Wisconsin is also federally recognized. Known as the "People of the Standing Stone", the Oneida Indian Nation is the largest employer in the central New York region today. Their enterprises include three casinos, hospitality, dining, recreation, and retail centers (oneidaindiannation.com, 2020). The Oneida Nation of Wisconsin's enterprises include seven convenience stores and three smoke shops, a golf course, and the Oneida Casino (Oneida Nation of Wisconsin, 2023).

## Health & Healing Then

Medicine men and women were from the Bear Clan, known as "Keepers of the Medicine". They used herbs and native plants to cure illnesses. The Oneida lived in balance with nature tending and preserving the Creator's gifts for future generations (oneidaindiannation.com, 2020).

## Health & Healing Now

Today, the Oneida provide high quality medical, dental, and behavioral health care for their people, specializing in diabetic and preventative health care for nearly 3,500 citizens. Their Behavioral Health Services and Pathways Case Management program includes mental health counseling as well as assessment, diagnosis, treatment planning, and ongoing therapy using varied approaches. These approaches include guided imagery, acupuncture, and art therapy (oneidaindiannation.com, 2020).

### Impact on Health of Interaction with White Culture Then

The Oneida believed in collaboration and cooperation when they allied themselves with the colonists during the Revolution. Over the next 200 years, land disputes dominated the Oneida relationship with White Culture. During that time, the Oneida became self-sufficient and rebuilt its community for success (oneideindiannation.com, 2020).

### Impact on Health of Interaction with White Culture Now

The Oneida Indian Nation has re-invested its gaming revenues to build job growth and tourism that benefits the entire region as well as the Nation itself. In 2022 the Nation donated $22,000 to the Muscular Dystrophy Association and $1,000 to the Feed Our Vets New Hope Mills Pantry. The Nation also sponsors a scholarship program for Nation Member students to attend college, graduate school, or trade/vocational schools. In Fall 2022, thirty-six Oneida students were enrolled in higher education programs, including Vocational (3 students), Associate degree (7 students), Bachelor's degree (15 students), Master's degree (5 students), Research PhD (4 students), and Professional Practice PhD (2 students). The program enables students to focus solely on their education and incentives are awarded for high academic achievement (oneideindian-nation.com, 2020).

## Onondaga

The Onondaga Nation is located south of Syracuse, New York. It is federally recognized and functions as an independent nation. Onondaga had two names "Keeper of the Central Fire" and "Wampum Keepers" to reflect the Nation's central location in the Iroquois Confederacy (Haudenosaunee). The economy is based on the Nation's tax-free smoke shop. The Onondaga  do not want a gaming enterprise as they believe it would be detrimental to their people (Onondaganation.org, 2023).

## Health & Healing Then

The Onondaga considered the maple the leader of all trees. The sugar maple sap was used for ceremonies and the willow as medicine for headaches. The American elm provided medicine. Medicinal plants were honored, and wampum made from clam shells was valued as a living history of the Haudenosaunee. Wampum designated leadership and when a speaker held a string of wampum, the people listening were respectful because that person spoke truthfully  (Onondaganation.org, 2023).

## Health & Healing Now

Today they focus on restoring the water of Onondaga Lake so it can be used for food and medicine. Wampum continues its importance and Faith Keepers continue to ensure that ceremonies giving thanks to the Creator and all of creation are still performed according to Onondaga tradition. These men and women determine when these ceremonies occur by using the lunar calendar. These ceremonies include Midwinter, Maple Sap, Planting, Bean, Strawberry, Green Corn, and Harvest Ceremonies (Onondaganation.org, 2023).

## Impact on Health of Interaction with White Culture Then

In the 1800s children were separated from their families and sent to either the Carlisle Indian School or the Thomas Indian School in Western New York (see Chapter 1). In 1850 the citizens of Syracuse petitioned New York State for a school on the Nation, and one has been there since that time and has been updated to serve the community (Onondaganation.org, 2023).

## Impact on Health of Interaction with White Culture Now

Salt mining from 1888-1987 polluted Onondaga Creek. Originally, it was crystal clear water. The underground salt layer resulted in mud boils in the water where trout no longer can live. The trout streams above remain clear, but the water flowing into the Nation is thick, brown, and contaminated from the silt draining into it. Onondaga Creek was a lifeline for the Nation when they settled here. Now, pollution will not allow the Onondaga to swim or fish. Onondaga Lake, once the most contaminated lake in the United States, is undergoing a clean-up as a Superfund site (Onondaganation.org, 2023). One bright spot is a group of volunteers calling themselves the Creek Rats. Beginning in 2001 or 2002, they began clean-up efforts on the 9-mile stretch from the border of the Onondaga Nation to Onondaga Lake. Their work has improved water quality in that area, but more must be done (Central NY News, 2022).

## Piscataway

The Piscataway Tribe lives in Maryland. The name originally was given as "the people who live on the long river with a bend in it" to describe their location on the Potomac. They refer to themselves as "The People" (Piscatawayindians.com, 2022). The Nation (Band/Clan) is state recognized. The Tribe's goal is to protect their identity, culture, traditions, and interests while establishing relationships with non-tribal entities. They seek advancement of their People through education, health, economic development, and social programs (Piscatawayconoy-tribe.com).

### Health & Healing Then

The Piscataway culture included the Seed Gathering in the early spring to awaken the earth from its winter sleep and prepare the soil for growing; the Feast from the Waters in the early summer that featured seafood; and the Green Corn Festival in late summer to celebrate the first corn of the harvest (Hamilton, 2018). Piscataway people spent significant time collecting herbal medicines (Tayac, 2019).

### Health & Healing Now

The Piscataway-Conoy Tribe's state recognition increased access to federal funds for housing, education, public health, and other programs to benefit tribal members. They continue to celebrate their culture with Festivals (Hamilton, 2018).

## Impact on Health of Interaction with White Culture Then

As the number of settlers increased, the Piscataway found themselves squeezed out of their tribal lands. Some tribal members chose to migrate and those who remained also lost identity as a people. They were counted in censuses as "mulatto" or "negro", regarded as outsiders in their communities, and suffered discrimination. They struggled to regain their traditions and cultural history. State recognition finally meant that the Piscataway are a distinct tribe with a long cultural heritage (Hamilton, 2018).

## Impact on Health of Interaction with White Culture Now

The Piscataway collaborated with environmentalists and community activists to prevent deforestation in 2019 that threatened the healthy ecosystem of Nanjemoy Creek which flows into the Potomac. The trees there oxygenate the District of Columbia and the unpolluted Creek supports wildlife, including a blue heron rookery (Tayac, 2029). The Piscataway-Conoy Tribe have also established a relationship with the Maryland Park Service to use Merkle and Chapel Point State Park to forge cultural connections with non-tribal members through ceremonies and education programs (Hamilton, 2018).

## *Seneca/Seneca-Cayuga*

The Seneca Nation was called "Keeper of the Western Door" and "Great Hill People" in their own language. They are federally recognized, and two tribes live in New York State-the Tonawanda Band of Seneca and the Seneca Nation of Indians. Other tribal members also live in Canada and Oklahoma and the Seneca Cayuga Nation in Oklahoma is also federally recognized. The Seneca Cayuga Nation's enterprises include two smoke shops, a gift shop, a lodge, and the Grand Lake Casino (Seneca Cayuga Nation, n.d.). The Tonawanda Band of Seneca are a traditional matrilineal tribe and Two Eagles Smoke Shop and Gas Mart on the Reservation sells tobacco and fuel products at discount prices (Two Eagles Smoke Shop, 2023). Today the Seneca Nation of Indians in New York State has multiple enterprises, including three casinos, an economic development company, a campground, an energy company, and gas and convenience stores that also sell tobacco and cigars. (sni.org, 2023).

## Health & Healing Then

The most important tradition for the Seneca Nation was the White Dog Ceremony. After killing white dogs as a sacrifice for their sins, they danced, threw ashes, and shot guns outside. After burning the dogs, they created tobacco incense smoke to cleanse themselves from their sins (senecanation.weebly.com).

## Health & Healing Now

Today, some Seneca use a white basket with sacred herbs in place of the white dog and still use tobacco incense. They also believe in the importance of dreams and fulfilling them. Their spirituality is strong (senecanation.weebly.com). The Seneca Nation Health System has three health care centers and provides services in five New York State counties and Warren County, Pennsylvania. The System offers preventive and primary care for acute and chronic illnesses to the Seneca Nation members. Services include well baby and child care, prenatal care, family health care, prevention screenings and ancillary support services. The System maintains collaborative agreements with local hospitals, agencies, and professionals in these communities (sni.org, 2023). Seneca Strong uses holistic healing, talking circles for men and women, and a Red Road to Wellbriety peer support to address drug and alcohol prevention and recovery (sni.org, 2023). The Seneca Cayuga Nation of Oklahoma also has multiple services for their tribal members. These include wellness, nutrition, victim services for domestic violence, substance abuse, and child welfare services (Seneca Cayuga Nation, n.d.).

## Impact on Health of Interaction with White Culture Then

The Seneca grew the Three Sisters-corn, beans, and squash- and the men were excellent hunters and fishermen. The Seneca did not suffer as much from their contact with White culture except for loss of villages and land in wars. Some accepted treaty terms to migrate westward. Others remained to develop their current homelands (sni.org, 2023).

## Impact of Health on Interaction with White Culture Now

The Seneca Nation Department of Emergency Management partners with other agencies to train emergency responders. The Seneca EMS helps support surrounding communities as well as Reservation members. The Early Childhood Learning Center meets or exceeds all Head Start and state health and safety codes and operates year-round for children from 6 weeks to 12 years of age. It is licensed by the New York State Office of Child and Family Services (sni.org, 2023).

## *Shawnee*

The Shawnee relocated to Oklahoma in the 1700s. They will be discussed with other tribes in that region.

## Susquehannock

The Susquehannock tribe no longer exists. They were called the Conestoga by the English and lived on the Susquehanna River mainly in Pennsylvania and New York State. Their name originally meant "people of the Muddy River" (Alexander, 2019).

## Health & Healing Then

The Susquehannock lived like other Iroquoian tribes by planting beans, maize, and squash and fishing and gathering shellfish in the summer before harvesting their crops (Alexander, 2019).

## Impact on Health of Interaction with White Culture Then

Initial interactions with White Culture were friendly. However, in the late 1670s the tribe suffered decimation from infectious diseases and warfare with their long-time enemies the Iroquois. By 1700 only 300 Susquehannock remained and the last of these were massacred by colonists in 1763 (Alexander, 2019).

## *Tuscarora*

The Tuscarora Nation has a federally recognized reservation in Niagara County, New York and has no official website (Wigle, 2014). The Tuscarora Nation of Indians is located in Windsor, North Carolina (skngov.com, 2020). The Tuscarora Nation of North Carolina has three bands in Robeson, North Carolina (Tuscarora Nation of North Carolina, 2023). The tribe migrated from New York originally to North Carolina and returned to New York State in the 1700s after defeat by the colonists. They relinquished their land in North Carolina and the state does not recognize the Tuscarora Nation of Indians there (Martin, 2016). Tuscarora means "hemp gatherers" (Native-languages.org, 1998-2020).

## Health & Healing Then

Tuscarora dietary practices were similar to other Iroquoian tribes. Their most vital crop was corn, but they also ate large game as well as crops they grew during the year. Tuscarora children also ate baby wasps picked from their combs as candy snacks. The Tuscarora used indigenous hemp for medicine and insulation and bloodroot plant as a dye (Martin, 2016).

## Health & Healing Now

Although the Tuscarora Nation in New York State has the Tuscarora Nation Health Center, the tribal members needed traditional medicine services at the Center. The University of Buffalo School of Nursing used grants from the Health Resources and Services Administration (HRSA) to expand student clinical sites, including the Tuscarora Nation Health Center. Students learned about how lack of access to heat, water, or food impacts primary care for these individuals. Telehealth technology expanded access to care and the result is more personalized, culturally sensitive, effective health care. Two University of Buffalo graduates currently are employed as nurse practitioners at the Tuscarora Nation Health Center (Anzalone, 2020).

## Impact on Health of Interaction with White Culture Then

In 1835 North Carolina classified Tuscarora as "mulatto". In 1863 when a yellow fever outbreak killed slaves who were building Fort Fisher, some Tuscarora were conscripted to continue the building. Three were beaten to death by a member of the Confederate Home Guard. In 1887 the Croatan Normal School was established to train future Indian teachers. Students were forced to learn revisionist history that defined their tribe as Croatan and erased reference to Tuscarora. In 1890 the tribe was listed as Indians in the North Carolina census, but the census papers were burned. In 1913 the tribe was designated as Cherokee and in 1916 their lands reverted to North Carolina as there were no designated Tuscarora. In 1956 Congress designated the tribe as Lumbee to prevent any threat of land claims. According to a Tuscarora chief, "We all went to school one day and they told us that we were going to be called "Lumbee" now. It confused us kids" (Tuscarora Nation of North Carolina, 2023). It took until 1984 for North Carolina to charter the Tuscarora Tribe of North Carolina (Tuscarora Nation of North Carolina, 2023; Tuscarora Tribe of NC, 2019).

## Impact on Health of Interaction with White Culture Now

Aside from conflicts and land losses, the modern Tuscarora in New York State were displaced, and 600 acres of their land was flooded to build a reservoir for the Niagara Power Project in 1958. Two fresh-water creeks in the reservation were dammed up. These creeks were the main fresh-water source for the tribe. Since that time the reservation has had a water crisis that is exacerbated by their location in the highest point of Niagara County. Well water tested positive for lead, harmful bacteria, total Coliforms, and E.coli. Tuscarora members were forced to purchase bottled water, and some formed the Tuscarora Water Drive to assist their neighbors. This effort continues today (Genco, 2021).

## Women in Native Society

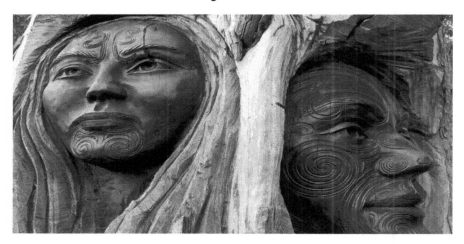

The role of women in native society was significant and many tribes in the Mid-Atlantic region were matrilineal (descended from the mother) and matriarchal (women in control of their community). The clan structure of the Iroquois Confederacy (Haudenosaunee) is an excellent example of matriarchal/matrilineal roles. Families began with a female ancestor and everyone living in her longhouse linked back to her. The Clan Mother was the head of each longhouse family and all her female descendants lived with her for their entire lives bringing their husbands with them. Her sons lived with her until marriage when they moved to their wife's house. They still were members of their mother's longhouse, and she would have their first loyalty. Family names and clans were passed down from mother to child. Marriage within the clan was not permitted. Women traditionally handled village concerns (haudenosauneeconfederacy.com, 2023). Clan Mothers served in social and political roles. They appointed the chiefs and served as the voice of the people. Chiefs were wise to follow their guidance. They also served as counselors providing advice and knowledge for the people (Oneida-nsn.gov, 2023).

This example reflects the importance and influence of women in many of these Native American tribes. Their role was essential for the health and viability of the tribe, and they were greatly respected for their ability and knowledge.

# Chapter 3
# Southern Tribes

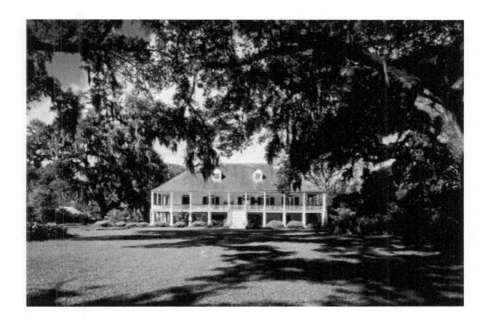

Tribes located in the Southeast United States were: Caddo, Catawba, Chickasaw, Choctaw, Creek, Cherokee, Powhatan, Quapaw, Saluda, Saponi, and Seminole.

## *Caddo*

The Caddo Nation is federally recognized tribe in Oklahoma today. The term Caddo means "real chief" and they had an agricultural economy (Perttula, 1951 [updated 10.8.2020]). Today, they are dedicated to preserving their culture and own convenience stores as well as an art gallery and Indian supply store (Caddo Nation, 2023).

### Health & Healing Then

The Caddo kept a perpetual sacred fire, and their ceremonies were based on crops and seasons. Healers used native plants and prayer to treat injuries, illnesses, and spiritual ailments. Emetics and herbal medicines were used for rituals. The Caddo were a matrilineal, clan-based society and spiritual leaders were called the xinesi. The xinesi communicated with the supreme god, led special rites, and served as religious leaders (Oklahoma Historical Society, n.d. & Perttula, 1952 [updated 10/8/2020]).

## Health & Healing Now

Indian Health Service provides annual funding for the Caddo Nation Community Health Program. Its staff members provide appointment scheduling for tribal members, medication pick-up and delivery, case management and screening, home visits, health education, and patient monitoring. All staff members are trained in first aid, CPR, and as First Responders for EMS (Caddo Nation, 2023).

## Impact on Health of Interaction with White Culture Then

The three Caddo Confederacies lived in Louisiana, Arkansas, Texas, and finally settled in Oklahoma after being uprooted as settlers moved into their lands. While in Texas, the Caddo were forced to move several times between 1847-1853 even though they had signed treaties. As an agricultural people, they suffered from hunger because they had to abandon their fields before harvesting crops. Some young men drank whiskey as their lifestyle deteriorated. They subsequently were removed from Texas to Oklahoma. On August 1, 1859 the Caddo began a move of 200 miles in heat over 100 degrees. They took only what they could carry and only the old and sick rode on wagons. Children and infants were carried, and the majority of the tribe walked. One person died during the journey and one baby was born (Caddo Nation, 2023). The first reservation schools were welcomed by the Caddo as a way to learn English and communicate better with White Culture. However, when students were sent to government schools, they were forbidden to speak Caddo and today few Caddo speak their own language fluently (refer to Chapter 1 for more details) (Caddo Nation, 2023).

## Impact on Health of Interaction with White Culture Now

Groundbreaking for a new child care center occurred on July 10, 2023. The facility will be designed by MASS Design Group and will be built by Arrowood Kakinah Enterprise, a Caddo Nation construction company. MASS Design considered the culture and community needs to create an energy-efficient design for classrooms, a cafeteria, a cultural center, and outdoor playground areas with planned trails. MASS received the 2020 Architecture Innovator of the Year from the Wall Street Journal for its commitment to healing and healthcare. In 2022 MASS received the American Institute of Architects Architecture Firm Award (Caddo Nation, 2023).

## *Catawba*

The Catawba Nation is located in South Carolina and is federally recognized. They were known as "people of the river" and negotiated with the state during the Removal Period to avoid moving west. That treaty gave them  new land in a more remote area for giving up 144,000 acres of land. The Governor thought the tribe had dissolved, but the Catawba were resilient and survived. Today, they own Two Kings Casino and are developing several business entities, including joint ventures (Catawba.com).

## Health & Healing Then

The Catawba had herb gatherers who practiced ethnobotany and used a large number of plants and herbs to cure multiple health conditions and diseases. They followed rules to gather, prepare, and administer these curatives successfully (Speck, 1944).

## Health & Healing Now

The Catawba Indian Nation's Special Diabetes Program promotes traditional foods and activity by establishing community gardens. Nearly 50% of tribal members over age 65 have pre-diabetes or diabetes and gardening increases access to vegetables and fruits that improves members' diets. The Program partnered with the Catawba Cultural

Center using a Centers for Disease Control and Prevention (CDC) grant for materials. Besides creating gardens at multiple sites, the Program has assisted 23 families with gardening help and offers advice and support to seniors and youth. These gardens help prevent and manage diabetes by creating a healthier community (nihb.org, n.d.).

## Impact on Health of Interaction with White Culture Then

The Catawba were skilled traders, but interactions with White settlers resulted in disease epidemics during the 1700s. Smallpox devastated Catawba villages for the fourth time in a hundred years, reducing the population by 1760 to less than 1,000. Originally the Catawba were farmers who fished and hunted on their tribal lands. As settlements increased, Catawba lands decreased reducing their ability live as they always had. They have rebounded from this and received $50 million from a land claim settlement with South Carolina (Catawba.com).

## Impact on Health of Interaction with White Culture Now

The Boys & Girls Club of Catawba Nation began in 2017 for middle and high school children with support from the Boys & Girls Club of America Native Services Division. In 2019 an elementary site was chartered. The Clubs create a positive, safe, and fun environment with opportunity to learn about tribal culture, healthy lifestyles, and character development. Grants supporting this initiative include Walmart Food Access Program, TRAIL Diabetes Prevention grant, Office of Justice Program Mentoring grant, Child Care Development Fund, and Tribal Youth Prevention grant. These Clubs promote growth and development of youth via social, cultural, physical, emotional, and intellectual components (Catawba.com).

## Chickasaw

Chickasaw were "Spartans of the Mississippi Valley" who were successful traders and farmers on their native lands. They were forced to relocate to Indian Territory during the Great Removal also known as the "Trail of Tears". The Chickasaw fought for the Confederacy in the Civil War and suffered hardships after that. However, the tribe produced successful ranchers and farmers and built schools, banks, and businesses in what is today Oklahoma. The Chickasaw Nation is federally recognized and is involved in enterprises and commerce to increase business opportunities for their citizens through economic development support, training, and business counseling for their entrepreneurs (Chickasaw.net, 2023).

## Health & Healing Then

The Chickasaw practiced holistic medicine. The "alikchi" or healer/medicine man was considered divinely selected and had vast knowledge. They focused on spiritual as well as physical diseases and used tea and herbal remedies. They were counselors and believed that everything has a spirit and nature, and the environment must be balanced. They followed sacred formula and used rattles and animal bones. Everything was done with the Creator's help and Chickasaw medicine was considered the most powerful of tribes in this area (Storytellers, 2023).

## Health & Healing Now

The Chickasaw Nation Let's Eat! Program provides meals for children ages 1-18 year-round. Qualifying families receive $60 of free food per child per month from May through July annually. The Chickasaw Health Information Center has multiple health resources. These resources include information about diabetes, cardiovascular disease, environmental health, community health and wellness, drug information, and medical conditions. Health researchers are invited to improve community health and wellness with agreements with the Chickasaw Nation Department of Health (Chickasaw.net, 2023).

## Impact on Health of Interaction with White Culture Then

Early interactions with White Culture were positive and involved trading. In the nineteenth century, the tribe was forced to relocate to Indian Territory and moved to what is now Oklahoma where they still reside. The move was traumatic, and the Chickasaws traveled hundreds of miles in extreme heat and cold. They suffered less than other tribes because they were able to pay for their own removal and select favorable seasons to travel. This saved numerous lives on the journey (Chickasaw.net, 2023).

## Impact on Health of Interaction with White Culture Now

The Chickasaw Lighthorse Police Department and seven of its officers were awarded a State of Oklahoma Citation of Recognition in 2023 for their actions with the Ratliff City Police and Oklahoma Highway Patrol to safely evacuate Ratliff City residents from wildfires in the area. They maintained and evaluated roads for visibility and fire risks to keep the roads safe for emergency use. They also maintained an evacuation center and staging area to provide other first responders a place for rest. The Chickasaw Nation has cross-deputation agreements with counties and municipalities to protect all citizens regardless of jurisdiction (Chickasaw.net, 2023).

## *Choctaw*

The Choctaw Nation is federally recognized and resides in Oklahoma today. The name Choctaw is derived from Chahta, a legendary tribal chief (native-languages.org, 1998-2020).The tribe originally lived in Mississippi and parts of Alabama and Louisiana (NPS.gov). Today they have a diverse business portfolio, including 8 casinos and several travel plazas. They seek new revenue-generating business opportunities to support services for the Nation's members (Choctawnation.com, 2023).

## Health & Healing Then

Stickball was used to mediate conflicts and continues today to teach family values and social structure. To prepare for the game, players prayed, fasted, meditated, danced, and rubbed their bodies with traditional medicines. Alikchi (spiritual leaders) guided players and drummers, paced the game, and celebrated major plays (Choctaw-nation.com, 2023). The medicine wheel was useful for ceremonies and prayer and the medicine circle was important in Choctaw culture. The medicine circle had a cross to represent the male spirit and a circle that represented the female spirit. Each part of the cross has a meaning. East means triumph; West means death; North means defeat; and South means happiness and peace (Varela, 2014).

## Health & Healing Now

The Choctaw Nation Health Services Authority provides services through a hospital and eight clinics within the reservation. Multiple services are available including meals for children in congregate sites; behavioral health services for children, adolescents, and adults; diabetes prevention and treatment; community health nursing; dental services; dermatology; a residential treatment center for women with or without children; and emergency care (Choctawnation.com, 2023).

## Impact on Health of Interaction with White Culture Then

After being displaced from their tribal homelands by treaty and by force, the Choctaw became the first tribe removed to Oklahoma in 1830. They walked the entire trip and many of them died during the travel. At least 3,000 native people died on this march (NPS.gov).

## Impact on Health of Interaction with White Culture Now

The Choctaw Nation Human Resources Department has a Total Rewards Department with concierge service connecting employees to their medical needs and using Bluetooth devices to monitor health conditions like diabetes and hypertension. Their total rewards packages prioritize employees' well-being and diversity, equity and inclusion software improve job postings and remove unintentional biases from position descriptions. In 2023 the Human Resources Department was awarded the Human Resources Director US (HRDUS) Innovative HR Team Award and recognized in 2022 at one of six Best Places to Work (Choctawnation.com, 2023).

## *Creek*

Today the majority of the Creek tribe live in Oklahoma, but they were originally from Alabama and Georgia (Carlisle, 1952). They are federally recognized as the Muscogee (Creek) Nation and the name Creek is from the English name for a river in their homeland (native-languages.org, 1998-2020). The Nation has established diversified successful business entities, including nine casinos and gaming establishments (Muscogee-nation.com, 2023).

## Health & Healing Then

A medicine man or woman had a pouch with medicines. Some were made from leaves, roots, or herbs. Pebbles, shells, and other objects were also included. Preparation was based on a traditional formula during the singing of a particular song. Many diseases were thought to be caused by animals. Four was a sacred number and to become a medicine man or woman, the person fasted four days and sang a song four days about the medicine, its properties, and its benefits. Each medicine must be learned in four days and the person had four months each year for four years to complete the education. The head medicine man was responsible for kindling the council fire, but medicine men and women only worked preparing and giving medicines.

The chief prophet (who might be a medicine man) prepared and administered war medicines. He was feared because he had power to cause or cure fatal illnesses. This medicine man could heal wounds by having the wounded man eat certain kinds of earth. Then, he applied clay or mud by crawfish to the wound and the patient was isolated so no woman with menses saw him. If this occurred, no cure was possible. Treatment of insanity was unique. The medicine man placed four clear pebbles in a cup of clear water, performed ceremonies, and sang certain songs. Then, he put some of the water in his mouth and spurted it violently on the head of the insane person and caused him to drink four times from the cup. Afterward, the medicine man could make the insane person do what he wanted and treated him in various ways until he was cured (Hewitt, 2039).

## Health & Healing Now

The Muscogee (Creek) Nation has numerous health programs. One of these is the Native American Caregiver Support Program where respite workers provide temporary relief to primary caregivers for aging, disabled, or sick community members. The Muscogee Nation Elder Services Department has services for the tribe's growing elderly population. Services are for citizens who are 65 or older, the frail or impaired, and for those in need. These services include lawn mowing, light maintenance, cleaning gutters, and cutting and delivering firewood (as schedule permits). Since social interaction is important, there is a monthly elders meeting, trips locally, and travel to cultural activities. The Elders Department shares information about community activities. The Social Services Department assists with unmet essential needs and provides referrals as needed (Muscogeenation.com, 2023).

## Impact on Health of Interaction with White Culture Then

After giving up some of their tribal lands to Americans, the Creeks passed a law in 1811 forbidding any more land sales. During the War of 1812 they were defeated and forced to vacate a large part of their territory. This impacted their ability to grow crops and depleted the game animals the Creeks depended on for their lifestyle. Ove the next 20 years many Creeks migrated west and in 1836, the remaining tribe members were forced to journey to Indian Territory (Carlisle, 1952).

## Impact on Health of Interaction with White Culture Now

In May 2023 the Governor of Oklahoma vetoed the Native American Regalia Bill. The bill would have permitted Creek graduates and those of other tribes to wear their tribal regalia to honor their accomplishments and academic achievements by paying tribute to their culture and heritage. His veto was overridden by the Oklahoma legislature and took effect July 1, 2023. This is a step toward restoring justice in the relationship between educational facilities and Native Americans (Black Horse, Bree; Kilpatrick Townsend & Stockton LLC, 2023).

## *Cherokee*

The Cherokee Nation are federally recognized and live primarily in Oklahoma. They have become prosperous in diverse businesses, including four casinos, tourism, and retail endeavors (Cherokee.org, 2023). The name Cherokee means "speakers of another language" (native-languages.org, 1998-2020).

## Health & Healing Then

Cherokee medicines included yarrow, black cohosh, American ginseng, and blue skullcap. They used the bark of the red maple for cramps and eye soreness; yarrow for healing wounds, hemorrhoids, and bowel concerns; roots of blue cohosh as an anticonvulsive and anti-rheumatic; black cohosh to treat coughs, colds, and rheumatism; witch hazel for colds, sore throats and fevers; root of goldenseal herb for cancer, dyspepsia, and as a tonic; the common rush plant as an emetic;  and infusions of blue skullcap root treated monthly menses and diarrhea (Setzer, 2018).

## Health & Healing Now

The Cherokee Nation Health Services is the largest health system that is tribally-owned in the United States. It has multiple health services that include two in-patient health facilities and nine out-patient health facilities. Public Health programs promote healthy lifestyles and services, including behavioral health, eyeglasses, crowns & bridges, hearing aids, HIV & Hepatitis C services, home health, neurology, and rehabilitation services. The Patient Experience Team ensures access to services for members living outside the Tribal Jurisdictional Service Area and Patient Benefit Coordinators are advocates for insurance benefits and utilization of resources such as Medicare and Medicaid (Cherokee.org, 2023).

## Impact on Health of Interaction with White Culture Then

The treaty with the Cherokee Nation during the Removal stated they would not be forced to move from their new home in Oklahoma Territory. When Statehood arrived, tribes' land was given to individual non-Cherokee owners. When Cherokees became state citizens much of their infrastructure was gone and a time of poverty began for the tribe. It took many years to regain their government and power (Cherokee.org, 2023).

## Impact on Health if Interaction with White Culture Now

In 2010 the Cherokee Nation began an initiative to combat obesity and tobacco use with  funding by the Centers for Disease Control and Prevention (CDC). The statistics indicated serious health concerns. About 66% of the Cherokee population is obese or overweight and this will affect 1 in 3 children in the community. About 29% of adult Cherokee citizens currently smoke, more than 12% use smokeless tobacco, and almost 29% of Cherokee high school students smoked a cigarette in the past 30 days. The Nation established biannual screenings for chronic diseases. To prevent obesity, they developed relationships between local farms and schools to provide healthy nutrition, required 150 minutes of physical activity each week in school systems, and offered fruit options in school vending machines. To reduce tobacco use, they fostered tobacco-free, smoke-free environments in schools and businesses. Cherokee members were referred to the 5 A's tobacco intervention program. The Nation partnered with organizations like the Northeast Regional Oklahoma Students Working Against Tobacco Abuse to educate community members about dangers of tobacco use. They required all contractors in businesses, casinos, hotels, and resorts to be tobacco-free so residents and visitors are not exposed to second-hand smoke (CDC.gov, 2010).

**Note:** Refer to Oklahoma Statues, Title 21 Section 1247 (11/1/2010) for details about Oklahoma Statutes on Smoking in Public Places and Indoor Workplaces which permits designated smoking rooms if enclosed and ventilated properly (ok.gov, 2010).

## *Powhatan*

Today eight Powhatan descended tribes have been recognized by the Commonwealth of Virginia. They are the Pamunkey, Mattaponi, Upper Mattaponi, Chickahominy, Eastern Chickahominy, Nansemond, Rappahannock, and Patawomeck tribes. Two of these—the Mattaponi and Pamunkey-- live on reservations and make yearly tribute to the Virginia governor based on previous treaties (Stebbins, 2012) The Pamunkey Tribe received federal recognition in 2015 and plans to build a resort and casino on land acquired from Norfolk. Their other enterprises include FedTribe (specializing in IT and  communications technology) and Pamunkey

Indian Enterprises-Professional Services (specializing in professional services needed for the Federal government). Each qualifies as a Native American Tribal 8(a) company and Small Disadvantaged Business (Pamunkey Indian Tribe, 2021).

## Health & Healing Then

The Powhatan tribe worshipped many spirits. The main spirit was Okee who had human form and was emulated. A female spirit guided those passing into the spirit world and the sun was integral to maintain life, home, and health. Special dwellings called Quiocosin in remote locations were only entered by a shaman or chief. The shamans lived there and served as spiritual advisors and doctors. They may enter a trance, perform rituals, or dances. Sacrifices to Okee, such as deer's blood or food, protected hunters or maintained the spirit's favor. Medicine, such as red puccoon root, healed patients and ended sickness by shamans with the spirits' help. There were also rituals when a boy becomes a man and when a chief dies to help him enter the spirit world. Dances in regalia represented the world and spirits, the harvest, and hunting season (Heutmaker, 2017).

## Health & Healing Now

Powwows continue today to celebrate the spirituality and culture of the People (Heutmaker, 2017). The Upper Mattaponi Tribe opened a health clinic in 2021 by purchasing an abandoned building and renovating it. Since physicians are limited in that area, the non-Native doctor and Native nurse practitioner treat the surrounding community as well as tribal members. Recently, they have expanded services to include home health care and are hiring more staff with plans for future clinics in Virginia (D'Angelo, 2022).

## Impact on Health of Interaction with White Culture Then

After Pocahontas' death in 1617, conflict occurred between the Powhatan tribe and the English settlers resulting in lost native lands. In 1647-1677, reservations were established, and tribute required from the Powhatan who lived there. In 1924 the Racial Integrity Act was passed which recognized only two racial classifications: "white" and "colored". The Powhatan and other tribes in Virginia didn't exist. Walter Plecker, head of Vital Statistics, was a white supremacist and follower of the eugenics movement. He called tribe members "mongrels" and his aggressive policies caused many tribal members to flee Virginia. Ironically, the Indian Citizenship Act of 1924 granted citizenship to all native Americans. The Racial Integrity Act was finally repealed in 1967, but it did a lot of damage in the years before then (Stebbins, 2012).

## Impact on Health of Interaction with White Culture Now

Lack of federal recognition of the Mattaponi Tribe resulted in ineligibility for the American Rescue Plan funds for housing, economic development, and infrastructure (Mattaponi Tribe, 2022). The Pamunkey Indian Tribe received a 3-year Species Recovery Grant in 2018 from the National Oceanic and Atmospheric Administration (NOAA) to study Atlantic sturgeon and their habitat, including collecting water quality data and developing a Pamunkey River Keeper position to continue this work and improve stewardship. They collaborated with researchers from Chesapeake Scientific with the goal of recovering the sturgeon population. The sturgeon played an important role in Pamunkey life for food, income, and as a rite of passage for the tribe's young men who rode on the sturgeons' back (NOAA Fisheries, 2020).

## *Quapaw*

The Quapaw Nation is federally recognized and lives in Oklahoma. The Tribe originated in Arkansas. The name 'Quapaw' means "downstream people" (native-languages.org, 1998-2020). The Quapaw Nation has multiple enterprises including the Downstream Casino Resort, the Quapaw Casino, an RV Park, convenience stores and gas stations, a cattle company, golf course, farmers market, fitness center and tribal museum (Quapaw Nation, n.d.).

## Health & Healing Then

The Quapaw had multiple clans although membership was inherited through the father (gentes). The clans were named for animals, natural happenings (e.g., thunder) or heavenly bodies. Tribal members believed they were descended from a common ancestor causing mutual obligation and strong sense of shared identity. The Quapaw had numerous ceremonies where each clan had specific duties. Some ceremonies were held at specific times that aligned with planting and harvesting. Others included naming ceremonies, curing rituals, marriages, and adoptions. Village leaders were advised by councils of male elders and consent of all village leaders was essential when decisions involved the entire tribe (Wilson & Sabo III, 2008).

## Health & Healing Now

Chat piles of mining waste have caused many health problems for tribal residents. These include respiratory infections, lung cancer, hypertension, high infant mortality, and high lead levels in children (Mobley, 2020 & Herrera, 2022).

Today, the Quapaw Nation uses the Community Health Representatives Program of Indian Health Services to provide health promotion and disease prevention services. Their responsibilities include home visits, monthly health screenings transport for medical appointments, medication set-up, case management, monitoring, and patient care, and wound dressings and checks. The program also provides an annual health fair for the community and tribal members (Quapaw Nation, n.d.).

## Impact on Health of Interaction with White Culture Then

Interaction with White culture resulted in the 1852 measles epidemic that killed 40 tribal members. From 1865-1868, relocation to the reservation in Oklahoma caused the tribe to be starving and desolate where they were reduced to eating roots to survive (Quapaw Nation, n.d.). The Quapaw Nation was also adversely impacted by the Tar Creek Superfund site. This area had mining for cadmium, lead, and zinc from the late 1800s to the late 1970s. It was added to the National Priorities list by the EPA in 1983. Surface water problems in Tar Creek had to be addressed to reduce contamination that could impact drinking water. Mining waste removal and cleanup of contaminated soil from residents' land led to residential relocation (epa.gov, 2023). Children had elevated blood lead levels and the community of Pilcher was known as the "most polluted town in America" (Herrera, 2022).

## Impact on Health of Interaction with White Culture Now

In 2012, the Quapaw Nation was awarded EPA funding and became the first Native tribe in the United States to lead and manage Superfund site cleanup. They began by cleaning up Catholic 40 property. This is a 40-acre property owned by the Nation that is culturally and historically significant to them. The EPA has awarded the Nation multiple cooperative agreements to clean up other restricted tribal lands. Their focus is cultural preservation, expansion of ranching, and agricultural use. They and the Oklahoma Department of Environmental Quality have cleaned up mining waste of over six million tons (epa.gov, 2023). Today, the Quapaw Nation wants to regulate contractors by developing environmental codes to regulate environmental cleanup inside the reservation (Herrera, 2022).

## *Saluda*

The Saluda tribe no longer exists. It was believed to be a small tribe in South Carolina which moved to Pennsylvania in the 1700s and affiliated with the Shawnee. (Access Genealogy).

## Health & Healing Then

No information available

## Impact on Health of Interaction with White Culture Then

No information available

## *Saponi*

There are three state recognized Saponi tribes in North Carolina. They are the Sappony in Roxboro; the Haliwa Saponi of Hollister; and the Occaneechi Band of Burlington. All are interested in preserving their heritage and culture and the well-being of their communities (sappony.org; obsn.org, 2021; & Haliwa-saponi.org, 2022).

## Health & Healing Then

The Saponi grew their own foods with a large number of vegetables. Their agricultural-based society was healthy, and they used home remedies and traditional root medicine healing methods (Gillis, 2021).

## Health & Healing Now

An interview with a Haliwa-Saponi woman discussed health issues impacting the tribe. Obesity rates are higher for tribal members than for White neighbors. When the Haliwa-Saponi grew their own food, most of their diet was vegetables and there was less obesity. When corporate farms bought out small farms, the community became dependent on processed foods instead of fresh fruit and vegetables. Food deserts were created because convenience foods took the place of grocery stores with fresh food. These were high in added sugars and lack of exercise and recreation programs resulted in obesity from childhood through adulthood. Tribes that are not federally recognized don't receive assistance from the Food Distribution Program and support on health issues is mainly educational from state funding. Many tribal members are reluctant to seek health care from local facilities and prefer home remedies and traditional medicine. Indian Health Services is unavailable to tribes without federal recognition. Many tribal members lack a primary care physician, health insurance, and can't access cost effective healthcare. They lack education and access causing poor health outcomes and higher death rates than Whites (Gillis, 2021).

## Impact on Health of Interaction with White Culture Then

As their native lands decreased, many Saponi joined other tribes in migrating. Those who remained intermarried with the settler community, resulting in an acculturated community. The Indian Reorganization Act of 1934 determined that "Indian" had to fit a stereotype and Saponi were not seen as "Indian". The development of agribusiness created dependence on food shipped from outside the community and food deserts developed that fueled obesity (Gillis, 2021 & obsn.org, 2021).

## Impact on Health of Interaction with White Culture Now

A Sappony Tribe member is employed by the North Carolina Commission of Indian Affairs as a Victim Advocate for Domestic Violence, Sexual Assault and Human Trafficking. She is available for all tribal members with concerns about these issues and is one of a number of such advocates in the State (sappony.org).

## *Seminole*

The Seminole Tribe of Florida and the Seminole Nation of Oklahoma are both federally recognized. The word Seminole means "separatist" or "runaway" (native-languages.org, 1998-2020). When the Removal came, the Seminoles fought back. Although more than 3,000 were moved west to Oklahoma, less than 1,000 remained. As women, children and elders were captured, many warriors went with them to keep their families together. The remainder stayed moving into the wetlands and became today's Seminole Tribe of Florida. The Seminoles there opened the first smoke shop in 1977 and created a revenue-producing enterprise. They subsequently opened the first high-stakes bingo hall resulting today in six casinos in Florida (semtribe.com/stof, n.d.). The Seminole Nation of Oklahoma after Removal were confined to the Creek Nation and subject to its laws. After a decade, they began to re-establish themselves and today own three casinos and other enterprises (sno-nsn.org, 2023).

## Health & Healing Then

When a death occurred, the entire family mourned four days and took herbs made by the medicine man on the fourth morning. They drank them with tea or washed with them. The medicine men used roots, animal parts and other natural ingredients to treat mental and physical illnesses. Traditional chants were also integral to the medicine men. Many believed that luck (good or bad); success or failure; safety and danger; right decisions and wrong decisions were influenced by medicine being applied (semtribe.com/stof, n.d.).

## Health & Healing Now

The Seminole Health and Human Services Department (HHS) is focusing on opioid overdoses in 2023. Community education is vital and Narcan accessibility is essential to deal with emergency situations. Narcan kits are available at the Seminole Police Department and the Tribe's EMS staff. Overdoses have involved Fentanyl and Cocaine and three people required treatment in intensive care in the past few months. Discussion is underway about additional locations for Narcan in the community. HHS is also promoting annual health exams and check-ups. Kidney, cardiac, hypertension, liver, obesity, and diabetes issues have increased. They are encouraging younger people to come routinely to increase prevention and early intervention and have increased their staffing to address these issues (Scott, 2023).

## Impact on Health of Interaction with White Culture Then

Interactions with White Culture resulted in loss of farmland and relocation within Florida to deep wetlands where they survived and thrived in a hostile environment (semtribe.com/stof, n.d.). The Treaty of 1833 merged the Seminoles in Oklahoma into the Creek Nation with loss of autonomy. The Treaty of 1845 enabled the Seminoles to have their own land and resolved conflicts between the tribes (okstate.edu, 1845).

## Impact on Health of Interaction with White Culture Now

The Advocacy & Guardianship Department supports at-risk children and families, including those in the Florida child welfare system. These Child Advocates collaborate with non-tribal county and state groups to protect children, develop parenting skills, recruit foster parents, and monitor placements under the Indian Child Welfare Act and other laws (semtribe.com/stof, n.d.). The Seminole Nation of Oklahoma provides victim advocacy services, court advocacy, utility and housing services, community outreach, and referral for additional resources. The court-mandated 52-week Batterer's Intervention Course focuses on breaking the cycle of violence and abuse and the Seminole Nation Domestic Violence Program provides classes for sexual assault victims and collaborates with a licensed counselor for additional services (sno-nsn.org, 2023).

## The Removal Period-Trail of Tears

This Photo by Unknown Author is licensed under CC BY-NC-ND

Each of the tribes profiled in this section was impacted by the Indian Removal Act of 1830. They had lived on their native lands for centuries until White culture arrived. Even if not adversarial, the native tribes and settlers didn't understand each other. To the tribes, the land was for everyone and must be cultivated for future generations. To the settlers, it was an opportunity to grow cotton as a cash crop regardless of the damage to the indigenous people who lived on it. In the early 1800s officials, including George Washington, believed that the best approach was to "civilize" the tribes by converting them to Christianity and making them act like the White settlers. Many members of the Cherokee, Creek, Choctaw, Chickasaw, and Seminole tribes embraced these new customs and were known as the "Five Civilized Nations".

This conversion didn't stop settlers from stealing, looting, and burning tribal towns and houses. They also murdered native people and stole native land (History.com Editors, 2023).

State governments in North Carolina, Alabama, Georgia, Florida, and Tennessee passed laws designed to limit tribal rights and take more territory from them. The Indian Removal Act gave the U.S. Government power to exchange tribal land in these states for land in the west that was obtained in the Louisiana Purchase of 1803. This Indian Territory was in today's State of Oklahoma (History.com Editors, 2023).

In 1831 the Choctaw were expelled from their lands and marched west in the winter without food, supplies, or any governmental help. Thousands of tribal members died on the journey that they called "a trail of tears and death". In 1836 15,000 Creeks set out on this journey and 3,500 died on the way. The Cherokee had signed a treaty in 1819 that their land would be forbidden to settlers forever. This treaty lasted less than 20 years and in 1837 the first 2,000 Cherokee voluntarily relocated by boat using rivers to go west. Less than 2 dozen died of this group. In 1838 more than 15,000 Cherokee were forcibly removed and more than 5,000 of them died of exposure, starvation, and disease (typhus, dysentery, cholera, and whooping cough) on their journey (History.com Editors, 2023).

The Trail of Tears is over 5,000 miles long and covers nine states: Alabama, Arkansas, Georgia, Illinois, Kentucky, Missouri, North Carolina, Oklahoma, and Tennessee (History.com Editors, 2023). Chickasaw, and Seminole tribes also made the trek which took several months on foot with only the elderly and sick able to ride in wagons or on horseback. There are graves-marked and unmarked-all along the Trail of Tears. On arrival in Oklahoma Territory, much of the land promised to the tribes in the treaties was taken away. This cultural genocide and forcible removal of entire indigenous nations is recognized by a memorial and official Historic Trail in Oklahoma and the largest tribal cultural center in the United States to honor indigenous people. In 2020 the Supreme Court recognized that almost half of Oklahoma is Native land. These are steps toward reconciliation and acknowledgement, but cannot make up for past wrongdoing (Mandewo, 2020).

It is worth noting that tribal removal also occurred in Northern states too where the Black Hawk War in 1832 opened millions of acres to White settlement in Illinois and Wisconsin displacing Native nations such as Sauk and Fox (History.com Editors, 2023).

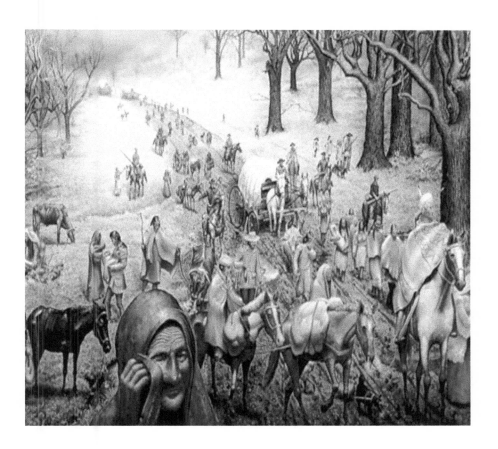

# Chapter 4
# Midwest Tribes

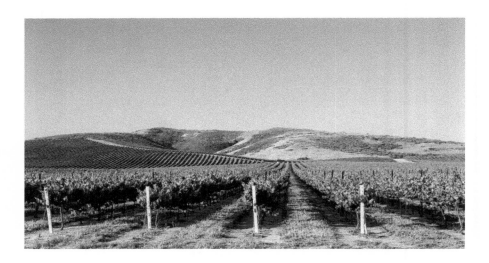

Numerous Native tribes lived in today's Midwestern states. They included: Blackfoot, Cahokia, Chippewa, Dakota, Fox, Ho-Chunk, Huron, Illinois, Iowa, Kaskaskia, Kickapoo, Menominee, Miami, Missouri, Odawa, Ojibwe, Omaha, Osage, Ottawa, Peoria, Potawatomi, Sauk( Sac), Shawnee, Wea, Winnebago, and Wyandot tribes.

## *Blackfoot*

The Piegan Blackfeet tribe live in Montana and other Blackfoot tribes live in Canada. They called themselves "Real People" and the term Blackfoot originated by Whites based on the color of their moccasins when first introduced to White culture. Some tribal members prefer Blackfoot rather than the plural term. The Blackfeet Nation is federally recognized and nearly 40% of the reservation is owned today by non-Blackfeet. In the later part of the 20th century, the Nation was awarded compensation from the United States for land losses in 1888 and for unfair federal accounting of tribal funds. These settlements promoted business development including the Glacier Peaks Hotel & Casino, Blackfeet Heritage Center and Art Gallery, Glacier Family Foods, Oki Communications, and

Blackfeet National Bank (the first tribally owned, full-service bank in the U.S.). This bank is now the Native American Bank and includes other tribes. Blackfeet Community College offers associate degrees and certificate programs to prepare tribal members for future success. The Blackfeet Nation has also negotiated a Water Compact and Settlement Act to ensure a reliable long-term water supply and potential water-related projects. They are also working with conservation groups to prevent further oil and gas drilling on their sacred land (Blackfeet Nation, 2023; Graetz, 2023; Hanes & Pifer, 2023).

## Health & Healing Then

The traditional Blackfoot Medicine Wheel has four quadrants of physical, spiritual, emotional, and mental health. Spirituality was essential for healing and all four were required for health (McTighe, 2018). The Blackfoot believed spirits were active in everyday life and illness was the result of an evil spirit in the person's body. Medicine men or women acquired knowledge via internship and learned to use visions to remove evil spirits. Herbs were used to treat smaller injuries or cuts. Traditionally, the medicine man or woman was paid through a gift of horses. (Hanes & Pifer, 2023)

## Health & Healing Now

The Blackfeet Nation have lost the staples of their diet. Most of their food came from buffalo and the rest came from bulbs, roots, eggs, wild berries, and vegetables. Today, the Blackfeet are less active and most of their diet is from processed purchased food that is high in sugar and calories. Alcohol consumption is also an issue and "has contributed to the rise of coronary heart disease, stroke, high blood pressure, cancer, diabetes, obesity, osteoporosis, dental caries, periodontal disease, and diverticular disease" (Malinowski, n.d.).

## Impact on Health of Interaction with White Culture Then

Like other tribes, the Blackfoot suffered significant population losses from epidemics of diphtheria and smallpox in the 1800s. Decimation of the buffalo by White hunters created dependency on government agents for food and essential supplies. As the buffalo were killed, the tribe suffered from famine and had to adapt to a new agricultural lifestyle. Between 1884-1910 Holy Family Mission, a Catholic boarding school, was established on the reservation. This was followed by a government boarding school and day schools. As previously described, these schools focused on assimilating Blackfoot students into White Culture by forbidding native language use and traditional customs (see Chapter 1). In the late 20th century, the Blackfoot language and cultural values were reborn to identify with Blackfoot heritage (Hanes & Pifer, 2023).

## Impact on Health of Interaction with White Culture Now

In March 2020, four people died in one week on the Blackfeet Reservation from fentanyl overdoses. Overdose deaths have disproportionately affected Native Americans making them the highest death rate of all racial groups and twice as many as White people from 2019-2021. The Blackfeet have less access to health care resources for addiction. The Indian Health Service (IHS) is chronically underfunded, and the local treatment center is not equipped to handle opioid withdrawal. There are only two detox beds in the local IHS facility and medication-assisted treatment is not available. Drugs such as methadone or buprenorphine are only available 30-100 miles away and this is prohibitive for daily or weekly dispensing. Tribal leaders requested help from the IHS Alcohol and Substance Abuse Program, but the agency prefers to supply medications for tribes to run their own programs. The Rocky Mountain Tribal Leaders Council (including the Blackfeet Nation) is collaborating with the Montana Healthcare Foundation on a feasibility study for a tribal-operated treatment center. The Blackfeet passed a resolution to support this initiative and declared a state of emergency in March 2022. The tribe has created a task force to identify both short- and long-term needs to address this issue. The tribal policy investigator leading the task force wants to train more people to administer Naloxone and for the tribe to have needle exchanges to reduce infections and HIV. A reorganization of the tribal health department is planned to provide drug addiction resources in one location. Poverty, housing, and food insecurity also must be addressed (Bolton, 2022).

## *Cahokia*

The Cahokia tribe lived in Illinois until the 1400s and is now extinct. They left the area due to over-population and natural disasters prior to arrival of White Culture and disappeared after that time (Mark, 2021).

### Health & Healing Then

No information available

### Impact on Health of Interaction with White Culture Then

No interaction with White Culture.

## *Chippewa (Ojibwe)*

Ojibwe call themselves "Original People" or "True People. The term Chippewa meant "puckered up" referring to the top of their moccasins (Milwaukee Public Museum, 2022). Several separate Chippewa (Ojibwe) tribes live in the United States. The Sault Tribe is federally recognized and lives in Michigan. Their business enterprises include a property management company, convenience stores, townhouse rentals, five Kewadin Casinos, and the Michigan Indian Press (Sault Ste. Marie Tribe of Chippewa Indians, 2023). The other federally recognized Chippewa tribe in Michigan is located in Saginaw. Their enterprises include a marina, an economic development company, a campground, a waterpark, a hotel (the Retreat), the Soaring Eagle Casino, and the Ziibiwing Cultural Center (sagchip.org, 1998-2023). The Minnesota Chippewa Tribe is federally recognized and consists of six bands on member reservations. It has casinos, gas and grocery stores, lodging, and RV park, and a community college within its six bands (Minnesota Chippewa Tribe, n.d.). The St. Croix tribe of Wisconsin is federally recognized. They have casinos, hotels, a campground, convenience stores, and commercial rental properties (stcroixojibwe-nsn.gov, n.d.) The Turtle Mountain Band of Chippewa live in North Dakota and are federally recognized. They have a loan program utilized by customers in multiple states and a community college (tmchippewa.com, n.d.). The newest federally recognized tribe is the Little Shell Tribe of Chippewa Indians of Montana. They promote native artists and sell products in Shop LS 574 (Montana Little Shell Chippewa Tribe, n.d.).

## Health & Healing Then

The Chippewa used plants for medicine, gathering those with medicinal properties. This knowledge was passed from generation to generation. Red Ceder and White Cedar were sprinkled on burning cinders to release their incense during ceremonies. Besides evoking good feelings, they encouraged spirits to enter ceremonies. Choke Cherry and Arrowhead (Swan Potato) were food sources and other plants supplemented the Chippewa's diet. New Jersey Tea roots relieved shortness of breath, bloating, and constipation. Bitterroot was a physic and Avens Root was used as an astringent to stop bleeding when applied to wounds (Ferris, 2021).

## Health & Healing Now

Each Chippewa tribe has a different approach to the tribe's current health care issues. The Sault Ste. Marie Tribe's Anishnaabek Community and Family Services manages 30 grant contracts for three mission areas: direct services for tribal members in financial, nutritional, and housing needs; child placement services for safety and well-being; and advocacy services for crime victims (Sault. Ste. Marie Tribe of Chippewa Indians, 2023). The Saginaw Chippewa Tribe has a unique approach to behavioral health-the Washing Away Ceremony for Community Healing. The ceremony is held in the Behavioral Health Lodge and people schedule 30-minute appointments to wash and release negative energy with support from two team members. It is designed to assist with grounding and balance (sagchip.org, 1998-2023). The Minnesota Chippewa Tribe's Human Service Division addresses elderly services, child welfare, nutrition education, tribal employment, and chemical dependency prevention and intervention (Minnesota Chippewa Tribe, n.d.). The St. Croix Tribe has a Behavioral Health Clinic that provides substance use and mental health treatment. Their approach to recovery assesses any co-recurring mental health and addiction issues together (stcroixojibwe-nsn.gov, n.d.). The Turtle Mountain Band has the 5th Generation Healing Center to provide support and education for alcoholism and drug abuse. Health education provides programs on prevention and healthy living as well as infant care and STD/STI awareness (tmchippewa.com, n.d.). The Montana Little Shell Tribe has a Chronic Disease Prevention Specialist who helps members with chronic diseases such as asthma, cancer, and diabetes find resources and monitors their progress. A personalized, unique "Prevention Prescription" has improved screening and chronic disease prevention outcomes by 37% (Montana Little Shell Chippewa Tribe, n.d.).

## Impact on Health of Interaction with White Culture Then

Contact with White Culture did not adversely impact the health of the Ojibwe (Chippewa).

Their alliance with the French and then the British forced them to lose lands and move westward as forests were cut for lumber and copper mines expanded. After reservations began, the Ojibwe (Chippewa) could no longer live by hunting and gathering and worked as lumberjacks for White companies and the Dawes Act of 1887 divided up reservations to encourage assimilation (Milwaukee Public Museum, 2022).

## Impact on Health of Interaction with White Culture Now

The Little Shell Chippewa Tribe has partnered with the Rocky Mountain Tribal Leaders Council and the Montana Tobacco Use Prevention Program to reduce tobacco dependence through education, support, and resources. This is a primary focus for their Chronic Disease Prevention Specialist, and they recommend use of the Montana Tobacco Quit Line which is staffed 5 AM to 11 PM every day with voicemail and returned calls (Montana Little Shell Chippewa Tribe, n.d.).

## *Dakota*

The Dakota Tribe (meaning "friend or ally") lives in Minnesota, where four communities are federally recognized, and one is not (Dakota Wicohan, 2020). The Dakota Wicohan is a nonprofit cultural resource center to share Dakota language, lifestyle, and outreach (Dakota Wicohan, 2020). The Shakopee Mdewakanton Sioux Community  has enterprises that include a natural foods store, a tribal garden, hotels, family entertainment centers, and two casinos (shakopeedakota, 2023). The Prairie Island Indian Community's enterprises include an elder and independent assisted living community, a golf course, a convenience store, and the Treasure Island Resort and Casino (prairieisland.org, 2023). The Upper Sioux Community's enterprises include a convenience store, a RV park and campground,   and the Prairie's Edge Casino Resort (uppersiouxcommunity-nsn.gov,   n.d.).   The   Lower   Sioux   Indian Community's enterprises include a golf course and the Junction Casino Hotel (lowersioux.com, 2023).

## Health & Healing Then

The Dakota used native plants for medicinal purposes. Rose Hips in teas and tonics treated coughs and colds. Echinacea had various uses, including treating pain in wounds, sores, and toothaches. Chokecherry was used in the Sun Dance. Leaves were put in a tea and the twigs were used as an offering. Sage root was an anti-convulsive and its leaves treated stomachaches. Jo-pye as a tea treated bladder, kidney, and gallstones. Yarrow was an antiseptic and dandelions were used in winter to prevent vitamin deficiency (stolaf.edu, 2020).

## Health & Healing Now

The Lower Sioux use the Family Spirit Program, the only evidence-based home visit program developed for Native American families. It is designed to support Native parents from pregnancy to three years after birth. The Community Health Nurse does home visits to increase parenting skills and knowledge, promote optimal development for children 0-3, ensure recommended health care and well-child visits, provide linkage to community services, and promote life skills and positive outcomes for children and parents. The program is recommended for at-risk mothers or those younger than 22 and a curriculum of 63 lessons is available (lowersioux.com, 2023). Upper Sioux Health Services provides support for tribal members with diabetes and has a Community Health Representative who does home visits, collaborates with health providers, and arranges health services for the community. Health Services also focuses on elderly tribal members by providing a home health aide to help with activities of daily living and ensuring that elders and disabled tribal members receive one meal per day through the Meal Site program. Elders may have the meal delivered to their home if they cannot do communal dining. Transportation to dental and medical appointments is a service by the Community Transportation Assistant (uppersiouxcommunity-nsn.gov, n.d.). The Prairie Island Indian Community has an ordinance on child welfare (1/1/2020) that considers the negative effects of intergenerational trauma related to boarding schools and removals of community children. Parents have experienced physical, emotional, cultural, and spiritual trauma and resulting addiction requires time and support for recovery. The Community strives to maintain the family unit whenever possible and provides services for children and families that include prevention, early intervention, and community alternatives before seeking residential treatment (prairieisland.org, 2023). The Shakopee Mdewakanton Sioux Community has a certified fruit orchard and organic vegetable garden. Wozupi ("garden" in Dakota) Tribal Gardens uses natural growing techniques, including no-till soil management, living mulches, cover cropping, intensive compost application, supporting the surrounding ecosystem, and controlling pests with beneficial insects. This supports land stewardship by the Community and their greenhouse and high tunnels extend the availability of fresh produce to nine months a year (shakopeedakota, 2023).

## Impact on Health of Interaction with White Culture Then

The United States breached the Treaty of 1851 and didn't provide food and services to the Dakota on their reservation. Local traders refused to provide food and the tribe faced disease and starvation. After the Dakota rebelled and lost, 1,200 women and children were force marched 120 miles to a concentration camp near St. Paul, Mn. where hundreds died from disease and starvation. The language and culture were considered illegal for four generations. Assimilation policies and boarding schools created multiple issues that the Dakota continue to address today— alcoholism, substance misuse, suicides, incarceration rates, and dropout rates (Dakota Wicohan, 2020).

## Impact on Health of Interaction with White Culture Now

The Prairie Island Indian Community is the largest employer in Goodhue County, Minnesota. Their well-paying jobs and benefits economically impact the area. More than 200 new businesses have been created to support gaming resort operations. For the past 34 years, the Prairie Island Indian Community has supported community and non-profit organizations by donating more than $24 million. Their charitable giving also includes health care, education, environmental awareness, and youth sports activities (prairieisland.org, 2023).

## *Fox*

The Fox tribe today is joined with the Sauk (Sac) tribe and there are three federally recognized Sac and Fox tribes: the Sac & Fox Nation of Oklahoma, the Meskwaki Nation of Iowa, and the Sac and Fox Nation of Missouri in Kansas and Nebraska. The name Fox is derived from Meskwaki or "people of the red earth" (Alexander, 2023). In 1730 after losing in battle to the French, Fox refugees joined the Sac tribe and they moved from Wisconsin to Iowa, Illinois, and Missouri until an 1804 treaty between both tribes and the United States. One group separated from the others and moved to Missouri where they became a distinct tribe. In 1856, Iowa allowed the Sac and Fox to live there, and the Meskwaki purchased land there in 1857. Remaining tribal members were removed to Oklahoma after a treaty in 1867 (Alexander, 2023). The Sac and Fox Nation of Missouri in Kansas and Nebraska's enterprises include a museum, a trading post, a truck stop, and the Sac and Fox Casino (sacandfoxks.com, 2023). The Meskwaki Nation's enterprises include a recreation center, a bank, an organic farm, several businesses, and the Meskwaki Bingo Casino Hotel (meskwaki.org, 2023). The Sac & Fox Nation of Oklahoma's enterprises include the Sac and Fox Casino and the Black Hawk Casino along with education incentives (sacandfoxnation-nsn.gov, 2023).

## Health & Healing Then

Frog medicine was used for creating an erection by applying pulverized bones of a frog into a powder and applying this mixture to the penis. When playing lacrosse, a Fox tribesman rubbed medicine on his stick and his body to gain power over his opponent. Sacred bundles protected the people from evil. The bundle couldn't be placed on the ground, but must be hung. An evergreen tree's leaves must be used in smoking a sacred bundle. The Fox had nature beliefs and manitous or spiritual powers. The Sun was a man and grandfather who gives light and warmth. The Moon was the people's grandmother who was kind. The Earth was the grandmother of the people and the trees who were grandfathers. An offering of tobacco should be made before cutting a tree and all parts of it should be used. Stars were great manitous, and most were people who have died and gone to live in the sky (Jones, 1939).

## Health & Healing Now

The Sac & Fox Nation of Oklahoma's Adult Protective Services provides protection for vulnerable tribal elders and incapacitated adults from neglect and abuse. They investigate reports of abuse or neglect, assess for risk of harm, and provide protective services, such as case management, collaboration with health care providers, and guardianship or protective placement (sacandfoxnation-nsn.gov, 2023). The Meskwaki Nation has multiple behavioral health services. These include screening, assessment, and treatment for mental health issues, alcohol and substance use issues, and crisis intervention services. Other screening and referrals involve gambling, tobacco use, and domestic violence (meskwaki.org, 2023). The Sac and Fox Nation of Missouri in Kansas and Nebraska also use "Honor the Circle. Honor Your Family." to prevent violence against Native women that covers ritual abuse, cultural abuse, coercion and threats, economic abuse, using children, minimize/lie/blame, emotional abuse, intimidation, isolation, and male privilege (sacabdfoxks.com, 2023).

## Impact on Health of Interaction with White Culture Then

The French sought to exterminate the Fox and nearly destroyed the tribe in 1728. Only the release of Fox tribesmen held as prisoners of war by other tribes and adopted captives saved the Foxes from extinction by 1731. This was when they took refuge with the Sauk (Sac), An epidemic in 1766 killed half the Sauk and Fox village inhabitants. As the tribes migrated to Kansas in 1842, deaths occurred and about 300 died of cholera in 1851 and of smallpox in 1852. When some of the tribe left for Iowa, they faced desperate financial conditions based on refusal by the U.S. Government to pay their annuities. This continued until 1867 when Fox in Kansas moved to Oklahoma (Jones, 1939).

## Impact on Health of Interaction with White Culture Now

Dealing with a loved one struggling with substance abuse is difficult in any setting. A member of the Meskwaki Nation described how teamwork can help an at-risk individual receive treatment via substance abuse committal. The process requires obtaining mental health or substance abuse committal papers or both with the assistance of the court house clerk. The magistrate then decides if treatment should be mandated. If the individual refuses, the Meskwaki Police or Tama County Police take the individual to detox at Covenant Emergency Department. The individual is treated respectfully throughout the process and a court hearing is held after detox is completed attended by the affected individual and the person who completed the committal papers. The process is informal with the best interest of the individual paramount throughout the journey. The tribal behavioral health staff is also a resource for family, so they understand that they are saving their loved one's life even if he or she is angry by the committal choice (meskawki.org, 2023).

## Ho-Chunk (Winnebago)

Ho-Chunk Nation is a federally recognized tribe known as "people of the sacred voice" who live in Wisconsin. Ho-chunk Nation was previously the Winnebago Nation. The tribe's enterprises include convenience stores, campgrounds, bingo halls, hotels, and casinos (ho-chunknation.com, 2023).

## Health & Healing Then

The Ho-Chunk people practiced specific group and personal rituals and taboos related to clan membership, vision quests, and life events. Breaking taboos and other incorrect behavior could cause illness. Elderly shamans used spiritual means and herbal medicines to cure illness. Their powers could be used for good or evil (Milwaukee Public Museum, 2022).

## Health & Healing Now

A community health assessment of the Ho-Chunk Nation was published in 2019 with the following results:

1.  There are income disparities between Ho-Chunk members and other Wisconsin residents with a larger percentage of Ho-Chunk households earning less than $25,000 annually. Many Ho-Chunk households support multiple family members.
2.  Issues affecting Ho-Chunk quality of life are low income/poverty, discrimination/racism leading to anxiety and depression, (45% of respondents) and domestic violence.
3.  Ho-Chunk participants stated that areas needing improvement are positive teen activities, child care options, more affordable housing, mental health support groups, more highly paid employment, and healthy food choices/healthy family activities.
4.  Participants stated that children need healthy relationships/ mental health, dental hygiene, and nutrition. Traditional Ho-hunk food would foster healthy living and community relationships.
5.  Environmental concerns included mold, clean drinking water, and mosquito/tick-borne diseases.
6.  Some Ho-Chunk communities need healthcare and fitness facilities that they can access without driving two hours (Suryanarayanan, 2019).

## Impact on Health of Interaction with White Culture Then

European diseases and warfare significantly reduced the Ho-Chunk tribe in the 1600s. They intermarried with other tribes to rebuild their population. Although the federal government tried several times to remove them from Wisconsin, they were finally allowed to remain. As many members converted to the Native American Church (Peyote Religion), religious differences disrupted tribal unity. Seasonal unskilled labor and tourist programs kept children from progressing in school to obtain better paying jobs (Milwaukee Public Museum, 2022).

## Impact on Health of Interaction with White Culture Now

A Ho-Chunk Nation Health Profile Report in 2023 used data from the Ho-Chunk Nation Department of Health and data from Wisconsin DNR and DHS as well as CDC and Wisconsin Electronic Disease Surveillance System (WEDSS) to report on tribal public and environmental health. The Environmental Health division provides car seat and bike helmets for injury prevention, free water testing and well construction if funding available, mold and radon inspections, foodborne/waterborne illness complaint inspections and testing, and resources to help with community hazards clean-up. Ho-Chunk sanitarians inspect tribal facilities and events to ensure public safety (Ho-Chunk Nation Department of Health, 2023).

## *Huron (Wyandot)*

The term Huron was given the tribe by the French and means "boar's head' referring to the men's roached hair. After losing to the French in 1748, the tribe settled around Sandusky, Ohio and became the Wyandot Tribe (accessgenealogy.com, 2023). Their story continues there.

## Health & Healing Then/Now

See Wyandot

## Impact on Health of Interaction with White Culture Then/Now

See Wyandot

## *Illinois (Peoria)*

The Illinois was a powerful, large group of tribes in 1673. They were almost extinct by 1832 and joined the Peoria tribe after warfare and disease had decimated their population (Illinois State Museum Society, 2000). Their story continues there.

## Health & Healing Then/Now

See Peoria tribe.

## Impact on Health of Interaction with White Culture Then/Now

See Peoria Tribe

## *Iowa*

The Iowa Tribe of Oklahoma and the Iowa Tribe of Kansas and Nebraska are both federally recognized. Iowa or Bah Kho-Je means 'people of the grey snow". The Iowa Tribe of Oklahoma has several tourism enterprises including the Native Marketplace, the Grey Snow Eagle House, an RV Park, and two casinos. They also hold Powwows annually (bahkhoje.com, 2023). The Iowa Tribe of Kansas and Nebraska's enterprises include a bee farm, a sanitation company, farm operations, a gas station and convenience store, and White Cloud Casino (Iowa Tribe of Kansas and Nebraska, 2023).

## Health & Healing Then

The Iowa tribe used plant-based medicine. Sweet flag, also called calamus, was a small root chewed to sooth an irritated or sore throat. Sweetgrass was in sacred bundles and was used for purification and attached to sacred items. White sage or prairie sage could be used as smoke to purify people and objects. It also could be used as medicinal tea to treat flu or a bad cold (Ioway Cultural Institute, n.d.).

## Health & Healing Now

The Iowa Tribe of Kansas and Nebraska's services include an Imagination Library providing free books for Native children from birth-age 5, eye glass vouchers, the senior citizens meal and  caregiver program, the Boys & Girls Club, the PEACE Program to prevent violence against women, and the Community Health Representatives Program which ensures access to health services (Iowa Tribe of Kansas and Nebraska, 2023). The Iowa Tribe of Oklahoma's services include social services for support with housing, food, clothing, and utilities, assistance for children, home care services for vulnerable adults, residential care if needed, burial assistance, and emergency funding for personal property damage (bahkhoje.com, 2023).

## Impact on Health of Interaction with White Culture Then

In 1803 a smallpox epidemic killed 100 men as well as women and children. This reduced the tribe from 1,100 to 800 people. In 1905, they were under the jurisdiction of the Kickapoo Boarding School (Access Genealogy, 2023). The Kickapoo Boarding School in Horton was affiliated with Presbyterian missionaries and children frequently ran away and were punished on their return according to a quote from the Department of the Interior 's 1899 report "A prompt returning of the runaways and a whipping administered soundly and prayerfully helps greatly toward bringing about the desired result" (Alatidd, 2022). In 1896, the school housed three children in one bed and exemplified "rampant physical, sexual, and emotional abuse; disease; malnourishment; overcrowding; and lack of health care in Indian boarding schools" (Alatidd, 2022).

## Impact on Health of Interaction with White Culture Now

The Iowa Tribe of Oklahoma's Victim Services Unit's Set Aside Program serves all community victims of every ethnicity. Their major focus is serving victims of drugged or drunk drivers, human trafficking, and elder abuse. Their programs are coordinated with local, state, federal, and tribal services. They also serve all community victims in their Sexual Assault Service Program and their Tribal Governments Program for victims of domestic violence, stalking, and dating violence. All three programs are supported by Department of Justice grants (bahkhoje.com, 2023).

## *Kaskaskia*

The Kaskaskia tribe no longer exists as a tribe. Their descendants are enrolled in the Peoria Tribe of Indians of Oklahoma (Peoria Tribe of Indians of Oklahoma, n.d.).

## Health & Healing Then

Shamans could be men or women who asked animal spirits for healing rituals and special medicines. The calumet tobacco pipe was used to ensure peace.(Warren, 2004).

## Impact on Health of Interaction with White Culture Then

Warfare and disease decimated the population and  cultural traditions were abandoned when they adopted European beliefs (Warren, 2004).

## *Kickapoo*

Three Kickapoo tribes are federally recognized and are located in Oklahoma, Kansas, and Texas. The Kickapoo Tribe of Oklahoma's enterprises include a travel plaza and two casinos (Kickapoo Tribe of Oklahoma, n.d.). The Kickapoo tribe of Kansas' major revenue source is the Golden Eagle Casino (ktik-nsn.gov, n.d.). The Kickapoo Traditional Tribe of Texas' enterprises include a convenience store and a casino and hotel (kickapootexas.org, 2021). Kickapoo means "those who walk the earth" (native-languages.org, 1998-2000).

## Health & Healing Then

The Kickapoo used a wide variety of plants for curing rituals. These rituals may be conducted by individuals, clan leaders, and members of bundle societies. The Woman's Dance and Buffalo Dance were associated with treatment of illness and infertility (everyculture.com, 2023).

## Health & Healing Now

The Kickapoo Tribe of Oklahoma Social Services department has several programs to identify unmet needs of tribal members and collaborates with government agencies and other tribal programs to reduce inequities and improve well-being. These services include the general assistance program for enrolled members, low-income housing energy assistance, school clothing allowance, and adult protective services (Kickapoo Tribe of Oklahoma, n.d.). The Kickapoo Tribe of Kansas has a fitness center, a diabetes prevention center, a senior citizens center, a child care program, a health center, and a food distribution program to benefit tribal members (ktik-nsn.gov, n.d.). The Kickapoo Tribe of Texas has a community wellness center, a health clinic, a New Beginnings Project to promote life changes, and New Hope, Healing Grounds to address alcohol and substance abuse, domestic violence, and parenting education to prevent child abuse (kickapootexas.org, 2021).

## Impact on Health of Interaction with White Culture Then

The Kickapoo tribe of Texas lived in poverty as recently as the 1980s, living under the international bridge at Eagle Pass before moving to a 123-acre reservation in 1987 on the outskirts of town. Under the bridge, they had no bathrooms, water or privacy and passersby insulted them and threw trash on them. In the 1990s they lived in poverty, and many were alcoholic or addicted to fumes of spray paint (Texas Monthly, 1997). The Kickapoo Boarding School in Horton, Kansas treated Kickapoo children harshly, whipping them when they ran away and forcing them to sleep three in a bed. In the 2022 report from the Department of the Interior and Bureau of Indian Affairs, this school was described as an example of "rampant physical, sexual, and emotional abuse; disease; malnourishment; overcrowding; and lack of health care in Indian boarding schools" (Tidd, 2022).

## Impact on Health of Interaction with White Culture Now

The Kickapoo tribe in Kansas has a water plant that is old and inadequate which is their only source of drinking water and has negotiated with government agencies to help rebuild the damaged dam on the Delaware River (ktik-nsn.gov, n.d.).

## *Menominee*

The Menominee Indian Tribe of Wisconsin is federally recognized and is dependent on funding by the Bureau of Indian Affairs and the Indian Health Service as it strives to develop economic opportunities. Its current business enterprises are the Menominee Casino and Resort, the Thunderbird convenience store, and a convention center and banquet hall (menominee-nsn.gov, 2023). Menominee means "wild rice people" (native-languages.org, 1998-2020).

## Health & Healing Then

The Menominee honored owls and found them a good omen. According to legend, a Saw-whet owl took a girl child to her home. When the child returned to her home as a woman, the owl gave her four bundles that each contained a substance with magic power. Each of these packets had different medicine and was tied with a different color. The packet tied with red was love medicine. The packet tied with yellow enabled its owner to get valuable gifts. The packet tied with black contained hunting medicine and the last packet was tied with any color and gave success in playing games. The owl also taught the woman a song to use with each bundle and showed her how to use the medicine. When she returned to her family, the medicines she brought taught the Menominee women to develop their complex system of medicine from herbs, plants, leaves, and barks (LaRock, n.d.).

## Health & Healing Now

Today, the Tribe provides services for addiction, including crisis assessment for opioid or mental health issues. As they work to address social issues, the Menominee Tribe continues to lack available housing and employment opportunities on the reservation. Their aging infrastructure is incapable of handling current demand for economic, occupational, educational, cultural, and housing for its citizens (Menominee-nsn.gov, 2023).

## Impact on Health of Interaction with White Culture Then

In the 1860s European diseases, such as dysentery and smallpox, killed hundreds of Menominee. In 1954 a Federal program called Termination ended tribal sovereignty and the reservation was eliminated in 1961. This ended all federal services and led to seriously declining tribal employment while increasing poverty and severely reducing basic services and health care. In 1975 the reservation was re-established (Milwaukee Public Museum, 2022).

## Impact on Health of Interaction with White Culture Now

The Menominee Tribe is aware how adverse childhood experiences (ACEs) have impacted tribal health and use Trauma-Informed Care initiatives in a program called Fostering Futures to address unhealthy behaviors. The historical trauma of land loss and boarding schools until the 1940s; generational trauma of family disruption and poverty; and personal trauma (abuse, neglect, domestic violence, family substance use, racism, incarceration, loss of loved ones) all contributed to child abuse and neglect, substance use, and other unhealthy behaviors. The statistics reflect how ACEs have resulted in health disparities in the Tribe and county.

1.  There are high rates of marijuana/synthetic marijuana use and prescription drug use.
2.  46% of adults in Menominee County smoke and 59% of high school students have smoked.
3.  40% of adults are obese and 50% of children are overweight or obese with 1 in 3 children obese.
4.  Child abuse and neglect rates were 5 times higher than the state average in 2012 and neglect has increased.

Fostering Futures is a Wisconsin initiative that integrates trauma-informed care to improve state citizens health and well-being using an interdisciplinary state wide approach. In 2015 the Menominee Tribe received the Robert Wood Johnson Culture of Health Prize for their efforts in education and community engagement. In 2016 the Tribe was asked to address the US Senate Committee on Indian Affairs and the Council on Native American Trauma-Informed Initiatives about their work addressing trauma in Indian Country (menominee-nsn.gov, 2023).

## *Miami*

The Miami Tribe of Oklahoma is federally recognized. The name Miami means "the downstream people". The Miami Nation Enterprises is the Tribe's business component and includes multiple companies, including contractors, fence builders, technology services, construction services, environmental and energy services, and the Prairie Sun and Prairie Moon

Casinos (miamination.com, 2023). There is also a Miami Tribe in Indiana that is not federally or state recognized. The Miami Nation of Indiana remained when the rest of the Tribe was removed to Oklahoma in 1846. They continue to seek federal recognition. Several local cemeteries are owned and operated by the Tribe, and they seek support from grants and donations to maintain their historic sites (miamiindians.org, n.d.).

## Health & Healing Then

Plant knowledge was essential for Miami food and medicine. Moss on the north side of trees was used as a poultice for cuts and bites. Any yellow flower helped sluggishness. Wild onion or wild garlic's root was mosquito repellant. Juneberry's root was a tonic. Dogbane was used to make sacred items. Wild ginger's root relieved colds. Milkweed was a salve for warts. Butterfly weed was a heart plant. Common boneset was used for broken bones and old-field blossom was smoked by the elderly and had strong medicinal properties. Orange jewelweed sap was used for bug bites, poison ivy, and nettle stings. Eastern cedar warded off bad spirits (Toupal, 2006).

## Health & Healing Now

The Miani Nation Department of Environmental Quality conducts mold and lead-based paint inspections water and soil sampling collection, and asbestos testing. The Indian Child Welfare Program identifies at-risk families and uses a client-centered and trauma-informed approach to treatment. The Child Care Development Funding Program is designed to provide available and affordable child care services so parents can gain employment and education to improve their lifestyle. The Nation also encourages tribal members to learn how to garden and grow food as well as fishing, hunting, and learning about edible plants (miamination.com, 2023).

## Impact on Health of Interaction with White Culture Then

The removal of the Miami in 1846 to Indian Territory reduced the tribe from 500 to less than 100 people. Forced assimilation made the Miami strive to reclaim their language, traditions, and culture (miamination.com, 2023).

## Impact on Health of Interaction with White Culture Now

The Myaamia Center recently received a grant from the Robert Wood Johnson Foundation to develop an assessment and evaluation protocol about past and current ideas of health within the Tribe. The collaboration between Miami University and the Miami Nation is funded by a three-year grant to link tribal well-being to language and cultural revitalization. They seek to develop a Myaamia Wellness Model to measure wellness in the tribal community and incorporate wellness and health topics into programming and educational materials. The Cultural Resource Office is involved to ensure the research serves the community and benefits will extend beyond the grant timeframe (miamination.com, 2023).

## *Otoe-Missouria*

The Otoe-Missouria Tribe lives in Oklahoma and is federally recognized. Originally, these were two distinct tribes with Otoe called Jiwere and Missourias called Nutachi. They have multiple enterprises to generate revenue that will fund tribal programs and services, provide employment for tribal members and provide community services. These enterprises include five Casinos, a cattle ranch, and a steakhouse, (Otoe-Missouria Tribe, n.d.). The term Missouri means "people of the river mouth" (Wikiwand, n.d.).

## Health & Healing Then

The Otoe and Missouria tribes used sacred bundles in war, hunting, and medicine. Otter skin pouches were used in the Medicine Dance and herbs were chewed and rubbed on the body to protect the wearer and another herb mixture to poison arrows against the enemy. Dried human forefingers in sacred bundles could revive an unconscious or fainting man. Sweetgrass was used as incense. Tattoo bundles contained pigments and tools for designs on faces and hands of Otoe men and women as sacred marks of honor. The Missouria tattoo bundle contained buffalo horn spatulas to rub in the pigment. The buffalo-skull shrine was used twice a year in a thanksgiving ceremony and dance (Harrington, 1913).

## Health & Healing Now

The Otoe-Missouria Tribe has six health programs. These include Public Health Nursing, Health Education and Nutrition, Mental Health and Substance Abuse, and Community Health Representatives. Services include home visits, substance abuse support groups, behavioral health counseling, health education, and transportation to medical appointments. Social Service focuses on victims of sexual assault and domestic violence. Youth programs include the after-school program and summer youth program. These programs are designed to develop leadership through cultural education, physical activity, and homework assistance (Otoe-Missouria Tribe, n.d.).

## Impact on Health of Interaction with White Culture Then

The Missouria Tribe lost many people to diseases like smallpox in the 1700s and went to live with their relatives the Otoe late that century, When White settlers squatted on the Tribe's land, the Otoe-Missouria were sent to a reservation in Nebraska where they were not allowed to hunt buffalo, treaties were broken, and food, medicine, and basic essentials were not delivered as promised. Children starved, sickness was prevalent, and mortality rates climbed. In 1881 they were moved to Oklahoma where they currently live. Their children were sent to boarding schools for assimilation. They learned English and were punished for speaking their own language. Some parents didn't teach their language to prevent their children from being punished and much of the Otoe-Missouria language was lost. Tribal elders today experienced the boarding schools and remember their trauma (Otoe-Missouria Tribe, n.d.).

## Impact on Health of Interaction with White Culture Now

The Otoe-Missouria Tribe is concerned about protecting the environment. In 1998, the EPA accepted their Tribal Master Plan and Tribal Quality Management Plan. The Tribe submits revisions annually for each document for review and approval. EPA grants help establish and maintain monitoring programs and results are reported to the EPA. The Water Pollution Control Program is funded through the Clean Water Act and provides financial support for maintenance of prevention and control of ground and surface water pollution. The Water Quality Technician has responsibility for water quality knowledge, using and maintaining monitoring equipment, record keeping, and reporting. The Department monitors the water's chemical condition, its physical condition, and biological measurements. Data and monitoring provide information about abrupt changes or long-term subtle changes in water quality (Otoe-Missouria Tribe, n.d.).

## Odawa

The word Odawa means "trader" and the Tribe was also known as Ottawa. Today, four Odawa (Ottawa) tribes are federally recognized. They are the Grand Traverse Band of Ottawa and Chippewa Indians, the Little River Band of Ottawa Indians, the Little Traverse Bay Band of Odawa Indians, and the Ottawa Tribe of Oklahoma. This section will discuss the three tribes living in Michigan. The Grand Traverse Band of Ottawa and Chippewa Indians has a business portfolio that includes the Eagle Town Market, the Turtle Creek Casino and Hotel, the Leelanau Sands Casino and Lodge, and the Grand Traverse Resort and Spa (Grand Traverse Band of Ottawa and Chippewa Indians, n.d.). The Little River Band of Ottawa Indians has enterprises that include the Little River Casino and Resort, a hotel and an event center (Little River Band of Ottawa Indians, 2023). The Little Traverse Bay Bands of Odawa Indians has enterprises including sustainable agriculture, an economic development corporation, and the Odawa Casino Resort (Little Traverse Bay Bands of Odawa Indians, n.d.).

### Health & Healing Then

The Odawa had four major spiritual practices during the 1700s and early 1800s to foster physical and spiritual health. The Midewiwin or Medicine Lodge ceremonies cured the sick using plant medicines, songs, and dances. The Wahbahnowin used certain medicines to help people's spiritual and physical health. Fire dances and sweat lodges were used and ceremonies sometimes lasted until dawn because the people believed that the morning star was a significant spirit. The Tchissahkiwin ceremonies sought contact with the spiritual world to receive help or information about a matter of importance or to predict the future. Spirits responded to questions from those seeking help. The Goosahndahwin ceremonies were also used to obtain remedies for illness. Wampum belts documented spiritual and historic events (Little Traverse Bay Bands of Odawa Indians, n.d.).

## Health & Healing Now

The Little Traverse Bay Bands of Odawa Indians' Community Health Department has several services for tribal members. The Community Outreach/Diabetes Program  provides diabetes education with home visits and nutritional counseling. The SDPI Healthy Heart (Mno Ode-Good Heart) is a special diabetes program to reduce the risk of cardiovascular disease. The Maternal Child Health Healthy Start Project reduces the risk of infant mortality by home visits, referral and follow-up services, health counseling for teens and families, childbirth education, transportation for provider visits, breastfeeding supplies, and incentives for health behaviors. Family Spirit provides services for expectant mothers, children from birth to age 5 and families. The Native Way Gym provides exercise classes, weight machines/equipment, and personal training to improve overall well-being and health (Little  Traverse Bay Bands of Odawa Indians, n.d.).   The Little River Band of Ottawa Indians' Family Services Staff provides the following services:  elder support, family and individual counseling, positive Indian parenting, victim services, individual/family self-sufficiency, and Indian Child Welfare Intervention and Reunification (Little River Band of Ottawa Indians, 2023).  The Grand Traverse Band of Ottawa and Chippewa Indians now offers virtual care through their Let's Heal program which is available on phones, computers, and tablets (Grand Traverse Band of Ottawa and Chippewa Indians, n.d.).

## Impact on Health of Interaction with White Culture Then

Beginning in 1870, the Odawa survived by growing crops on the land they had left and working in the lumber industry. As White settlers came to the reservation, the Odawa people lost power in local affairs and although education increased, few Odawa graduated from high school. The Catholic Boarding School at Harbor Springs taught Odawa children, but they only learned English, not their own language. Some Odawa children were sent to other boarding schools like Mount Pleasant and Carlisle in Pennsylvania. As tribal members became Christians a Christian first name was added to the Odawa family name and was also sometimes used as a last name changing the Odawa family name (Little Traverse Bay Bands of Odawa Indians, n.d.).

## Impact on Health of Interaction with White Culture Now

The Grand Traverse Band Conservation Department provides Great Lakes and Inland Enforcement for commercial and subsistence fishing and inland fishing, gathering, hunting and trapping in enforcement agreements with other member tribes in the Chippewa Ottawa Resource Authority. The Department participates in eight mandatory Joint Law Enforcement patrols annually and in at least four Joint Law Enforcement Committee meetings per year. They also must qualify semiannually with department-issued firearms and attain a minimum of forty hours of training in Conservation Enforcement annually. The Department also is "on call" duty for 24 hours for enforcement activity for Great Lakes Waters and Treaty Ceded Waters in  42 Michigan counties (Grand Traverse Band of Ottawa and Chippewa Indians, n.d.).

## *Ojibwe*

The federally recognized Ojibwe tribe is known as the Red Lake Band of Chippewa Indians in Minnesota. Ojibwe are "original people" or were called "puckered" relating to their style of moccasin (native-languages.org, 1998-2020). The Tribe began developing its infrastructure in the late 1900s to include improved housing, sewer, water, and roads. The Economic Development Department is helping Tribal members establish businesses and expanding the Tribe's economic base  (Red Lake Nation, 2023). They also recently opened the first adult-use cannabis dispensary this August after recreational marijuana was legalized in the State of Minnesota (Herrington, 2023).

## Health & Healing Then

The Ojibwe believed every plant was medicine and required the proper medicine lodge ceremony. The peyote lodge members chewed and swallowed peyote buttons of a cactus as a narcotic to see visions. The Ojibwe knowledge of plants was superb, and they understood proper times for gathering. The medicine man had the proper dream after fasting and went through a rigorous training course. Songs were essential to digging medicine roots. Tobacco was placed in the soil where the root was removed. Skin problems were treated with poultices and lotions while internal diseases were treated with medicinal teas. The medicine man could make bad medicine too. Some of the medicinal plants were:

1. Box elder where the inner bark made an emetic;
2. Red maple-where the bark as a tea treated sore eyes;
3. Mountain maple-also used to treat sore eyes;
4. Arrow-head-used as a remedy for indigestion;
5. Smooth sumac-used for throat inflammation;
6. Staghorn sumac-used to stop hemorrhage; and
7. Spreading dogbane-used as a tea for women to cleanse their kidneys during pregnancy (Smith, 1932).

## Health & Healing Now

Red Lake Nation has several programs in place for the health of their Tribal members. These include:

1. Emergency Medical Services;
2. Medical Transportation Services;
3. Meal delivery to disabled and elderly Tribal members;
4. Community Health Nursing Services;
5. Clinic Services;
6. Nutrition Services/Mental Health/Social Ser4vices;
7. Diabetes Services; and
8. Optometry/Dental Services (Red Lake Nation, 2023).

## Impact on Health of Interaction with White Culture Then

The Ojibwe suffered from epidemics of smallpox and other illnesses. Moving from their traditional lifestyle to permanent settlement resulted in a poorer lifestyle and a high rate of communicable diseases such as Trachoma and tuberculosis. Further land loss occurred along with lack of health care. From 1989-1991, anti-treaty groups like Stop Treaty Abuse protested against Ojibwe spearfishing within treaty rights. There were verbal threats, racial slurs, stoning, and gunfire. Two anti-treaty groups used slogans that said "Save a Deer, Shoot an Indian" and "Save a fish, spear a Squaw" (Roy, n.d.).

## Impact on Health of Interaction with White Culture Now

The Red Lake Nation is experiencing the same health concerns as other Native tribes. Diabetes, obesity, chemical dependency, fetal alcohol syndrome, suicide, and accidental death are current health issues (Roy, n.d.). Realizing that education is a path to a better future, the Tribe established Red Lake Nation College, a two-year community college. The College offers an Associate in Arts for liberal education and an Associate in Applied Science in Social and Behavioral Sciences. It is accredited by the Higher Learning Commission and recognized by the Department of Education enabling graduates to transfer to four-year colleges and universities. The College also has courses for non-degree students who wish to increase their knowledge (Red Lake Nation College, 2022).

## *Omaha*

The Omaha Tribe of Nebraska is federally recognized. The name Omaha means "go against the current" (native-languages.org, 1998-2020). The Tribe has provided assistance to its members from the American Rescue Plan Act and COVID Relief Package (Omaha Tribe of Nebraska, 2023). The Tribe purchased a grocery store, restaurant, and gas station in 2021 to provide fresh foods on the reservation, provide economic development and create local jobs. They are renovating and updating the store and restaurant, which will benefit tribal members without transportation (Dockter, 2021 [updated May 24, 2023]). In addition to their BlackBird Bend Casino, the Omaha Tribe has opened a second casino called Lucky

77. Currently Lucky 77 is a class 2 gaming facility, but the Tribe is seeking a compact with Nebraska to include class 3 games and sports betting there (Hofmann, 2023).

## Health & Healing Then

Omaha buffalo medicine men sang special songs for treatment along with using water and roots for healing. After compounding roots from his medicine pouch, he put bits of root in his mouth and took a mouthful of water. Then, he spit the root and water into the wound while others continued the song which demonstrated the power of his vision. Buffalo doctors were a society that only treated wounds. After treatment, the injured person was helped to rise at dawn and take four steps toward the east to meet the sun and greet the return of life. After four steps the song of triumph was sung ending the medicine incantation. After completing treatment, the medicine men entered a sweat lodge and bathed. After this, the medicine men received their fees, including horses, robes, necklaces, blankets, eagle feathers and other valued items. Two of their roots to heal wounds were the root of the hop vine and the root of the Physalis viscora (La Flesche, n.d.).

## Health & Healing Now

The Omaha Tribe were successful farmers before much of their land was taken. Today, few Omaha can farm much of their remaining land and have become dependent on government commodities, and processed, store-bought food instead of fresh vegetables. This has resulted in a significant increase in chronic diseases such as obesity and diabetes (Miewald, 1995).

## Impact on Health of Interaction with White Culture Then

When White settlers arrived, they brought smallpox with them that killed almost 90% of the Omaha Tribe (Omaha Public Schools, 2014). Assimilation also affected the Omaha Tribe in the late 19th century. The Genoa Indian Industrial School was the first Indian boarding school in Nebraska in 1884. The Superintendent had no experience managing a school and funds were inadequate for supplies or building maintenance.

Food supply shortages and lack of fuel, medical, cleaning, and school supplies was reflected in fluctuating financial government support. Some parents tried to reclaim their children and runaways were an issue. In July 1885, he warned his supervisor about a situation where several female students were bathing in a creek near a railroad bridge. Train workers taunted them and attempted rape. When they were arrested, the court released them because White men shouldn't be charged with evidence from Indians. In his final report in 1885, he wrote about poor conditions in reservations and Indian camps and that Native girls were subject to kidnapping and prostitution (Fanta, 2022).

## Impact on Health of Interaction with White Culture Now

Project Hope is partnering with the Omaha Tribe in a long-term initiative to prevent suicides among Omaha youth. Suicide is a serious public health concern on the reservation. It is the second leading cause of death for Native American young adults and adolescents. This project will use evidence-based curriculum and models for prevention and intervention strategies. Reasons for suicide are difficult to address, including depression, substance use, and disruptive behaviors and attitudes. Partnerships are vital and prevention will be coordinated between the two reservation schools, local prevention programs, and all entities within the Omaha Tribe. Community education, trainings, and cultural gatherings will identify suicide ideation criteria and approach clinical and public awareness strategies. At-risk youth will be referred for treatment using the Columbia University Teen Screen. Schools will be offered the American Indian Life Skills Development Curriculum for grades 9-12. An equine therapy program (EAGALA) will be used to improve mental health for groups, families, and individuals (SPRC.org, 2020).

## *Osage*

The Osage Nation is federally recognized and is located in Oklahoma. The name Osage means "middle water" (native-languages.org, 1998-2020). The Nation's enterprises include two convenience stores, the Osage Casino Hotel, and the Skyline Event Center (Osage Nation, n.d.).

## Health & Healing Then

Osage Big Moon Peyotism required ritual maintenance of a fire for the ceremony which lasted all night. The sacred properties of firewood enhanced the social relationships and spiritual benefits to the community. The firewood must be slow burning without sparks which could harm those sitting close to the fire. Smoke should also be reduced. The fire was considered a grandfather and was sacred. The favorite wood was red oak and slippery elm and white ash may be substituted. After the peyote ceremony, coals from the fire might be used to conduct a cedar ceremony by producing a smoke incense to bless and cleanse a home after a death or during times of spiritual or physical distress (Swan & Simons, 2014).

## Health & Healing Now

In 2020 a health survey of Osage members across the United States was published and the health status of those on the reservation was much worse than those living elsewhere. According to the survey, socioeconomic conditions there have worsened over the previous ten years. These risks "include poverty, obesity, smoking, binge drinking, diabetes, hypertension, heart disease, physical disability, high cholesterol and psychological distress such as depression" (Shaw Duty, 2021).

## Impact on Health of Interaction with White Culture Then

The Osage headright began in the late 1800s when the Osage were driven out of Kansas and purchased land in Oklahoma. In 1906 the Government allotted Osage land with two provisions. Land could only be distributed to Osage Nation members and mineral rights would be owned collectively by the Osage Nation. Each Osage received an equal share of profits from mineral rights called a headright. Private companies leased land to drill and paid a percentage of profits into a trust managed by the Bureau of Indian Affairs. The Bureau was to distribute payments from the trust to the headright holders. Oil made the Osage Nation rich and attracted conmen and swindlers. The Government created a system of guardianship by non-Osage to monitor tribe members who were considered incompetent to manage their money. This racist system allowed White guardians to pay themselves and give the Osage a small allowance. There were instances of White people marrying into the tribe, even by force, to become their guardians and kill them for their headrights. This was known as the Osage Reign of Terror and occurred throughout the 1920s. The system has been amended since then, but financial mismanagement and lack of transparency by the Bureau of Indian Affairs resulted in a $380 million settlement in 2011 for headright holders. About one quarter of all headright payments go to non-Osages and class action suits continue to fight for indigenous rights (Kesler, Aronczyk, Romer, & Rubin, 2023).

## Impact on Health of Interaction with White Culture Now

In 2021 the Osage Nation requested community input about building an Outdoor Health Complex in Pawhuska, OK. The new health complex will be available to everyone in Osage county (Shaw Duty, 2021). In 2022 the Pawhuska City Council voted unanimously to shut down an area for the Osage Nation to build the complex on an old railroad right of way that has been a dumping ground. The Nation is to build a new street connecting the neighborhood nicknamed The Bottoms to access from the neighborhood. A representative of the Pawhuska Fire Department said that the new street will lead to faster response times in emergencies. "The complex will have two regulation softball fields and a baseball field, all with synthetic surfaces, basketball courts that can be converted to pickleball or tennis with the change of nets, three sand volleyball courts, a soccer field, football field, outdoor stage, an urban garden, walking trails, horseshoe pitches, batting cages and two concession stands" (Red Corn, 2022). Pawhuska citizens believe the community will greatly benefit from the complex and that removal by the Nation of about three feet of soil poisoned by toxins will also improve the environment. The Osage Nation is continuing to seek additional grants, but has obtained funding and technical support from some Federal sources, oil companies, and sporting associations in Oklahoma and nationally. The Nation plans soil remediation and planting clover on the right of way to feed honeybees they are raising. Their goal is to get people more active and away from drugs by being in a safe environment to move, walk, or run and be healthier (Red Corn, 2022).

## *Ottawa*

The Ottawa Tribe of Oklahoma is federally recognized. The term Ottawa is from Odawa and means "traders" (native-languages.org, 1998-2020). Their enterprises include the Otter Cove Diner and Gift Shop, the Adawe Travel Plaza, the Otter Stop, and the High Winds Casino (Ottawa Tribe of Oklahoma, 2021).

### Health & Healing Then

Each spring the Ottawa held a feast of thanksgiving and prayer to celebrate the end of winter with singing and dancing. This was followed by the feast for the dead by singing, eating and throwing part of the food into a fire. Weapons and utensils were buried with the dead, and they were treated with reverence (Pokagon 1898 collection, 1998-2020).

### Health & Healing Now

The Indian Child Welfare Department of the Ottawa Tribe of Oklahoma has several programs to support Ottawa children. Indian Child Welfare strives to preserve families by supportive family services. When this is not possible, they work with DHS and other providers in the foster care system to address family problems for safe reunification. When adoption is needed, they support adoptive families to ensure children's well-being. Culture Keepers seeks to provide guardians and foster parents so Ottawa children can access Ottawa culture. This is also a resource for non-Native foster families who are foster parents or guardians for Ottawa children. The School Assistance Program provides funding for school supplies and clothes for Ottawa children from 4 years old through 12th grade in the current school year. An application is required, and the family must live within 50 miles of the Ottawa Tribal Office. "Ottawas Care 4 Ottawas" is an opportunity for Tribal members to sponsor an Ottawa child in foster care with gifts (Ottawa Tribe of Oklahoma, 2021).

### Impact on Health of Interaction with White Culture Then

600 members of the Ottawa Tribe of Oklahoma first relocated to Kansas in 1837. Climate differences between Kansas and Ohio, exposure, and

malnutrition resulted in more than 300 deaths in the first two years. By the time they moved to Oklahoma in 1867 only about 200 tribal members existed. After originally attaining federal recognition, the Government decided the Ottawa Tribe had no purpose and terminated them in 1956. The next 22 years were difficult before the Ottawa again received federal recognition as the Ottawa Tribe of Oklahoma (Oklahoma Indian Tribe Education Guide , 2014).

## Impact on Health of Interaction with White Culture Now

The Ottawa Department of Environmental Protection works under the EPA General Assistance Program and Clean Water Act grants. It is also funded by the Bureau of Indian Affairs for Natural Resource Damage Assessment and Restoration. This funding helps the Ottawa and other impacted tribes study how they have been affected by the Tor Creek Superfund site's mine waste and develop plans to restore lost or damaged resources (Ottawa Tribe of Oklahoma, 2021).

## *Peoria*

The Peoria Tribe of Indians of Oklahoma is a federally recognized tribe who are descendants of the Illinois tribe. The tribe's enterprises include the Buffalo Run Casino and Resort, the Buffalo Run Hotel, and the Peoria Ridge Golf Course (Peoria Tribe of Indians of Oklahoma, n.d.). Peoria means "he comes carrying a pack on his back" (Oklahoma Historical Society, n.d.).

## Health & Healing Then

The Illinois tribe used a shaman for serious injury or illness. The shaman could be a man or woman with access to supernatural powers for healing. The shaman used a gourd rattle and appealed to his or her personal manitou to diagnose the problem and use healing rituals or special medicines. Medicinal plants might be applied to the affected body part and the shaman might suck on the area to remove the offending manitou. A root was used to treat snakebites and other plants were used to cure the patient. Boiled root of basswood was used to treat burns, and boiled root or bark of white oak treated wounds. Powdered root of white ginger relieved childbirth pain and sumac was an antidote for diarrhea (Illinois State Museum Society, 2000).

## Health & Healing Now

The Peoria Tribe of Indians of Oklahoma just completed their one-year anniversary in 2023 of the Tribal Opioid Response Program Peer Recovery Support Services. This program has attained several milestones:

1. 44 Naloxone training kits distributed;
2. 60 Fentanyl testing strips obtained from partners;
3. 60 Fentanyl testing strips distributed to the testing community;
4. 39 people trained in key community sectors;
5. 17 people trained to provide prevention and education for schools;
6. 457 children educated about prevention and engaged in activities about consequences related to opioid and/or stimulant misuse;
7. 1,022 people educated in prevention and outreach activities about consequences of opioid and/or stimulant misuse;
8. 5,022 people educated via media campaigns about consequences of opioid and/or stimulant misuse; and
9. 7 community members connected to treatment and recovery services (Peoria Tribe of Indians of Oklahoma, n.d.).

The Tribe also sponsored and facilitated Talking Circles, Warrior Down, White Bison Medicine Wheel, and Twelve Steps for Men and Women. They also provided recovery support for several tribal members dealing with cannabis, opioids, cocaine, alcohol, and inhalants (Peoria Tribe of Indians of Oklahoma, n.d.).

## Impact on Health of Interaction with White Culture Then

The Illinois contracted deadly European diseases for which they had no immunity. Smallpox epidemics occurred about 1704, 1732, and 1756 that were deadly to tribal members (Illinois State Museum Society, 2000).

## Impact on Health of Interaction with White Culture Now

The Peoria Tribe is working with the Tar Creek Trustee Council on the Neosho Bottoms Mussel Restoration Project. In 2022 the Tribe did preliminary survey work to determine suitable sites on the Spring and Neosho Rivers to support mussels. In 2023 goals include selecting a survey team, finalizing strategies, making a second river survey trip, obtaining permission from landowners, acquiring final permits, and collecting Fatmucket brood stock. They must ensure there is adequate food for the federally-protected Neosho Mucket (a freshwater clam) to help with water clean-up. The Peoria Tribe has partnered with Missouri State University to raise the muckets for release and assist in the species' recovery for the future (Oklahoma Wildlife Department, n.d. and Peoria Tribe of Indians of Oklahoma, n.d.).

## *Potawatomi*

There are seven federally recognized Potawatomi tribes located in Oklahoma, Kansas, Wisconsin, Michigan, and Indiana. Potawatomi means "firekeepers' (native-languages.org, 1998-2020).

| State | Tribe(s) | Enterprises |
|---|---|---|
| **Oklahoma** | Citizen Potawatomi Nation | Enterprises include grocery stores and gas stations, the Grand Casino Hotel and Resort, the Firelake Casino, Firelake Gulf Course, bowling center and ball fields, the Firelake Arena and Grand Event Center, a gift shop, restaurants, a tribally-owned bank and a radio station (Citizen Potawatomi Nation, 2023). |
| **Kansas** | Prairie Band Potawatomi Nation | Enterprises include an economic holding company, PBP Entertainment Corporation, and the Prairie Band Casino and Resort (Prairie Band Potawatomi Nation, 2023). |

| State | Tribe(s) | Enterprises |
|---|---|---|
| **Wisconsin** | Forest County Potawatomi Community | Enterprises include a business development corporation, two casinos and hotels, and Greenfire Builders (Forest County Potawatomi Community, 2023). |
| **Michigan** | Hannahville Indian Community | Enterprises include HOPE (Hannahville Opioid Prevention & Education), the Hannahville Indian School, Hannahville Health Center Pharmacy, and the Island Resort & Casino (Hannahville Indian Community, n.d.). |
| | Match-e-be-nash-she-wish Band of Pottawatomi Indians (Gun Lake Tribe) | Enterprises include Gun Lake Investments, Noonday Market, the Gun Lake Casino, restaurants, a campground, and a sports bar (Gun Lake Tribe, 2017). |
| | Nottawaseppi Huron Band of the Potawatomi | Enterprises include an economic development company, a general store, and the Firekeepers Casino Hotel (Nottawaseppi Huron Band of the Potawatomi, 2022). |
| **Indiana/Michigan** | Pokagon Band of Pottawatomi Indians | Enterprises include an investment company and Four Winds Casinos [3 in Michigan and 1 in Indiana] (Pokagon Band of Potawatomi, 2023). |

## Health & Healing Then

The Potawatomi believed that every medicine plant had a song and a spirit, and it was necessary to address the spirit of the medicine. The four most important plants were sage, tobacco, cedar, and sweetgrass. Curing occurred in the preventive stage. Medicine people smelled medicine before seeing it and certain plants could only be gathered at certain times of the year. Wood from a tree struck by lightning was powerful medicine. They named every plant, shrub, flower, and tree that was indigenous to their homeland and treated the land respectfully. Before gathering plants, they offered tobacco and prayed, sang, and spoke to a plant before waiting for the plant to share instructions on its use. Medicines from a bog or swamp were good and could purify the blood. Cranberries were used to cure STDs and hemlock in small amounts could induce abortion by an experienced midwife. The poison ivy plant was used to treat poison ivy infection. Root of sweetgrass could be used in small amounts to heal and was believed to cure cancer. It was also important after healing to return to the medicine plant and thank it with thanksgiving songs (Toupal, 2006).

## Health & Healing Now

In 2022 three Potawatomi Bands (Pokagon Band, Gun Lake Tribe, and Nottawaseppi Huron Band) hosted a March for Missing and Murdered Indigenous People in Grand Rapids, Michigan. They and other indigenous people around Michigan came together to remember missing and murdered loved ones and to raise awareness of this crisis. Marchers, some a painted red handprint on their faces, carried signs and poster with powerful messages: "We will remember", "Inaction is a Powerful Choice" or "No More Stolen Sisters". There is limited data about these rates of violence, but the available studies paint an alarming picture:

1. In 2020, homicide was the third leading cause of death for indigenous women between ages 10-24 and the fifth for those between 24 and 34;
2. In 2020, homicide was the third leading cause of death of indigenous men between 15-24 years and the fourth for those between 25 and 34 years;
3. 9,571 indigenous people (5,295 women and 4,276 men) were reported missing in 2020 by the FBI National Crime Information Center;
4. Older studies documented that violent victimization affected indigenous women 1.2 times more than White women and indigenous men 1.3 times more than White men with 4 in 5 indigenous people experiencing violence during their lives (2016). A 2008 study funded by the National Institute of Justice found

that indigenous women are 10 times more likely to be murder victims than any other race (Dresslet, 2022).

This March was repeated in 2023 and the Tribes donated $8,000 to support indigenous domestic violence victims (Nottawaseppi Huron Band of the Potawatomi, 2022). The Nottawaseppi Band also has joined the Michigan Health Information Network Shared Services to share health data and improve quality of care for their members (Nottawaseppi Huron Band of the Potawatomi, 2022). The Hannahville Indian Community's Community Health Department has an in-home services program for personal care, respite care, homemaker assistance, screening services, medication management, and medical transportation. They also offer tobacco treatment, nutritional resources, cancer navigation, diabetes support, and the Healthy Start/Family Spirit Program (Hannahville Indian Community, n.d.). The Gun Lake Tribe also has a tribal health center that provides routine, urgent, and chronic care for all ages with cultural awareness, spirituality, and community-focused care (Gun Lake Tribe, 2017). The Pokagon Band opened a health clinic, the Mshkiki Community Clinic, in 2021 that serves low-income patients, including non-Natives. The Clinic provides dental care services in addition to routine clinic services (Pokagon Band of Potawatomi, 2023).

It's appropriate to close this section with another walk-the 6th Annual Recovery Walk sponsored by the Forest County Potawatomi Community. 2023 is the fifth year of this event to raise awareness and give strength to people suffering with addiction. The walk is 10-12 miles and ends where a wellness fire burns to greet them for prayers and healing. People of all ages in the community and county come together to support and help anyone fighting the addiction battle (Forest County Potawatomi Community, 2023).

## Impact on Health of Interaction with White Culture Then

In 1838 the Governor of Indiana ordered the removal of the Potawatomi Tribe, and 859 tribal members were force marched 660 miles to today's Kansas. Their leaders were shackled in back of a wagon and there were only a few horses for people and supplies. More wagons didn't arrive and the majority, even elderly and weak, had to walk. They walked in oppressive heat without adequate water. The pace of the march and the adverse conditions affected their health and most days someone, usually a child, died and were buried in hurriedly dug graves with no opportunity to mourn their loss. More than 40 people died on this journey that the Potawatomi called the Trail of Death (Citizen Potawatomi Nation, 2023).

## Impact on Health of Interaction with White Culture Now

The Prairie Band Potawatomi Nation Police and Fire participated in an active shooter exercise at Royal Valley High School with multiple other emergency agencies in  February 2023. Many area first responders from emergency medical services and law enforcement trained together and worked seamlessly as a team during the exercise. School staff and students also participated providing real world urgency for the responders (Prairie Band Potawatomi Nation, 2023). In January 2023, Citizen Potawatomi Nation's domestic violence program, House of Hope, hosted a new Jump Start Day with vendors, breakout sessions, and resources from organizations across the county. Realizing that domestic violence is not an isolated issue, community resources dealing with poverty, homelessness, health issues, and addiction came together to face these problems and share information. In addition to this partnership, House of Hope asked a hair salon operator to give free haircuts since many people lack funds for these. She gave 16 haircuts and helped participants feel good about themselves. Small breakout sessions talked about safety planning, smudging, and cultural knowledge. Response was so positive, that Jump Start Day will become an annual January event (Citizen Potawatomi Nation, 2023).

## *Sauk (Sac)*

The Sac (Sauk) tribe today is joined with the Fox tribe and there are three federally recognized Sac and Fox tribes:  the Sac & Fox Nation of Oklahoma, the Meskwaki Nation of Iowa, and the Sac and Fox Nation of Missouri in Kansas and Nebraska. The name Sauk (Sac) means "people of the yellow earth" (sacandfoxks.com, 2023). In 1730 after losing in battle to the French, Fox refugees joined the Sac tribe and they moved from Wisconsin to Iowa, Illinois, and Missouri until an 1804 treaty between both tribes and the United States. One group separated from the others and moved to Missouri where they became a distinct tribe. In 1856, Iowa allowed the Sac and Fox to live there, and the Meskwaki purchased land there in 1857. Remaining tribal members were removed to Oklahoma after a treaty in 1867 (Alexander, 2023). The Sac and Fox Nation of Missouri in Kansas and Nebraska's enterprises include a museum, a trading post, a truck stop, and the Sac and Fox Casino (sacandfoxks.com, 2023). The Meskwaki Nation's enterprises include a recreation center, a bank, an organic farm, several businesses, and the Meskwaki Bingo Casino Hotel (meskwaki.org, 2023). The Sac & Fox Nation of Oklahoma's enterprises include the Sac and Fox Casino and the Black Hawk Casino along with education incentives (sacandfoxnation-nsn.gov, 2023).

## Health & Healing Then

The Sauk always carried their medicine bundles and valued them highly. They used the contents to cure the sick and never went to war without them (Jones, 1939). The bundle also contained medicine that acted as a love charm and other medicine that assisted in childbirth. Songs were important when using the bundle. Curing medicine countered any negative effects on the user (Harrington, 1914).

## Health & Healing Now

See Fox Tribe comments

## Impact on Health of Interaction with White Culture Then

An epidemic in 1766 killed half the Sauk and Fox village inhabitants. As the tribes migrated to Kansas in 1842, deaths occurred and about 300 died of cholera in 1851 and of smallpox in 1852 (Jones, 1939). The Sauk boarding school experience was described by the experience of two Sauk boys sent to the St. Regis Seminary in Missouri in 1824. Although the boarding school was not a long-term facility (closing in 1831), the boys housed there worked in cornfields, had their hair cut, adopted White names, and lost their cultural identity. Their names have been lost to history. They did forced labor and were beaten and whipped by Jesuit priests (Hays, 2022).

## Impact on Health of Interaction with White Culture Now

See Fox Tribe comments

## *Shawnee*

There are three federally recognized Shawnee tribes in the United States: the Shawnee Tribe of Oklahoma, the Absentee Shawnee Tribe of Indians of Oklahoma, and the Eastern Shawnee Tribe of Oklahoma. The term Shawnee means "southerner" (native-languages.org, 1998-2020). The Shawnee Tribe's enterprises include a Cultural Center and the Golden Mesa Casino (Shawnee Tribe, n.d.). The Absentee Shawnee Tribe of Indians of Oklahoma's enterprises include an economic development authority, the Food Pantry, a workforce development program, and two Thunderbird Casinos (Absentee Shawnee Tribe of Indians of Oklahoma, 2021). The Eastern Shawnee Tribe of Oklahoma has the following enterprises: an RV Park, a recycling center, Shawnee Skies Training Center & Shooting Complex, the Outpost Casino, and the Indigo Sky Casino & Resort (Eastern Shawnee Tribe of Oklahoma, 2022).

## Health & Healing Then

Sacred bundles' contents and rituals were important to the Shawnee and their welfare (bigorrin.org, n.d.). The Shawnee and other tribes believed that there was a connection between the body, the mind, and the spirit and that they all had to be in balance to achieve health. The body was capable of healing itself using natural medicine Odell, 2017-2023).

## Health & Healing Now

The Eastern Shawnee Tribe has developed a food distribution program based on 2021 data that Ottawa County residents have a poverty rate of 20.4%, higher than average Oklahoma and U.S. residents. Eastern Shawnee families who meet financial criteria receive supplemental foods monthly from distribution sites, including Items to make three complete meals and recipes for use with them. At least one recipe is geared for youth so they can participate in food preparation. Items are selected carefully, and supplemental items are included for holidays. Tribal employees and volunteers assist with sorting and bagging groceries and over 100 families receive this support with $100-$120 spent per family monthly (Eastern Shawnee Tribe of Oklahoma, 2022).

The Absentee Shawnee Tribal Health System's Native Connections addresses behavioral health needs of youth from ages 12-24 by reducing substance abuse/trauma, mental illness, and suicidal behavior (Absentee Shawnee Tribe of Indians of Oklahoma, 2021). The Shawnee Tribe of Oklahoma plans a trauma support group that will meet every other week for two hours with discussions based on shared reading and experiences to promote healing and increase resiliency (Shawnee Tribe, n.d.).

## Impact on Health of Interaction with White Culture Then

The Shawnee Tribe suffered from European diseases in the 1600s. After multiple relocations and aggression and abuse by White settlers, they split into three Shawnee communities and remain that way today. The Shawnee Indian Mission Manual Labor School was established in 1839 as an Indian boarding school. There may be Shawnee children buried on the grounds there and the Shawnee Tribe considers it a sacred site and an important historic landmark (Shawnee Tribe, n.d.).

## Impact on Health of Interaction with White Culture Now

The Eastern Shawnee Tribe conducts a water monitoring program under an EPA grant for the Clean Water Act. This includes fish collection and laboratory analysis checking for contaminants related to mining and mining waste. Their results are compared annually and made public via a nationwide database and report to the EPA. Grand Lake where testing occurs is part of the Tar Creek watershed and fish are tested for lead. Mercury results have improved and have not exceeded consumption guidelines for several years. Contaminants are still present in water and fish, but the monitoring program has been effective in documenting improvement over time (Eastern Shawnee Tribe of Oklahoma, 2022).

## *Wea*

The Wea Tribe of Indiana is a state recognized tribe and was considered part of the Miami Nation. Wea is a shortened version of the tribe's original name meaning "place of the whirlpool" (Wea Indian Tribe of Indiana, 2005-2020). Today's Wea Tribe of Indiana uses grants and entitlements to preserve the tribe's culture and traditions (Wea Indian Tribe of Indiana, 2005-2020). The federally recognized Miami tribe is part of the Peoria Tribe of Oklahoma (Ohio History Central, n.d.).

### Health & Healing Then & Now

See Miami or Peoria

### Impact on Health of Interaction with White Culture Then

Disease, especially smallpox, was responsible for many deaths and the introduction of whiskey by the White traders resulted in more deaths (Wea Indian Tribe of Indiana, 2005-2020).

### Impact on Health of Interaction with White Culture Now

The Wea Tribe of Indiana seeks donations to address health and education needs of tribal members (Wea Indian Tribe of Indiana, 2005-2020).

## *Winnebago (Ho-Chunk)*

The Winnebago Tribe of Nebraska is federally recognized. Winnebago is from an Algonquian word that means "smelly water" (Native-languages.org, 1998-2020). The tribe operates Ho-Chunk, Inc., an economic development company. Ho Chunk, Inc. operates the WarHorse Casino, a housing and construction company, a trading group for Native American products, a real estate investment company, and a marketing/public relations firm (winnebagotribe.com, 2023).

### Health & Healing Then

The Winnebago people practiced specific group and personal rituals and taboos related to clan membership, vision quests, and life events.

Breaking taboos and other incorrect behavior could cause illness. Elderly shamans used spiritual means and herbal medicines to cure illness. Their powers could be used for good or evil (Milwaukee Public Museum, 2022).

## Health & Healing Now

The Winnebago Tribe of Nebraska participated in Indigenous Lactation Training for lactation counselors in 2023. The training emphasized that breast milk is medicine with multiple benefits, including bonding with the infant. Breast feeding is a cultural practice and the first traditional food (winnebagotribe.com, 2023). The Tribe has also implemented interventions to reduce type 2 diabetes and obesity from 2014-2019. They used the CDC's community health assessment tool and employed six evidence-based practices to improve health in both these areas. Interventions included:

1. allowing community health representatives access to Indian Health Services electronic health records;
2. considering a tribal sugar-sweetened beverage tax;
3. starting an infant and childhood obesity prevention health education program;
4. adopting a healthy foods and beverages policy;
5. participating in CDC's Diabetes Recognition Prevention Program; and
6. improving pedestrian safety and built environment (Alonzo, Decora, & Bauer, 2019)

This is an ongoing process where respectful collaboration and community support and engagement have enabled progress toward the Tribe's health goals (Alonzo, Decore, & Bauer, 2019).

## Impact on Health of Interaction with White Culture Then

European diseases and warfare significantly reduced the Ho-Chunk tribe in the 1600s. They intermarried with other tribes to rebuild their population (Milwaukee Public Museum, 2022). When the Winnebago were displaced to South Dakota, they fled at night to Nebraska where economic opportunities and population decreased through the 1960s (winnebagotribe.com, 2023).

## Impact on Health of Interaction with White Culture Now

Ho-Chunk, Inc. is a tribal development agency that is committed to the Winnebago people, but also has benefitted residents across Nebraska. The company employs more than 1,000 non-Natives and has reduced poverty, increased median household income, removed housing barriers, and invested in education, scholarship, and internship programs. Ho-Chunk, Inc. is now a leading regional employer in Nebraska, Iowa, and South Dakota (winnebagotribe.com, 2023).

## *Wyandot (Huron)*

The Wyandotte Nation is in Oklahoma and is federally recognized (Wyandotte Nation, 2022). The Wyandot Nation of Kansas is state, but not federally recognized (Wyandot Nation of Kansas, 2013). The Wyandotte of Anderdon Nation in Michigan is also state recognized (Wyandotte of Anderdon Nation, n.d.). The Wyandot tribe began after the fall of the Huron Confederacy and included remnants of those tribes (Wyandotte Nation, 2022). The term Wyandot means "islanders" or "dwellers on a peninsula" (touringOhio.com, 2023), The Wyandotte Nation's enterprises include   an economic development corporation, four convenience stores/gas stations, four casinos and two hotels, a technology company, and telecommunication products (Wyandotte Nation, 2022).

## Health & Healing Then

The Huron recognized three types of illness: those due to natural causes that were cured by natural remedies, those caused by the sick person's desires of the soul that were cured by supplying these desires, and those caused by witchcraft that were cured by removing the spell. Cures might be dreamed, or a medicine man might diagnose the illness. Potions or emetics might be used or poultices or scarification. The medicine man might blow on the area of pain or incise the skin, and suck out the blood. He always carried his bag of herbs and drugs. An apothecary carried his drugs and a tortoise shell for the ritual. The Huron valued Oscar (possibly wild sarsaparilla) to heal wounds, ulcers, and other sores. A root known as ooxral (Indian turnip) removed phlegm from old people and was also used to clear the complexion. It was first cooked in hot ashes. Sweats were used and injuries, such as wounds, were treated with natural remedies. If a cure was not achieved, a supernatural cause was suspected (Tooker, 1961).

## Health & Healing Now

The Wyandotte Nation of Oklahoma's Bearskin Healthcare and Wellness Center is a community healthcare clinic and fitness center that also provides outreach events to promote tribal health. Services include optometry, dental, audiology, laboratory services, and telehealth visits. The Nation also is seeing increased numbers of victims of domestic violence and sexual assault. The Wyandotte Nation's Family Violence Prevention Program advocates for victims in the justice system (Wyandotte Nation, 2022).

## Impact on Health of Interaction with White Culture Then

In the 1600s a smallpox epidemic killed half the Wendat tribe (Wyandotte of Anderdon Nation, n.d.). In 1763 the British used rum as a weapon against the tribe and a recipe for Indian Trade Whiskey is in the Kansas City Museum. Whiskey was used when negotiating treaties and many tribesmen became addicted to alcohol (Wyandot Nation of Kansas, 2013).

## Impact on Health of Interaction with White Culture Now

Bearskin Health and Wellness Center is also open to the public and accepts patients of all ages. Wyandotte Nation also hosts an Environmental Festival annually which educates students about the environment, environmental issues, and solutions. In 2023 eight northeast Oklahoma tribes participated along with students, teachers, and paraprofessionals from Wyandotte public schools. The Planning and Natural Resources Department also recycles tires at a tire collection event twice a year (Wyandotte Nation, 2022).

## Tribal Gaming

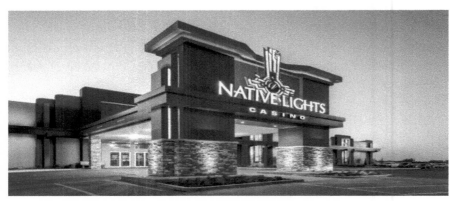

Many of the tribes have casinos as major income sources. How did this occur and how does it function?

In the 1970s some tribes began using bingo as a way to obtain funds to support tribal members and government. Some state governments were also seeking to increase state revenues by state-sponsored gaming. By the mid-1980s, many states authorized charitable gaming and some states sponsored state-operated lotteries. While tribal and state governments were interested in sponsoring gaming, control was an issue. Tribal governments wanted to conduct gaming independently without state regulation. In 1987 the Supreme Court ruled that tribal governments could establish and regulate gaming operations independently from state regulation as long as the state permitted some form of gaming (California v. Cabazon Band of Mission Indians, 480 U.S. 202).

Congressional hearings followed this decision that resulted in passage of the Indian Gaming Regulatory Act of 1988 (Public Law 100-497; 25 U.S.C. 2701). The Act (IGRA) compromised between tribal and state interests. States could require compacts with tribes for Class III gaming and tribes maintained full authority over Class II gaming. To ensure federal general regulatory oversight, the National Indian Gaming Commission was established as the primary federal agency (NIGC.gov, 2022).

Here is a synopsis of gaming:

| Class | Definition | Regulation |
|---|---|---|
| Class I | Traditional social and Indian gaming for minimum prizes | Authority over Class I gaming is vested in tribal governments. |
| Class II | The game of chance known as bingo and other games similar to bingo, including non-banked card games played against other players, not the House (excludes slot machines or electronic reproductions of any Class II games) | Tribal governments conduct, license, and regulate Class II gaming if the state where the tribe is located permits such gaming. The tribal government must adopt a Commission-approved gaming ordinance as the primary regulator. |
| Class III | The definition is broad and includes all types of gaming that are not Class I or Class II. These games include slot machines, craps, blackjack, roulette, and any electronic reproductions of any games of chance. | The following requirements must be met before conducting Class III gaming:<br>1. The form of Class III gaming must be permitted in the state where the tribe is located;<br>2. The state and tribe must have a compact approved by the Secretary of the Interior or regulatory procedures have been approved by the Secretary;<br>3. The tribe must adopt a tribal gaming ordinance that has been approved by the Chair of the NOGC.<br>This regulation is only for tribal gaming. Non-tribal gaming is regulated by state authorities. |

(NIGC.gov, 2022)

## The Role of the National Indian Gaming Commission (NIGC)

The NIGC's Mission is "to (1) promote tribal economic development, self-sufficiency, and strong tribal governments; (2) maintain the integrity of the Indian gaming industry; and (3) ensure that Tribes are the primary beneficiaries of their gaming activities" (NIGC.gov, 2022).

The Commission uses regulatory tools, such as training, public education, technical assistance, and enforcement to ensure regulatory compliance while respecting the responsibilities and capabilities of each tribe and ensuring gaming integrity. The NIGC monitors and regulates gaming activity in more than 520  gaming enterprises that are licensed by about 250 federally-recognized tribes in 29 states. The Commission inspects establishments, does background investigations, monitors tribal gaming activity, analyzes audits of Class II and some aspects of Class III operations, and investigates Indian Gaming Regulatory Act violations. It works with tribal regulatory agencies to review and approve gaming ordinances and management agreements. The NIGC provides extensive education and technical assistance to tribal leaders, tribal gaming commissions, and gaming operators.

The NIGC may take enforcement action for non-compliance, including civil penalties and temporary closure orders. Criminal concerns are referred to the appropriate tribal, state or Federal authorities. The Commission is also alert to any "corrupting influences by non-tribal government entities" (NIGC.org, 2022).

The Act empowers the Commission to cover its operating costs by assessing and collecting fees on tribal gaming revenues. These fees are "now capped at 0.809 percent of the industry's gross revenue" (NIGC.gov, 2022). It also receives payment for conducting background investigations and fingerprinting costs by potential contractors. Although the Commission is an independent regulatory agency in the Department of the Interior, the Agencies work together to ensure effective implementation of the Act and regulation of the gaming industry. The Commission maintains a trust relationship with Indian nations by having meaningful consultation with them prior to changing policies or regulations with tribal implications. The NIGC also focuses on timely and respectful responses to issues (NIGC.gov, 2022).

The Commission has a Chair and two Associate Commissioners. Only 2 of the 3 Commissioners may belong to the same political party and at least two Commissioners must be enrolled tribal members. The Commission has four areas of emphasis to be "more engaged and accountable to the Indian gaming industry and Indian Country" (NIGC.gov, 2022). These areas are:

1.  Industry Integrity-protect tribal gaming to create jobs, infuse tribal programs, and explore and strengthen tribal relationships with neighboring communities;
2.  Agency Accountability-meet public expectation for good governance and administrative processes that support effective and efficient decision-making that protects tribal assets;
3.  Preparedness-help tribes plan for risks to gaming assets that include natural disasters/public health/safety emergencies, need for modernization, and enhancing gaming operation and regulatory workforces; and
4.  Outreach-"ensure well-informed Indian gaming policy development through diverse relationships, accessible resources, and government-to-government consultation" (NIGC.gov, 2022).

In 2018 the NIGC hosted a conference to review 30 years of the Indian Gaming Regulatory Act and the Chairman of the NIGC, Jonodev Osceola Chaudhuri, shared the following comments:

"The future of Indian gaming is not yet written and policy-makers would do well to build on the self-determination principles that have powered the successes of the last 30 years. In evaluating the gains made over the last 30 years, we at the NIGC, as regulators, have seen the inarguable benefit of supporting tribal decision-making wherever possible so that the primary regulators of Indian gaming—the Tribes themselves—can pursue effective economic development tailored to their unique histories and landbases consistent with IGRA's policy goals and regulatory framework" (NIGC.gov, 2022).

## The Pandemic

The Pandemic affected Indian gaming as well as other business across the United States. In 2021 some tribes and gaming stakeholders responded about how they dealt with the Pandemic by supporting a sense of community. In rural Cattaraugus County, New York, the Seneca Nation and local leaders conducted a series of  COVID vaccination clinics for county residents at the Seneca Allegany Resort & Casino's Events Center. This was described by a member of the Seneca Nation, Kevin Nephew, President & CEO of the Seneca Gaming Corporation:

"For me, hosting the vaccination clinics at Seneca Allegany underscored not only the important role our properties play in the communities where we're located, but it also reinforced the sense that we are all in this together, and that we are going to come back stronger as a community. As President & CEO, I look forward to building important connections, not only within the Seneca community, but with our neighbors, team members and guests each and every day" (NIGC.gov, 2022).

# Chapter 5
# Great Plains Tribes

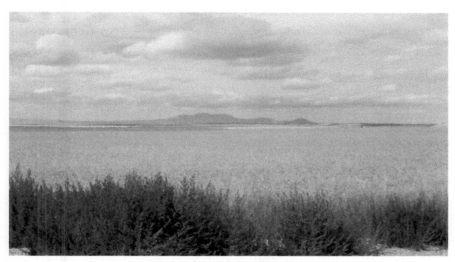

Tribes living on the Great Plains included the Arapaho, Arikara, Assiniboine, Cheyenne, Comanche, Crow, Gros Ventre, Hidatsa, Kiowa, Lakota, Lipan Apache, Mandan, Pawnee, Plains Apache (or Kiowa Apache), Plains Cree, Plains Ojibwe, Ponca, Sarsi, Nakoda (Stoney) and Tonkawa.

## *(Northern) Arapaho*

The Southern Arapaho Tribe was discussed as the Cheyenne-Arapaho Tribes of Oklahoma. The Northern Arapaho Tribe is located in Wyoming and is federally recognized. The term Arapaho is derived from a Pawnee word for "traders" (Native-languages.org, 1998-2020). Their enterprises include royalties from oil and gas leases, the Wind River Casino, the Little Wind Casino, and Arapaho Ranch. Until 2019, third party developers recovered natural resources and paid the Tribe royalties. Most of the proceeds didn't directly benefit tribal members. At that time, the Northern Arapaho and Eastern Shoshone Tribes created the Wind River

Energy Commission to control this operation and ensure these natural resources benefitted their members (Northern Arapaho Tribe, n.d.).

## Health & Healing Then

Respect was awarded to elders, especially those who had religious authority or medicine. The major festival annually was the eight-day Sun Dance ceremony where dancers fasted and painted their bodies before being attached to the Sun Dance pole by small skewers in their skin. If they showed no sign of pain during the ritual, they would receive a vision from the Great Spirit. Ceremonies included those for life transitions. Highly sacred ceremonies took place in a special tipi or a sweat lodge and included secret elder ceremonies, fasting, offerings, sweats, and prayers to the Flat Pipe, the original being on earth through which the Arapaho communicated with all sacred beings and forces. Before the reservation, the Arapaho had a sacred society of seven "Water-Sprinkling Old Men" who held daily ceremonies in the sweat lodge. After relocation to the reservation, they had a smaller group-the Four Old Men-with authority over religious life. Women also owned seven sacred bundles for their quillwork and there were medicine men with powers for prophecy, curing, and spiritual guidance (AAANativeArts.com, 1999-2023). Plant knowledge was used to cure illness and for ceremonies. Yarrow was used as a poultice for sores and Sweet flag cured stomach ailments (The Plant Lady, n.d.).

## Health & Healing Now

Although the Northern Arapaho have focused on reviving cultural traditions and language, oral storytelling is declining due to fewer elders and native speakers who are proficient in the language. Rituals are ignored or lost, and young people are not fluent in Arapaho dialects. The Tribe still faces limited opportunities, unemployment and financial issues (University of Colorado, n.d.). According to the 2016-2020 American Community Survey, 16.8% of Wind River residents live below the poverty threshold and the unemployment rate is 5.4%. Health care and social assistance is the largest area of employment (15.36%) (Northern Arapaho Tribe, n.d.).

## Impact on Health of Interaction with White Culture Then

The early Arapaho Tribe were nomadic buffalo hunters. When White gold hunters and settlers arrived in the Arapaho traditional hunting grounds, treaties resulted in the Northern Arapaho moving to the Wind River Reservation in Wyoming to live with their traditional enemies, the Eastern Shoshone. Rations were short for both tribes (AAANativeArts.com, 1999-2023). As hunting decreased, the Tribe began farming and ranching earn a living. Children were frequently sent to mission or boarding schools where they lost their language and traditional cultural customs. Reservation lands were sold, and allotments limited available land for farming. Economic opportunities were limited, and unemployment was high (University of Colorado, n.d.).

## Impact on Health of Interaction with White Culture Now

The Northern Arapaho are concerned about possible environmental exposures. A pilot study indicated exposures and additional study is planned to address radon exposure indoors and uranium and heavy metals in soil, A Community Advisory Board has been created. Its members from the Northern Arapaho community have expertise in environmental, health, and education aspects of the project. They are collaborating with members of the National Institute of Environmental Health Sciences research team from the University of Utah to assess environmental exposures on the Reservation and better understand the current respiratory status of tribal members by studying environmental risk factors that impact respiratory outcomes. An alliance between the Tribe and the Rocky Mountain Tribal Epidemiology Center is proposed for further research. Repeated surveys will examine feedback about changes to improve environmental health. Funding for this initiative began in 2021 and expires in 2024 (niehs.nih.gov, 2021).

## *Arikara (Sahnish)*

The Arikara are one of three affiliated tribes called the MHA Nation who live in central North Dakota. The other two tribes are the Mandan and Hidatsa. The MHA Nation is federally recognized, and each tribe maintains their own traditions. The Arikara call themselves Sahnish which means "the original people from whom all other tribes sprang". Today, the MHA Nation owns Four Bears Casino and Lodge and is seeking additional employment options for tribal members. Revenue comes from government enterprises, grants and programs. Much of their income comes from oil and gas development through the People's Fund (MHA Nation, 2018).

## Health & Healing Then

Sahnish priests belonged to the Medicine Lodge, which included nine distinct powerful societies. Sweat lodges and baths were used to prepare for ceremonies. Societies were able to heal, and the tribe was expert in using medicinal herbs. They grew an herb that was a special tobacco and tobacco was used in multiple ceremonies and prayers. When a medicinal plant was dug up, it was first addressed respectfully, asked to give itself for healing, and begged to have mercy on the sick person. The Sahnish were experts on healing wounds who also aided other tribes in wound care. Their Buffalo Society could set bones and could cauterize difficult wounds to heal them (indianaffairs.ND.gov, 2002).

## Health & Healing Now

Today, many Sahnish conduct their religious ceremonies using seven existing sacred bundles. The most important of these is "Mother Corn" to help the tribe live well in the world with the sacred bundles (indianaffairs.ND.gov, 2002). The MHA Nation paid to build the Good Road Recovery Center for residents to treat drug addiction in 2018. The Center incorporates customs and tradition in residential recovery and a transitional living center. The MHA community has been overwhelmed with illegal drugs from Mexican cartels that include heroin, cocaine, fentanyl, and methamphetamines. Substance abuse is prevalent in native tribes, especially when traditional families and values are eroded. The Center uses cultural techniques to help their clients. The day begins with meditation and participants burn sage, cedar, and sweetgrass. They use their hands to brush the smoke over their bodies-a process known as smudging. Smudging cleanses the mind and removes negative energy. The traditional 12-Step program includes uniquely native traditions. Participants use sweats and off-site equine therapy. Women have classes on native traditions by sewing quilts and ribbon skirts. Men use traditional methods to make drums Since the Center opened in 2018, its clients continue to increase (Warren, 2021).

## Impact on Health of Interaction with White Culture Then

Early interactions with White Culture caused four bouts of smallpox that left the people weak and killed about half their population. After this, they joined the Mandan and Hidatsa. In the mid-1870s, Indian agents withheld rations on reservations if families didn't send their children to school. Children at Fort Berthold attended either the Fort Stevenson Boarding School or C.L. Halls' Congregational Mission School. Many children were shipped to schools like Carlisle Indian School in Pennsylvania or Hampton Institute in Virginia. They wore uniforms, were forced to speak English, and given Christian names. Some lost their own names and heritage completely (see Chapter one for additional details). The agents also exploited the tribes by encouraging the sale of tribal lands and cheating on provisions. In 1946 the Army Corps of Engineers began construction on the Garrison Dam which resulted in loss of 94% of the tribe's farmlands and displaced 80% of the people with devastating effects. The project's specifications were altered without Congressional approval to protect Williston, ND and avoid interfering with irrigation projects. Nothing was done to protect the tribes who offered an alternative site that was rejected by the Corps (MHA Nation, 2018).

## Impact on Health of Interaction with White Culture-Today

Lake Sakakawea separates MHA communities and there is only one bridge that crosses the lake. Residents have long drives to access scattered communities. This causes difficulty when delivering medicine or trying to get quick lab results. Driving 98 miles from the Nation's main clinic to the satellite clinic takes 1.75 hours. If the Lake can be crossed, the distance is only 40 miles. MHA has obtained a grant to test drone delivery of specimens and medications. They are collaborating with the University of North Dakota's School of Aerospace Sciences and drone medication delivery will begin in 2024 in partnership with the University of Michigan-affiliated Michigan Medicine and Zipline, a drone delivery company based in California. The drones must fly in blustery winds and subzero temperatures. Being able to obtain same-day test results and reducing travel time are positive implications of the drone delivery system. Drones are being tested that will carry up to 55 pounds and test flights are planned for summer 2023 with approval from the Federal Aviation Administration (FAA) for longer distance flights. Drone flights in severe weather will be tested later in 2023. The University of North Dakota's aerospace program sees applicability to other rural areas in the state. MHA leaders are also interested in drone use to monitor pipelines, collect air quality samples, and use infrared sensors to detect oil field leakage of methane and other carcinogen-causing gases such as benzene and hydrocarbons. They also considering a land use study and training students as drone pilots to have their own skilled workforce for drone applications (Springer, 2023).

## Assiniboine

The Assiniboine and Sioux comprise the Fort Peck Tribes described under Lakota/Sioux in this chapter. Their current enterprises are located there. Assiniboine means "stone boilers" and their name for themselves is Nakona or Nakonabi meaning "the friendly people" (FourStar [Wamakashka Doba Inazhi], 1992-2003). Assiniboine (Nakota) are also part of the Fort Belknap Indian Community in Montana with the Gros Ventre (Aaniiih) tribe discussed later in this chapter (Fort Belknap Indian Community, 2023).

### Health & Healing Then

The family was important to the Assiniboine and religion was foundational. The first story of the Assiniboine was about Inkdomi who was on a raft when the world was water. He and four other beings discovered land beneath the water and from the mud, he made land and man. The first woman appeared from the man's leg and Inkdomi married her. All Assiniboine were descended from this union, and all have since been related to each other as family. A tribal name was given to each infant by someone who was a pipe carrier so the Creator and all the spirits would know the child who would receive protection throughout life. When a girl became an adolescent, she received a woman's name, and a maternal aunt taught her tribal rules and the woman's role. When a boy became an adolescent, he had to pass certain tests. Then, he fasted and completed the religious rituals of the Wotijaga or Medicine Lodge. After that, he received a man's name. Religious ceremonies were part of tribal identity (Shanley, 1999). A variety of plants were used medicinally. Some of these included:

1.  purple prairie clover-treatment for measles, heart disease, and stomach conditions;
2.  Moench purple coneflower-used for snakebites, rabies, gunshot wounds, and to reduce inflammation;
3.  boxelder leaves-drank as tea for stomach problems; and
4.  lavender hyssop-drank as tea for cardiac fatigue and cold symptoms (Magee, 2004).

## Health & Healing Now

See  Fort Peck Tribes under Lakota/Sioux

## Impact on Health of Interaction with White Culture Then

The Assiniboine people were friendly and willing to help anyone in need. White traders took advantage of Assiniboine hospitality and gave them blankets and gifts carrying smallpox. The Tribe suffered from smallpox epidemics three times and half the people died as a result. Other tribes then took their land and abused their women, children, and elders. As White culture increased, many Assiniboine decided to learn the White man's ways, educate their children, and assimilate into White society, leaving the Tribe forever (FourStar, 1992-2003).

## Impact on Health of Interaction with White Culture Now

The Fort Peck Tribes have a tribal policy that allows law enforcement to put members in jail or juvenile detention for threatening or attempting suicide. In 2021 two to four charges per week resulted in incarceration due to lack of facilities and mental health workers. The reservation has a suicide rate that in some years has been six times the national average. Non-tribal individuals are put in a hospital with a police guard until an evaluation can occur. There is only one IHS mental health specialist on the reservation and she sees 2-5 emergency cases a week. Since IHS doesn't have its own transportation, family members must bring the patient or transportation funds are requested from the tribe. Open positions are available, but are difficult to fill (KFF Health News, 2021). In 2023 the Fort Peck Tribes are beginning a suicide prevention research study in collaboration with Washington State University and are seeking volunteers (Fort Peck Tribes, 2023).

## Blackfoot

See Chapter 4

## Cheyenne

The Cheyenne are divided into two tribes-the Northern Cheyenne in Montana and the Southern Cheyenne in the Cheyenne and Arapaho tribes of Oklahoma. Cheyenne means " people who speak in a strange tongue". Both tribes are federally recognized. In the mid-19th century, the tribes split. The Northern Cheyenne became keepers of the sacred Buffalo Hat Bundle and Southern Cheyenne were keepers of the four Sacred Arrows (Hirst, 2020). The Northern Cheyenne are employed in power and construction companies, local schools, and the federal and tribal government. Chief Dull Knife College is an accredited 2-year school providing associate degrees and vocational education (Northern Cheyenne Tribe, 2013). The Southern Cheyenne own the Lucky Star Casino located in six communities. They also operate and manage the Cheyenne and Arapaho Farm and Ranch Program with over $1 million in farming assets (Cheyenne and Arapaho Tribes, 2022).

### Health & Healing Then

Men and women used herbs for healing and used an animal claw or bear tusk to stir liquid medicine. Bark Medicine (Balasamorrhiza sagittate) healed headaches and stomach discomfort. Chewing the root was used for toothache and sore throat. A tea of the root was good for fever and boiled small pieces of root in an infusion helped ensure an easy delivery. Black Sagebrush was used for cramps and dysentery by drinking a tea with the leaves and stem ground fine. A pinch of the powder in a cup of water should stop the bleeding and cramping. Poison ivy was treated by Poison Weed medicine (Astragalus nitidus) where the leaves and stems were ground to a powder and sprinkled on the afflicted skin when it had a watery appearance. Bear-berry was used as a diuretic. Other plant medicines were used for chest colds, increasing nursing mothers' milk supply, and paralysis (Bird Grinnell, 1905).

## Health & Healing Now

The Cheyenne and Arapaho Department of Health has multiple programs to address serious medical and mental issues experienced by tribal members. These programs include the Diabetes Wellness Program and the Health Education Program. Diabetes services focus on preventing or delaying diabetes onset while preventing complications by promoting physical fitness, improving nutrition, providing foot and vision care, and managing the disease. The Health Education Program provides outreach to help tribal members lead healthier lives with better nutrition, improved physical activity, and tobacco prevention and education (Cheyenne and Arapaho Tribes, 2022). The Northern Cheyenne are also experiencing issues with alcohol, drugs, and violence in their community (Northern Cheyenne Tribe, 2013).

## Impact on Health of Interaction with White Culture Then

Reservation life for both tribes was difficult with disease, lack of food and housing, problems with ration disbursement, and dependency on the federal government (Hirst, 2020).

## Impact on Health of Interaction with White Culture Now

The Lame Deer Wastewater Treatment Facility experienced untreated wastewater overflows around its collection system and lagoon. Many overflows flowed into Lame Deer Creek. Since 2017, the Northern Cheyenne Tribe and representatives from the Northern Cheyenne Utilities Commission (NCUC), EPA, Department of Justice, Indian Health Service, and federally-funded technical assistance providers helped the NCUC complete major infrastructure improvements to its collection system and lagoon. This workgroup continues to help the NCUC develop their managerial and operational capacity. Since this project began, there has not been an overflow in the collection system and lagoon. The Clean Water Act and National Pollutant Discharge Elimination System are now in compliance to protect residents' health and the environment (EPA.gov, 2021).

## Comanche

The Comanche Nation of Oklahoma is federally recognized. The name Comanche means "The People" and they are also known as "Lords of the Plains". Their enterprises include four casinos and tribal smoke shops (Comanche Nation, 2023).

### Health & Healing Then

The Comanche believed that all animals, plants, trees, mountains, rocks, and other natural resources had spirits or souls. They trusted in Manitou, the Great Spirit. Their ceremonies were similar to other Native tribes and included the sweat lodge, vision quest, and Sun Dance. A calumet with tobacco was passed from person to person at all holy functions and was used to confirm a peace settlement. It also offered prayers and petitions in religious services. They believed they were guided and protected by the spirits in all their endeavors (The American History.org, 2022). Comanche ethnobotany included Prairie Broomweed as a poultice for eczema and skin rashes, Little Bluestem Grass to treat syphilitic sores, and Crested Prickly Poppy as a salve for sore eyes (The Plant Lady, n.d.).

### Health & Healing Now

The Comanche Nation Prevention and Recovery programs provide education, prevention, and treatment for tribal members returning from incarceration or suffering from  long-term substance abuse. Their programs are designed to be culturally and educationally beneficial to youth and young adults by outreach that addresses suicide awareness and alcohol/substance abuse. The Nation also has a diabetes program and the Comanche Tribal Elders Program to provide caregivers for fragile elders (Commanche Nation, 2023).

## Impact on Health of Interaction with White Culture Then

Diseases like smallpox and cholera greatly reduced the Comanche population by the 1870s. The Federal Government began moving the Comanche to the Oklahoma reservation in the 1860s and promised them schools, churches, and annuities as well as stopping the buffalo hunters who were killing the herds the Comanche depended on for food. The government failed to stop the buffalo hunters and, when they attacked hunters in 1874, the Comanche were driven by the Army unto the reservation which was further reduced with 160-acre allotments (Weiser, 2021).

## Impact on Health of Interaction with White Culture Now

In 2022 the Comanche Nation received a $487,000 grant from the Federal Transit Administration to add an ADA-accessible van to ensure transportation of residents to necessary appointments and treatments. This required new dispatch and operator software, employee salaries, fuel costs, and maintenance fees. The Nation is to report on progress annually and the service beneficiaries are Comanche County and surrounding rural communities. This grant is effective until 2023 (GovTribe.com, 2022).

## Crow (Apsáalooke)

The Crow or Apsáalooke Nation is a federally recognized tribe in Montana. The name Apsáalooke means "children of the large-beaked bird" (tribalnations.mt.gov, n.d.). Their enterprises include a market, a restaurant, a marina, and a tour company (crow-nsn.gov, 2023). One coal mine operates providing employment and royalty income for tribal members. They also maintain a buffalo herd of about 300 and Little Big Horn College (tribalnations.mt.gov, n.d.).

## Health & Healing Then

Medicine bundles were received in visions and dreams to heal wounds. Snake effigies and otter skin in bundles were powerful medicine bundles. Buffalo power was used to heal wounds. Medicine bundles also treated women's diseases and cured barren women. Stomach kneading relieved indigestion. Crow medicine bundles were fairly small and compact with a limited number of sacred objects and usually one major one that served a specific purpose (Wildschut & Ewers, 1960). Plants used for medicine included milkweed to treat sore, achy joints and big-seed biscuitroot to ease labor pain and reduce cold and flu symptoms (Magee, 2004).

## Health & Healing Now

Apsaalooke Healing is the accredited program to help tribal members recover from alcoholism and drug abuse through out-patient treatment and referral for in-patient care if needed (crow-nsn.gov, 2023). A Crow woman and a researcher from Montana State University began a small project in 1996 to get Crow women to increase cancer screenings. The project was successful, and they founded non-profit Messengers for Health, which was nationally recognized in 2018 for leading community-based participatory research. Community members and researchers are equal partners and Messengers for Health now studies chronic disease. Crow people suffer from chronic diseases like diabetes, substance use, obesity, depression and the two women found that mental health must be addressed before people can change behavior. They designed a program where elders who are managing chronic illness themselves mentor support groups where people can grow and learn together (nimhd.nih. gov, 2019).

## Impact on Health of Interaction with White Culture Then

Relationships with White explorers and  fur traders were good, but over 20% of the tribe died from smallpox and other diseases. The Crow lived by hunting buffalo and as the buffalo herds disappeared, they were forced to return to farming on the land that remained (montanakids.com, 2020).

## Impact on Health of Interaction with White Culture-Today

Crow elders are important to the tribal community because they share oral history and preserve the tribe's cultural history. Alzheimer's disease and other related dementias impact Native Americans as well as other U.S. populations. A Crow tribal member serves as lead community researcher and tribal liaison for a collaborative study with the Northern

Arizona University Southwest Health Equity Research Collaborative to improve early detection of dementia in the Crow tribe. The research team is diverse and examines protective factors such as spirituality, cultural values, family unity and behavioral traditions common to Native Americans. Their purpose is to develop a predictive model for dementia. They are starting with a cultural concept called Baakalaaxdeete or "have a good memory" in the Crow language and seek to identify early and accurately Crow tribal members at risk for dementia. The project is in its beginning stages and the partnership between the researchers and the Crow tribe should help the community reduce risk factors and "have a good memory" as long as possible (nau.edu, 2023).

## Gros Ventre/Nakoda (Assiniboine)

Gros Ventre or Aaniiih are part of the Fort Belknap Indian Community with the Nakoda (Assiniboine) and are federally recognized. Their name in their own language is "white clay people" and Gros Ventre is French for "big belly" (native-languages.org, 1998-2020). Nakdta is "the generous ones". Their major industry is agriculture on small cattle ranches and farms (Fort Belknap Indian Community, 2023). Their major business enterprise is the Island Mountain Development Group (IMDG) which was established in 2009. This company's diversified holdings include real estate, financial technology, construction, information technology, government contracting, and a community development financial institution ((Island Mountain Development Group, 2023).

### Health & Healing Then

The Gros Ventre believed in a supernatural being called "the One Above" as the ultimate source of life. Tribal keepers cared for two medicine bundles-the Flat Pipe Bundle and the Feathered Pipe Bundle. Keepers received special training and made prayer-sacrifice vows. The Sun Dance was central to religious ceremonies. The Gros Ventre also created the Grass Dance which was conducted in a multi-sided building with a hole in the roof. It was central to their cultural traditions (Little Missouri Cultural Heritage Project, 2018). White Prairie Aster was used to stop bleeding and as an eyewash. The Prairie Coneflower treated fever, stomach pain, poison ivy, and rattlesnake bites. The Gumbo Lilly reflected the environment around it and treated toothache, uterine prolapse, and sores (University of Montana, 2023).

## Health & Healing Now

The Aaniih Nakoda College's medicinal garden has  more than 60 plant species that have been used as medicines for generations. In 2020 the Indian Health Service (IHS) began seeking applicants for two traditional healers at the Fort Belknap IHS Hospital. Traditional healers can treat illnesses and diseases that require lifestyle changes. This includes heart disease, diabetes, and domestic violence issues. These traditional healers are not licensed or certified and can help with mental, physical spiritual, and emotional needs of tribal members. They also can serve as patient advocates by educating hospital staff about cultural sensitivity and traditional health practices. By using traditional treatments like blessings, sweats, and ceremonies, they can connect patients with tribal culture to support their healing. Medicinal plants are also important to regain health knowledge that was in danger of being lost (Akridge, 2020).

## Impact on Health of Interaction with White Culture Then

Around 1754, the Gros Ventre had their first contact with White traders and their first exposure to smallpox (Fort Belknap Indian Community, 2023.  In the 1780s, multiple smallpox outbreaks caused many deaths. In 1837 the tribe lost 200 members to smallpox although this was less than other tribes. As White settlers increased, Gros Ventre territory became smaller and the buffalo they depended on for food decreased. They were reduced to seeking annuities at Fort Belknap for food and supplies. The government tried to move them to Fort Peck, but they refused and were allotted a small reservation to share with the Nakoda (Assiniboine) at Fort Belknap (Little Missouri Cultural Heritage Project, 2018).

## Impact on Health of Interaction with White Culture Now

Gold mining at Zartman-Landusky mines a quarter century ago used large amounts of cyanide to remove gold from ore. Cyanide is lethal to humans in small amounts. A study to determine health impacts from 1996 was never done. Today, asthma, emphysema, diabetes, and thyroid problems have impacted the Fort Belknap tribes, especially children. Lead poisoning and chemical burns from swimming in water from the mining area have also been reported (Klauk, 2023). The Tribes have dealt with surface and groundwater pollution for more than 20 years and a mineral withdrawal order to stop approval of new mining claims expired in October 2020 for a 48-hour period before it was reinstated for 20-years. During that time ten new mining claims were filed by Blue Arc and processed. The new order also reduced the covered area by 842 acres. In 2021, Blue Arc applied to the Montana Department of Environmental Quality for a mineral exploration license at Zortman which was opposed by three environmental groups and the Fort Belknap Indian Community (Eggert, 2021). In 2022 the Montana Department of Environmental Quality cited Blu Arc for exploring mining without legal permits at eight locations on four properties and levied a maximum fine of $500K. No environmental review was done, and the exploration disturbed 0.6 acres of land that was being remediated. The Fort Belknap Indian Community and conservation organizations continue to oppose additional mining in this area of the reservation (Great Falls Tribune, 2022).

## Hidatsa

The Hidatsa are one of three affiliated tribes called the MHA Nation who live in central North Dakota. The other two tribes are the Mandan and Arikara (Sahnish) The MHA Nation is federally recognized, and each tribe maintains their own traditions. The Hidatsa call themselves "willows". A Sahnish name for the tribe is "people of the water". Today, the MHA Nation owns Four Bears Casino and Lodge and is seeking additional employment options for tribal members. Revenue comes from government enterprises, grants and programs. Much of their income comes from oil and gas development through the People's Fund (MHA Nation, 2018).

### Health & Healing Then

Tribal and personal bundles possessed the spiritual world, and this power could be used for good or evil. Healing was also described as strong medicine or power. Fasting, vision experiences, and self-torture could control power. Men and women with special medicine bundles used songs and rites as medical and religious experts to heal wounds or assist with childbirth. Priests were older men who were responsible for important clan and tribal bundles. Their function was to maintain harmony between supernatural spirits and forces and the tribe. Ceremonies included the Sun Dance, the Red Stick buffalo-calling ceremony, and the Big Bird rainmaking ceremony. Hidatsa traditional medicine combined practical knowledge and supernatural intervention to treat injuries. The healing process used symbolic healing, sacred songs, and sweat baths. Death was usually related to supernatural causes and violations of ritual prescriptions (everyculture.com, 2023).

## Health & Healing Now

See Warren reference under Arikara Tribe.

## Impact on Health of Interaction with White Culture Then

The smallpox epidemic of 1837 was the second time this disease impacted the Hidatsa. Survivors of three Hidatsa villages became a single village until they unified with the Mandan in 1845 for social and economic survival (MHA Nation, 2018).

## Impact on Health of Interaction with White Culture Now

See Springer reference under Arikara Tribe.

## *Kiowa*

The Kiowa Tribe is located in Oklahoma and is federally recognized. The name Kiowa means "principal people" (native-languages.org, 1998-2020). Their enterprises include the Kiowa Casino, Indian City Screen Printing, Kiowa Construction, and the Kiowa Gift Shop (Kiowa Tribe, 2023).

## Health & Healing Then

The Kiowa respected the sun, stars, and other members of the constellations as well as natural phenomena like the cyclone. Animals and birds like bison, bear, and eagle were sacred. The Sun Dance was conducted annually and was a significant ritual. Other rituals included the sweat lodge ceremony for purification and the pipe ritual where the Calumet was filled with tobacco and passed from one participant to another (Tribe Facts, 2018). Some Kiowa practiced the Ghost Dance between 1890-1916 as followers of the peyote religion (Oklahoma Historical Society, n.d.). Many plants were used medicinally. Here are a few examples. The Western Buckeye was brewed and drank as an emetic. Giant Ragweed was used to wash sores and drank as a tea to cure slow healing sores. Prairie Sage was rolled up, chewed, and swallowed for stomach issues. It also treated lung conditions. Mexican Mugwort leaves were chewed to soothe sore throats (umt.edu, 2004).

## Health & Healing Now

The Kiowa News has information for tribal members about blood pressure and diabetes along with a recipe for healthy nutrition. The Kiowa Community Health Representatives serve as liaisons between the Kiowa people and the Indian Health Service to provide health education and promote disease prevention. The Kiowa Administration on Aging provides multiple services to tribal members. Its primary function is providing nutritional services in congregate sites and via home delivery if needed. Elder participation has increased in the past couple of years to an average of nearly 200 meals per day. The Kiowa Tribe Teen Prevention Network provides substance abuse and mental health services to lessen suicidal behavior among Kiowa youth to age 24. The program collaborates with school districts to provide life skills classes based on the American Indian Life Skills curriculum. Training on drug/substance use prevention and suicide prevention is also available. Outside service referrals are done for mental health counseling (Kiowa Tribe, 2023).

## Impact on Health of Interaction with White Culture Then

From 1868-1901, the government tried to make Kiowa into ranchers and farmers. This effort was unsuccessful because of drought conditions and inadequate annuity funds in lean times. Forced allotment resulted in smaller per capita payments from leased land after 1901. Federal Indian policies fostered dependency and rural Kiowa lived in poverty before World War II (Oklahoma Historical Society, n.d.).

## Impact on Health of Interaction with White Culture Now

The Missing & Murdered Indigenous Women & Girls (MMIW) has a Kiowa Chapter founded in 2020. The first year, they examined 30 cases. The majority of these were related to domestic abuse although several included kidnapping and runaways. This number increased to 60 in 2021 and 80 in 2022. Currently in 2023 there are 90 cases, some of which include young boys and men. The Chapter provides community assistance and outreach. It collaborates with outside organizations, including the 2023 Miss Indian Oklahoma who publicizes their efforts. MMIW-Kiowas Chapter also maintains a Facebook site to share information (Kiowa Tribe, 2023).

## *Lakota*

There are seven federally recognized Lakota tribes in the U.S. Lakota means "ally or friend" (native-languages.org, 1998-2000). Although part of the Sioux confederacy, some Lakota prefer not to use the word Sioux because it is a derogatory term from the Ojibwe meaning "little snakes" (native-languages.org, 1998-2000). The Assiniboine and Sioux tribes are known as Fort Peck Tribes and live in Montana. They seek economic development with investors through workforce preparedness and manage a small Casino (Fort Peck Tribes, n.d.). The Cheyenne River Sioux Tribe lives in South Dakota and works to promote public health initiatives, community development, and manages the 7th Generation cinema (Cheyenne River Sioux Tribe, n.d.). The Lower Brule Sioux Tribe's enterprises include the Lakota Foods popcorn company, the Golden Buffalo Casino and Motel, hunting and fishing on the reservation, and an annual Powwow and Rodeo (Lower Brule Sioux Tribe, 2019). The Oglala Sioux Tribe also lives in South Dakota and owns and manages the East Wind Casino (Oglala Sioux Tribe, 2022). The Rosebud Sioux Tribe of South Dakota owns and manages the Rosebud Casino, hotel, RV park, and fuel plaza (Rosebud Sioux Tribe, 2023). The Standing Rock Sioux Tribe in South Dakota owns and manages the Prairie Knights Casino and Lodge, the Grand River Casino and Resort, and promotes tourism with an annual Powwow (Standing Rock Sioux Tribe, n.d.). The Lower Sioux Indian Community of Minnesota has a cultural department, a health clinic, a recreation center, and an office of economic development (Lower Sioux Indian Community, 2023).

## Health & Healing Then

Lakota tribes practiced natural medicine and believed that medicines are people you invite into your body and that you should welcome them by talking with them and welcoming them. In other words, they should be treated like a spirit being. Ancient Lakota doctors or medicine men treated the spirit as well as the body. They used a variety of leaves, roots, and herbs as well as singing and dancing to create healing potions. Their purification (today's detoxification) cleansed both body and spirit. Every medicine man had different gifts and visions to cure the sick. They believed that they did not heal, but welcoming the medicines to the body and asking for their help was essential for healing to occur (native-net.org, 2005-2020).

## Health & Healing Now

Fort Peck Tribal Health provides health education, environmental health, animal control, diabetes services, end stage renal disease dialysis, and medically necessary transportation (Fort Peck Tribes, n.d.). Cheyenne River Sioux Tribe Support Services provides cash in emergencies, emergency lodging and heating, elderly stipends, school clothing assistance, funeral assistance, food vouchers, and college grants (Cheyenne River Sioux Tribe, n.d.). The Lower Brule Sioux Tribe Community Health Representative Program provides homemaker services, case management, patient care monitoring, patient transport, interpreter services, and advocacy. It also is a vocational rehab site and N.E.W. job training program (Lower Brule Sioux Tribe, 2019). The Standing Rock Sioux Tribe's Nutrition for the Elderly Program has multiple services. These include caregiver programs, case management, assisted living, meals, elder abuse prevention programs, home modification and repair, respite care, and transportation (Standing Rock Sioux Tribe, n.d.).

## Impact on Health of Interaction with White Culture Then

The early 1880s caused the Lakota suffering from annihilation of the buffalo which they depended on for food. Over 300 Assiniboines died of starvation in 1883-1884 due to shortages of medicine and food during severe winter weather. There were frequent changes of agents and few improvements in services (Fort Peck Tribes, n.d.). Starvation also impacted other Lakota/Sioux tribes and forced assimilation to white culture occurred. When dams were authorized on the Missouri, two Acts in 1954 and 1962 took the bottomland of the Missouri River valley and almost all the economic, social, and cultural base of the Lower Brule Sioux Tribe. 22,296 acres were lost, one town (Lower Brule) was underwater, and 69% of the residents lost their homes. Lake Sharpe and Lake Francis as reservoirs were created and these waters continue to eat away the land, and cultural sites., Cemeteries had to be moved. Forests, fishing grounds, and hunting sites were flooded causing economic deprivation (Lower Brule Sioux Tribe, 2019).

## Impact on Health of Interaction with White Culture Now

The Oglala Sioux Tribe, Rosebud Sioux Tribe, and the Cheyenne River Sioux Tribe joined together in 2022 to take control of healthcare for their citizens. This enables the Great Plains Tribal Leaders Health Board to use the Oyate Health Center by adjusting services as needed without waiting for Indian Health Service offices or Washington, DC to make decisions. This change increases local decision-making authority, decreases wait times, and expands behavioral health services (NewsCenter1 Staff, 2022).

## *Lipan Apache*

The Lipan Apache Tribe of Texas is state recognized. They are known as "The Light Gray People" (Lipan Apache Tribe, 2023). The Tribe conducts two Powwows a year in the spring and fall. Their focus is on preserving their culture, traditions, language, and history ( Lipan Apache Tribe, 2023).

## Health & Healing Then

The Lipan Tribe honored their ancestors-their Grandmothers and Grandfathers. Nopalito and Yucca plants provided food, medicine, and for daily needs. The buffalo represented the hunt and knowledge that the Creator will provide for the people. The Sacred Hoop of Life had four directions: East (black), West (yellow), South (blue), and North (white). The pathway from East to West was sacred to the Lipan people (Lipan Apache Tribe, 2023). The buffalo were integral to the Tribe and other Native communities. Their grazing was essential to prairie ecology. Some plants only sprouted in their hoofprints, and others seeded through their dung (Baddour, 2022).

## Health & Healing Now

As a state recognized tribe, the Lipan Apache Tribe is not entitled to Indian Health Services' benefits. The tribe is currently pursuing federal recognition. The Tribe is a voting member of the National Congress of American Indians which facilitates health provisions of the Affordable Care Act and Indian Health Care Improvement Act (Lipan Apache Tribe, 2023). The Texas Buffalo Project has returned bison to Lipan land and fifteen of them were introduced to children at a summer camp as they learned about their heritage (Baddour, 2022).

## Impact on Health of Interaction with White Culture Then

The Lipan people struggled to survive throughout the late 1800s. Smallpox took a toll and food shortages forced the Tribe to scatter in small groups from Texas to Mexico. People of all ages were marked for extermination, and they survived by moving from place to place (Lipan Apache Tribe, 2023).

## Impact on Health of Interaction with White Culture Now

The Lipan Cemetery in Presidio, Texas-Cemeterio del Barrio de los Lipanes- is a sacred burial ground to the Lipan Tribe. As settlement in the area increased, homes were built around_it, rocks were taken from the site, and it was reduced to a fraction of its original size. Many in the area did not realize it was a burial site and the property was jointly owned by the city of Presidio and Presidio County. Parts of the mound were eroding and building a fence around the area would cost between $40,000-$60,000. The cemetery was designated a Texas State Antiquities Landmark, and the city and county couldn't manage the cemetery or fund the needed fence. In late 2021, both agreed to transfer the property back to the Lipan Tribe because the Tribe could file for grants to absorb the cost (Kaur, 2021). The Tribe has successfully raised funds for the protective wall and continues to seek additional funding for the site. MASS Design Group designed the wall structure. The Tribe has partnered with Big Bend Conservation Alliance to construct the protective wall which should be finished in late 2023 (Lipan Apache Tribe, 2023).

## Mandan

The Mandan are one of three affiliated tribes called the MHA Nation who live in central North Dakota. The other two tribes are the Arikara (Sahnish) and Hidatsa. The MHA Nation is federally recognized, and each tribe maintains their own traditions. The Mandan call themselves "the People of the First Man". Today, the MHA Nation owns Four Bears Casino and Lodge and is seeking additional employment options for tribal members. Revenue comes from government enterprises, grants and programs. Much of their income comes from oil and gas development through the People's Fund  (MHA Nation, 2018).

### Health & Healing Then

The Mandan People wore multiple symbolic tattoos to commemorate important personal events that were often celebrated in sacred ceremonies. They believed in Animism where the universe and all natural objects possessed souls or spirits. Their rituals included the Sweat Lodge and Sun Dance ceremonies and the Vision Quest. Young men were cleansed in a sweat lodge, followed by a solitary exposure within a day and night. Then, they had skewers shaped like sharp animal claws embedded in their flesh and, when removed, the scars showed they had completed their Vision Quest. The tribe also used the Calumet or sacred ceremonial pipe filled with tobacco for sacred ceremonies (Alchin, 2017).

## Health & Healing Now

See Warren reference under Arikara Tribe.

## Impact on Health of Interaction with White Culture Then

Smallpox reduced the Mandan population to only 125 in 1837. They combined with the Arikara (Sahnish) and intermarried with them. Only a few full-blooded Mandan were left, and their culture was changed (MHA Nation, 2018).

## Impact on Health of Interaction with White Culture Now

See Springer reference under Arikara Tribe.

## *Nakoda (Stoney)*

See Assiniboine & Gros Ventre

## *Pawnee*

The Pawnee Nation was originally from the Great Plains and today lives in Oklahoma. It is federally recognized, and the word 'Pawnee' means "Men of Men" (Pawnee Nation, 2023). The Nation's enterprises under the Pawnee Tribal Development Corporation include Teepee Smoke Shop & Casino, StoneWolf Casino and Wolf SportsGrille, Pawnee Trading Post Casino, and Arrow Stop Travel Plaza (Pawnee Tribal Development Corporation, n.d.).

## Health & Healing Then

Cedar was used in prayer and ceremonies as a token of peace and the morning star symbolized the place where God lived (Pawnee Nation, 2023). Pawnee religious practices were connected to the natural world and Pawnee burned juniper leaves as a prayer smoke offering. In the Pawnee Hako Pipe Ceremony, needle grass (Pawnee hairbrush) was gathered to represent Toharu, the covering of the earth. Toharu's power gave food to animals and men so they could be strong in life. Plants also were used for medicinal purposes that included:

1. eastern redcedar as a cold remedy and cough medicine;
2. cattail to dress burns and prevent chafing of infants;
3. smooth sumac as remedy for dysmenorrhea and dysentery;
4. jack-in-the-pulpit or Indian turnip for treating headaches and rheumatism; and
5. common sunflower taken by women who became pregnant while still nursing so the infant wouldn't become sick (Ledford, 2012).

## Health & Healing Now

The Pawnee Nation's Health & Community Services Division has two departments. The Health & Prevention Department provides case management, health education, monitoring of at-risk individuals, and advocates for individuals and families to access comprehensive health services. The Department is also responsible for the Diabetes Program, the Substance Abuse Program/Suicide Prevention Initiative/Tribal Opioid Response, and the Fitness Center. The Social Services Department is responsible for domestic violence programs, family services, food distribution, emergency assistance, and services for elders and disabled individuals (Pawnee Nation, 2023).

## Impact on Health of Interaction with White Culture Then

An industrial boarding school planned for the Pawnee in Nebraska closed in 1875 because the tribe was scheduled to be removed to Indian Territory (now Oklahoma) in 1876. When the tribe arrived, schools were not ready. Two day-schools opened in 1876 that would teach students English and elementary education before sending them to boarding schools. The Pawnee Boarding School finally opened in Fall 1878. It was overcrowded with inadequate, poor quality water. In 1889, 39 girls shared 13 beds. The sewer system was also inadequate. In the following years, a Boys' Dormitory, commissary, and carpenter shop were built. Further construction included classrooms, offices, and a gym. The boarding school operated until 1958 and was returned to the Pawnee Nation in 1972 (Asylum Projects, 2021). Pawnee students could not speak their language, observe traditions, or practice religious ceremonies. They called the boarding school "Gravy U' because of the gravy served at each meal (Pawnee Nation, 2023).

**Impact on Health of Interaction with White Culture Now**

Today, the former boarding school houses the Pawnee Nation College a two-year school that prepares students to enter the workforce or attend a four-year school. The school received nonprofit status in 2006 and offers associate degree and certification programs. The College assists the Pawnee Nation in renovating the former boarding school to honor the indigenous students who attended Gravy U (Pawnee Nation College, n.d.). It also offers American Indian Studies courses.

## *Plains Apache (or Kiowa Apache)-currently Apache Tribe of Oklahoma*

The Apache Tribe of Oklahoma (formerly known as the Plains Apache/Kiowa Apache) is a federally recognized tribe in Oklahoma. Apache means "enemy" (native-languages.org, 1998-2020). The Tribe's enterprises include the Golden Eagle Casino, a business committee to enhance tribal members skills, and the coming Trading Post Casino (Apache Tribe of Oklahoma, 2023).

**Health & Healing Then**

The Apache Tribe tried to act as peacemakers as treaties reduced tribal lands and epidemics of cholera and smallpox occurred. Tribal elders were respected for their knowledge and experience. Their spiritual life centered on four sacred medicine bundles and the importance of being in harmony with nature. They joined the Sun Dance and harvested plants and buffalo. They strived to continue their cultural traditions by giving children names to honor either an ancestor or a special event. Other ceremonies included the Blackfoot Dance to honor warriors and the Rabbit Dance where children received an Apache name (Apache Tribe of Oklahoma, 2023). Plains Apache used a variety of plants for medicinal purposes. Teucrium or Canada germander was called "fever medicine" and used to treat diarrhea, abdominal discomfort, menstrual cramps, and childbirth and miscarriage afterpains. Puffball treated skin ailments by rubbing the powder into sores Mountain cedar was used medicinally and in ceremonies (Jordan, 2008).

## Health & Healing Now

The Apache Tribe of Oklahoma Injury Prevention Program developed a program from 2017-2019 to prevent injuries from falls and motor vehicle accidents among tribal residents in Caddo County. They used the following interventions:

1.  Fix hazards in tribal elders' homes that could cause falls;
2.  Coordinate elders' eye screenings;
3.  Review elders' medications that could increase fall risk;
4.  Hold car seat safety events by providing car seats and education on usage;
5.  Observe and record car seat and seat belt use by community members; and
6.  Train Child Passenger Safety Technicians.

2020 statistics showed progress:

1.  26 homes checked for fall hazards;
2.  163 fall hazards fixed in homes;
3.  277 child safety seats provided and installed in vehicles;
4.  110 Child Passenger Safety Technicians trained; and
5.  200K community members informed via media campaigns (apachetribe.org, 2020).

## Impact on Health of Interaction with White Culture Then

The reservation years were very difficult for the Apache Tribe. Government policies discouraged religious ceremonies and traditions. Kinship and family were disrupted when children were placed in boarding schools, forbidden to speak their language and had their names changed to English ones. Here is a quote from one of those children: "When my father took me to school from the camp, I had long hair and was dressed in buckskin. They took off my buckskin. My hair was long and braided...They took scissors and cut the braids off and gave them to my father. The superintendent came in...He said my name was going to be James" (Apache Tribe of Oklahoma, 2023). As the buffalo were killed by hide hunters, there were food shortages, and they were forced to rely on limited government rations. The government wanted them to become farmers, but insects, drought, and lack of education didn't make them successful. 160-acre allotments reduced their lands significantly because remaining land was opened to White settlement (Apache Tribe of Oklahoma, 2023).

## Impact on Health of Interaction with White Culture Now

The Injury Prevention Program described above partnered with Safe Kids Worldwide to provide car seat education and resources. Tribal representatives also attended Oklahoma Traffic Safety Coalition meetings and installed a billboard to reach multiple people daily. The Apache Tribal Princess collaborated with the Injury Prevention team to record radio Public Service Announcements. The program has seen a nearly 65% increase in child safety seat use to a current rate in 2020 of 79% (apachetribe.org, 2020).

## *Plains Cree*

The Plains Cree are part of the Chippewa Cree Indians of the Rocky Boy's Reservation in Montana and are federally recognized. Rocky Boy meant "stone child", but was incorrectly translated into English. The tribe call themselves Ne-Hiyawak or "those who speak the same language". Their enterprises are primarily agriculture and livestock with some wheat farming and pole and post production. The Tribe also has a small ski area, Bear Paw Ski Bowl, that is staffed by volunteers. (mt.gov, n.d.).

## Health & Healing Then

The Cree used a variety of herbs and plants for health. Fire Root/Bitter Pepper Root was used for coughs. The bark of Juniperus communis was used as a poultice for wounds by cutting a stick into pieces about four inches long, boiling it until the outer bark could be easily removed, scraping the inner bark and beating it between two stones until it was pulpy and then applied to the wound. Red Willow Bark could be used as an emetic for coughs and fevers. Poplar Bark could also treat coughs. Service Tree was a treatment for pleurisy and inflammatory diseases.

Bitter Tea was a tonic that cured diarrhea. Leaves and barks were always chewed before being applied to wounds (Holmes, 1884).

## Health & Healing Now

The Chippewa Cree Tribe Human Services Division has several programs to meet tribal members' needs. These include Temporary Assistance to Needy Families, Tribal Child Support, Social Services, Tribal Vocational Rehabilitation, and Office of Victim Services (Chippewa Cree Tribe, 2011-2019).

## Impact on Health of Interaction with White Culture Then

Plains Cree suffered in smallpox epidemics in the late 18th century when they were known as the Parkland Cree. Most of them were vaccinated in 1838 when another smallpox epidemic struck, and they survived that epidemic. As the buffalo herds disappeared, the Cree in Montana joined the Chippewa on the Rocky Boy's Reservation (Meyer, 2011).

## Impact on Health of Interaction with White Culture Now

Stone Child College is a tribally-controlled community college by the Chippewa Cree Tribe that was founded in 1984. Tribal leaders wanted a college that would preserve their culture and prepare tribal members for post-secondary education. Stone Child College is accredited by the Northwest Commission on Colleges and Universities. It is listed in Accredited Institutions of Higher Learning. The College is committed to serving the needs of the community and has computer-equipped classrooms and financial aid and scholarships are available for students (Stone Child College, 2022).

## *Plains Ojibwe*

See Ojibwe in Chapter 4

## *Ponca*

There are two federally recognized Ponca tribes in Nebraska and Oklahoma. The Ponca Tribe of Indians of Oklahoma operates the Fancy

Dance Casino as a revenue source for the Tribe. The Ponca Tribe of Nebraska operates the Prairie Flower Casino along with a tribal museum and has a herd of 100 buffalo. The word 'Ponca' has multiple meanings from "that which is sacred" to "sacred Head" or "gentle Leader" (Holmes, 2011).

## Health & Healing Then

The Ponca practiced the sacred pipe religion and believed in an all-powerful creator, Wakonda. They modified the Sun Dance to add emphasis on fertility and gathered herbs and wild plants for healing and food (Ritter, 2011). Some of the medicinal plants used by the Ponca were Wormwood for burn dressings; Sagewort for gastrointestinal issues; Calamus for coughs and colds; Chokecherry as an antidiarrheal; and Thymeleaf Sandmat to increase milk production in nursing mothers (Gilmore, 1919).

## Health & Healing Now

The Ponca Tribe of Indians of Oklahoma has a Tribal Opioid Response Program that addresses addiction to pain medication and combines Medication-Assisted Treatment with Case Management and therapy to holistically address needs-physical, spiritual, and emotional. Support and skills coaching are vital to success. This program is partnered with the Tribal Opioid and Stimulant Response Prevention Program that focuses on substances used, recovery support, and a prevention campaign. Their Behavioral Health Program provides counseling to encourage growth and well-being. Multiple services are offered including trauma-informed therapies for domestic/family violence. The Hope and Recovery Center is a 60-day residential facility for alcohol and drug treatment for those tribal members 18 or older who have completed a 5-day detox and are willing to receive psychosocial and physical evaluation (Ponca Tribe of Indians of Oklahoma, 2022). The Ponca Domestic Violence Department of Nebraska provides advocacy services, emergency placement, referrals, case management, transportation, and other services for survivors during a crisis. They serve victims of stalking, domestic violence, human trafficking, elder abuse, and sexual assault (Ponca Tribe of Nebraska, 2023).

## Impact on Health of Interaction with White Culture Then

The Ponca had a smallpox epidemic in 1800 which significantly reduced their population. As White settlers entered Ponca territory and squatted on fertile bottom land fields, the chiefs signed treaties which drastically reduced Ponca homelands. From 1856, the Ponca were unable to hunt buffalo and often faced starvation. The Fort Laramie Treaty of 1868 gave the Ponca Reservation to the Sioux in error. The government wouldn't correct this mistake and in 1876 an Indian bureau agent took 8 chiefs, some who were elderly, to what would become Oklahoma to look at sites for a new reservation that were not suitable for agriculture. The chiefs didn't want any of the sites and asked to return home. The agent became angry and left them in the middle of winter without food or funds to find their way home. When they arrived home, they found that the government had issued an order in April 1877 to forcibly remove the Poncas. This long march began in May 1877, resulting in suffering and deaths. When they finally arrived in Oklahoma in July 1878, many had malaria and little food because they hadn't been able to plant and cultivate crops. Some of the Ponca eventually ended up in Nebraska and poverty and diseases affected both tribes. In 1962, the U.S. Congress decided to terminate the Northern Ponca Tribe in Nebraska and removed them from federal programs and land holdings. It took until 1990 for the Tribe to be restored as federally recognized  and much of the Tribe's cultural heritage was lost during that time (Holmes, 2011 & Ponca Tribe of Nebraska, 2023).

## Impact on Health of Interaction with White Culture Now

Ponca Health Services and tribal volunteers participated in the Heartland Pride Parade in Omaha in July 2023 with other Nebraska businesses and community organizations.  CHI Health Center of Omaha hosted a follow-up event where businesses and community organizations could showcase products and interact with the community (Ponca Tribe of Nebraska, 2023).

## *Sarsi*

See Blackfoot

The Sarsi are located in Canada today. After 1790 they arrived on the northwestern Plains and were rapidly assimilated into the Blackfoot tribe. They do not exist as a separate tribe today in the United States (Brasser, 1991).

## Sioux

See Lakota

## Nakoda (Stoney)

See Gros Ventre

## Tonkawa

The Tonkawa Tribe is federally recognized and lives in Oklahoma. They call themselves "real people" and are also known as "civilized people" (Tonkawa Tribe of Oklahoma, 2022 & native-languages.org, 1998-2020). Its enterprises include the Tonkawa Indian Casino West, the Native Lights Casino, two smoke shops, and Red Pipe LLC, a business services entity (Tonkawa Tribe of Oklahoma, 2022).

### Health & Healing Then

The Tonkawa Tribe used dances in their ceremonies. These included the "wolf dance" to celebrate the origin of the Tonkawa where only men participated. In the "deer dance", both men and women ate the red bean of the wild mesquite plant. The "wild hog dance" required men and women to eat the bulb of a plant that may have been peyote. Their "sun dance" did not look into the sun or practice the torture of other tribes. Their funeral rites were elaborate. Friends and relatives sat in a circle around a dying person and sang and talked until the death occurred. Then, the person's face was painted yellow, the hair was cut, and the person was wrapped in robes. Valued possessions were often buried with the body and the tribe mourned for three days. No singing was permitted, and three women walked all night crying for the deceased person. After this time, a smoking ceremony was conducted (The Historic Round Rock Collection, 1991).

## Health & Healing Now

The Tonkawa Tribe administers federally funded services and programs to support tribal health. These programs include child/adult education, housing support, transportation, child care, community health, and diabetes care (Tonkawa Tribe of Oklahoma, 2022).

## Impact on Health of Interaction with White Culture Then

Tonkawa bands were decimated by smallpox in 1779 which killed half the tribe. Further diseases and warfare reduced the bands into a single tribe. They became poorer and in 1830 were described as "ill-clad people, dirty, and disgusting…most often [they] go naked and they suffer greatly from hunger" (The Historic Round Rock Collection, 1991). The Tonkawa "Trail of Tears" began when they were sent from Fort Griffin, Texas by railroad in 1884 to winter at the Sac-Fox Agency in Oklahoma. A child was born on the trip and named "Railroad Cisco". In the spring of 1885,  the Tribe was moved again, traveling 100 miles by wagon and fording rain-swelled rivers through axel-deep mud  from severe spring rains. They finally reached their present home on June 30th.

## Impact on Health of Interaction with White Culture Now

In 2022 the Tonkawa Tribe obtained a set-aside project grant from the Office for Victims of Crime to provide support and resources to crime victims and survivors (OVS, 2022) The program provides assistance with locating emergency shelter and medical services, court advocacy, crisis intervention, safety planning, and counseling referrals (Tonkawa Tribe of Oklahoma, 2022). They are part of the Native Alliance Against Violence which is Oklahoma's only coalition for tribal domestic violence and sexual assault that serves federally recognized tribes with their programs Native Alliance Against Violence, 2023). The Tonkawa Tribe has a sexual assault program providing case management, advocacy, safety planning, referrals, support services, protective order assistance, and traditional healing (Tonkawa Tribe of Oklahoma, 2022).

## Violence Against Native Women

In this section, many of the tribes are engaged in protecting indigenous women (also children and men) from kidnapping, sexual violence, trafficking, and potentially murder. The statistics for indigenous people are frightening and have been noted in some tribal health information about today's health. This is not just a regional issue. It is national in scope and affects multiple tribes throughout the country.

The Coalition to Stop Violence Against Native Women states that 4 out of 5 Native women experience violence and the murder rates for Native American women are more than 10 times the national average. This is alarming since Native people only consist of 2% of the U.S. population. Violence against Native women is centuries old from the time they first interacted with White culture and continues today. Many Native women live in rural areas where law enforcement is not easily accessed, and help may not be readily available (Native Hope, 2022).

Human trafficking is also epidemic in many Native communities. Large events, like the Sturgis Motorcycle Rally in South Dakota, illustrate the potential for sex trafficking. The state is home to nine Native American reservations, more than any other state. Native women and children are higher risk for trafficking than any other racial group. The U.S. Attorney's Office states than more than 40% of residents trafficked in South Dakota are Native women. The state itself only has 8% Native residents. Traffickers seek vulnerable victims and generational trauma exists in Native communities. This coupled with discrimination, oppression, and societal inequities makes Native women vulnerable. Although most bikers are well mannered tourists, Sturgis is a large gathering lasting a week and it also attracts human traffickers. Children are also sought by predators and South Dakota has two major highways that deliver victims of sex trafficking across the country. These interstate highways (I-90 and I-29) are part of what is known as the "Midwest Pipeline". In 2022 six arrests for sex trafficking occurred from undercover stings by the Division of Criminal Investigation. Victims ranged in age from 12 to 15 years, and it will take a lifetime for women and children who have experienced sex trafficking to attempt to heal from the abuse they have suffered (Native Hope, 2022).

Although law enforcement and government officials are trying to address sex trafficking, the public must also be aware of indicators and report suspicions promptly by calling 911 or the National Trafficking Hotline. Victims of sex trafficking may exhibit the following signs of abuse:

1.  Avoidance of eye contact and seems afraid;
2.  Not able or allowed to speak for herself/himself;
3.  Anxious, particularly around law enforcement;
4.  Unable to say where she/he is staying;
5.  Her/his story has numerous inconsistencies; and
6.  She/he shows signs of physical or mental abuse (Native Hope, 2022).

Native Hope continues to partner with the West River Human Trafficking Task Force and the SOAP (Save Our Adolescents from Prostitution) Project, which provides prevention education, advocacy, outreach, and mental health counseling for survivors nationally (The SOAP Project, n.d.).

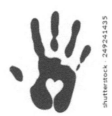

The Missing and Murdered Indigenous Women (MMIW) Red Hand over the mouth is the symbol of a growing movement to give voice to missing Native women and girls who cannot speak for themselves. It also stands for silence of law enforcement and the media about this crisis. Only 22% of Native Americans live on reservations and many others move between tribal and state lands. Reporting policies, jurisdictional issues, and lack of communication and cooperation between agencies make tracking missing Native women difficult. Poverty, lack of housing, and homelessness are contributing factors. Murder is the third leading cause of death for Native women. It is not only women who are affected. Men, boys, the elderly, and even infants are vulnerable, with the youngest victim less than one year old and the oldest 83-years old according to Urban Health Institute reports. 82% of Native men will be victims of violence during their lifetime and Native children will more likely experience trauma than their non-Native peers. Although the Urban Health Institute statistics are from 2016, the number of missing and murdered Native people continues to increase (NIWRC.org, 2023 and Native Hope, 2022).

This is an epidemic in tribal communities and urban settings where Native people live. May 5th annually is the National Day of Awareness for Missing and Murdered Native Women and Girls (MMIWG). It was established in

2017, but violence against Native women continues and "reflects the intersection of genocide, colonization, and violence against women, including but not limited to domestic violence, sexual assault, forced sterilization, and trafficking" (NIWRC.org, 2023). In 2023, it expanded to become a National Week of Action (May1-May 7) to campaign for action for missing and murdered Native women.

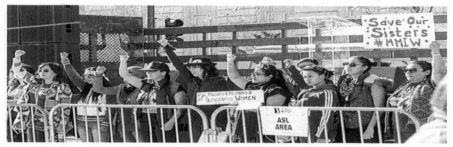

This Photo by Unknown Author is licensed under CC BY-SA

*No More Stolen Sisters! (Native Hope, 2022)*

Today, the MMIWG focus is on asking policymakers at all levels to address reforms that include:

1.  reauthorization of the Family Violence Prevention & Services Act (FVPSA) to provide federal funding for immediate shelter and supportive services. FVPSA;
2.  adjustment of the FVPSA funding formula to increase the amount received by tribes from 10% to 12.5%;
3.  provision of technical assistance and training to tribes by nonprofit tribal coalitions;
4.  permanent funding of the Native American Violence Hotline;
5.  increased access of tribes to the National Missing and Unidentified Persons System;
6.  required reports on tribal law enforcement needs;
7.  improved law enforcement officer applicants by background checks from the Bureau of Indian Affairs; (BIA)
8.  creation of a grant program to support coordination of efforts in missing and murdered persons' cases and sexual assault cases;
9.  evaluation of evidence collection, handling and processing; and
10. ensure access to culturally appropriate wellness and mental health programs by tribal police and BIA officers (NIWRC.org, 2023).

Violence against Native women is preventable, but it will take a concerted effort at all levels to achieve it.

# Chapter 6
# Rocky Mountain Tribes

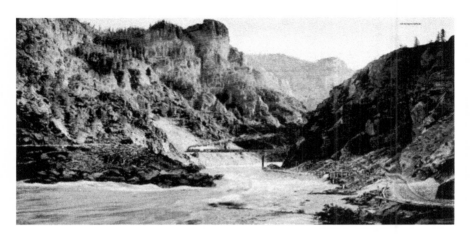

Tribes living in the Rocky Mountains included the Arapaho, Apache, Blackfoot Confederacy, Northern Cheyenne, Chippewa-Cree, Coeur D'alene, Crow, Goshute, Kiowa Ute, Paiute, Shoshone, Confederated Salish and Kootenai Tribes, and Ute.

| | |
|---|---|
| *Arapaho* | See Chapter 5 |
| *Apache* | See Chapter 5 & 7 |
| *Blackfoot (Confederacy)* | See Chapter 4 |
| *Northern Cheyenne* | See Chapter 5 |
| *Chippewa -Cree* | See Plains Cree Chapter 5 |

## Coeur d'Alene

The Coeur d'Alene Tribe is federally recognized and located in Idaho. Their original name was Schitsu'umsh which means "The discovered people" French fur traders called them Coeur d'Alene or "Heart of the Awl". Their enterprises include:

1. the Coeur d'Alene Casino;
2. the Tribal Development Corporation (grocery businesses, farming and agriculture, hardware and lumber supplies, and automotive services; and
3. Red-Spectrum Communications (internet and communication services ) (Coeur d'Alene Tribe, n.d.).

## Health & Wellness Then

The Coeur d'Alene Tribe had a shaman-man or woman- who coordinated burial of the dead, hunting rituals, or used their powers in healing ceremonies or ceremonials. Illness was caused by an object being shot into the individual or soul loss which was untreatable. The shaman used songs and a 'sucking tube' to remove the object. Prayer preceded gathering berries and roots. One root gathered in the late fall was the "water potato". In the summer, men and women fasted and sought visions to receive spiritual power. The Winter Medicine Dances (Jump Dances) were the conclusion of the year's spiritual cycle where the shaman treated the sick and blessed dance participants to bring them health and well-being (Frey, n.d.).

## Health & Wellness Now

Addiction is impacting families on the reservation and the Tribe is focused on providing youth with support, resources, and holistic care to break the cycle of addiction, crime, abuse, and poverty in the community. They have created a safe place-the Coeur Center-where at-risk children can play and learn to build healthy relationships through holistic wellness and healing. It is open to all community residents and is a prevention center as well as a recreation center. In 2014, 35.64% of youth on the reservation ages 10-24 were positive for depression. The Coeur Center is designed to address the social determinants of health, provide mental and behavioral health services, and have specialists and classes to help families deal with addiction and return to health (Coeur d'Alene Tribe, n.d.).

## Impact on Health of Interaction with White Culture Then

The Coeur d'Alene population was decimated by smallpox epidemics in 1831 and 1850. As Whites began to settle in their lands, they convinced the Coeur d'Alene Tribe to take in other tribes. In 1888 the tribes suffered from a scarlet fever and measles epidemic. The Coeur d'Alene Tribe fared better than the others because they had a doctor who quarantined the sick (worldhistory.us, 2018). In the 1970s-1980s, tribal members could only get healthcare at a run-down Indian Health Services (IHS) Clinic. Snow blew under the doors in the waiting room and anything beyond basic care required a trip to hospitals more than 45 minutes away on treacherous roads in the winter. Fragmented care with poor continuity went on over 15 years. Ambulatory care facilities in four surrounding counties didn't provide care on a sliding fee scale basis to medically underserved residents. Due to non-payment of medical bills by the IHS, tribal members were often turned over to collection agencies for payment (Coeur d'Alene Tribe, n.d.).

## Impact on Health of Interaction with White Culture Now

In the late 1980s, the Tribe developed a plan to create "a community-based rural health outpatient care delivery system" by partnering with the city of Plummer. They began by opening a facility to provide health services for everyone in need, including non-Native residents (Coeur d'Alene Tribe, n.d.). Today, the Marimn Health clinic is a federally qualified community health center where eligible patients are treated on a sliding fee scale, and no one is refused service. This includes non-Native community residents. The partnership between the Tribe and City of Plummer may have been the first joint venture between a city municipality and tribe to provide health care for all residents. They began by securing federal and state funding. They also obtained a designation from the Idaho Governor's office as a Medically Underserved Population which was accepted by the USPHS. They receive limited funding from the Bureau of Primary Health Care to continue providing care on a sliding fee basis. Today, 30% of their patients qualify for this program (Coeur d'Alene Tribe, n.d.).

## *Crow*

See Chapter 5

## *Goshute*

There are two federally recognized Goshute Tribes: the Confederated Tribes of Goshute in Nevada and Utah and the Skull Valley Band in Utah (Goshute Indian Tribe, 2023 & Utah.gov, 2023). Goshute means "desert people" (Utah American Indian Digital Archive, 2008). The Skull Valley Band of Goshute Indians of Utah is small, consisting of approximately 31 people (Native Ministries International, 2022). In 1976, they built a rocket motor testing facility that is leased to Hercules, Inc. and seek other income sources (Utah.gov, 2023). The Confederated Tribes of Goshute tried agriculture unsuccessfully and now manage an elk herd and profit from hunting permits (Utah.gov, 2023).

### Health & Wellness Then

Early Goshutes' health practices included numerous plants and some animals. Rattlesnake oil was used to treat rheumatism by rubbing it on the affected organ. If a person had a persistent nosebleed, he/she would take some of the nasal blood and pour it on a red ant's nest where it was eaten by the ants. Then, the hemorrhage would stop. The arrowroot would be mashed or chewed up into a paste to treat a bullet or arrow wound. Colds, coughs and bronchial infections were treated by boiling cedar leaves in water and drinking the decoction hot. Sage-brush leaves were used to treat fevers and could also treat coughs, colds, and other ailments (Chamberlin, 1911).

### Health & Wellness Now

Health issues affecting the Goshutes today include obesity, diabetes, and hypertension. The combination of diabetes and hypertension also causes a greater risk of retinopathy. Food and nutritional insecurity contribute to obesity from lack of access to nutritious high-quality food (Hicks et al, 2020).

## Impact on Health of Interaction with White Culture Then

The Goshute Tribe maintained a perfect ecological balance in the limited resources of their homeland. Permanent White settlements disrupted this balance and reservations had Indian agents who tried to assimilate the Tribe into White culture and promoted agriculture which was unsuccessful in their desert lands. Unemployment and poverty became constant problems (Utah American Indian Digital Archive, 2008).

## Impact on Health of Interaction with White Culture Now

The Goshutes own and operate Sacred Heart Healthcare on the Confederated Tribes of the Goshute Reservation (founded in 2012) that cares for all underserved people in local communities. Their Circle of Care philosophy is based on their tradition of healing and includes coordination, communication, and exploring all options for health. Their four locations provide primary care, behavioral health care, physical therapy, dentistry, optometry, podiatry, nutrition services, and a substance use recovery program. There also is a specialized pain management program for patients with chronic pain (Sacred Circle Healthcare, 2021).

## *Kiowa-Ute*

See Kiowa in Chapter 5

## *Kootenai*

The Kootenai Tribe of Idaho is federally recognized. Another Kootenai Tribe is part of the Confederated Salish and Kootenai Tribes on the Flathead Reservation in Montana and is also federally recognized. The Kootenai Tribe of Idaho will be discussed here. Kootenai means "water people" (native-languages.org, 1998-2020). Their enterprises include the Kootenai River Inn Casino & Spa and the Twin River Resort for RVs and camping (Kootenai Tribe of Idaho, 2022).

## Health & Healing Then

Kootenai healers were mostly women in the Crazy Owl Society. They were to prevent epidemics by obeying the spirits. The spirits would come to a powerful woman, and she would sing. Other women in the Society would join her as she circled all camp lodges to treat them, After this, she would lead the group to strike trees, then run to the west. After a council, they would adjourn. The Kootenai Shamans' Society consisted of all the medicine people. Dances also contributed to spiritual health. The Blanket Dance was a meeting with spirits to seek help from them. The Sun Dance focused on success in hunting and bonding within the tribe. The Grizzley Bear Dance was held to pray for abundant food. The Fir Tree Dance was held in times of famine to bring game back to the land. No ceremony was associated with death. The deceased was quickly buried by two people and spouses would cut their hair for mourning (Ojibwe, 2015).

## Health & Healing Now

Health outreach and education are available for immunizations, diabetes, substance abuse, and smoking prevention. The Tribal Health Clinic provides on-site primary care and counseling services. Increased immunization rates have resulted in better health outcomes. Education is also important to the Kootenai Tribe. Youth are supported after school with a homework tutor/mentor and members seeking higher education are supported with funding for tuition, supplies, fees, and books. The Tribe also provides support for members seeking alternative career choices (Kootenai Tribe of Idaho, 2022).

## Impact on Health of Interaction with White Culture Then

Diseases for which they had no immunity killed Kootenai tribal members. These diseases included smallpox, measles, diphtheria, tuberculosis and alcohol. When Idaho revoked tribal rights to hunt and fish, the tribe had to leave its native land to survive. Few tribal members received land allotments in the 1930s. The Kootenai struggled to survive and in 1964, the 67 remaining members declared war peacefully on the United States and publicity finally gave them 12.5 acres and their economic development improved (Kootenai Tribe of Idaho, 2022).

## Impact on Health of Interaction with White Culture Now

Conservation of natural resources is a tribal priority. Since 1989, the Tribe has coordinated with federal and state agencies to prevent extinction of the Kootenai sturgeon and serves as co-manager of the Kootenai River System. They also have projects to identify factors affecting native resident wildlife and fish and to address them through restoration actions that are ecosystem-based. The Kootenai River Habitat Restoration Program is a 10 to 15 year project to restore a 55-mile stretch of the Kootenai River (Kootenai Tribe of Idaho, 2022).

## *Paiute*

There are multiple federally recognized Paiute tribes in California, Nevada, Oregon, Arizona, and Utah. The term Paiute means "influenced by the Ute" (native-languages.org, 1998-2020).

| State | Tribe(s) | Enterprises |
|---|---|---|
| **California** | Bishop Paiute Tribe | Enterprises include a business development program, a water commission, an RV park, a restaurant and deli, and the Wanaaha Casino (Bishop Paiute Tribe, 2022). |
| | Cedarville Rancheria-Northern Piute Tribe | Cedarville Rancheria owns and operates a fueling station with public scales (Cedarville Rancheria, n.d.). |
| | Fort Bidwell Indian Community | The Fort Bidwell Indian Community's major enterprise is agriculture (UVE, 2023). |
| | Fort Independence Indian Community of Paiute Indians of the Fort Independence Reservation | Enterprises include the Oak Creek Travel Plaza, the Oak Creek Dispensary (Cannabis and CBD), and the Oak Creek Casino (Fort Independence Indian Reservation, 2020). |
| | Utu Gwaitu Piute Tribe of Benton Paiute | The Benton Paiute Reservation has an economic development |

| State | Tribe(s) | Enterprises |
|-------|----------|-------------|
|  | Reservation | corporation and operates the Benton Station Café, a gas station, convenience store, and restaurant (Benton Paiute Reservation, 2023). |
| **Nevada** | Paiute-Shoshone Tribe of the Fallon Reservation and Colony | Enterprises include Stepping Stones Youth Facility, the Community Learning Center Cultural Program, and the Fallon Tribal Health Clinic (Fallon Paiute-Shoshone Tribe, n.d.). |
|  | Lovelock Paiute Tribe of the Lovelock Indian Colony | Enterprises include the Johnson-O'Malley Youth Program, the Tribal Elders Program, a Housing Authority, and Social Services (Lovelock Paiute Tribe, n.d.). |
|  | Las Vegas Tribe of Paiute Indians | Enterprises include the Tribal Smoke Shop (largest cigarette retailer in the U.S.), the Las Vegas Paiute Resort and Golf Course, and the NuWu Cannabis Marketplace (Las Vegas Paiute Tribe, n.d.). |
|  | Shoshone-Paiute Tribes of the Duck Valley Reservation | Enterprises include a Day Care Center, Tribal Environmental Protection Program, the Sho-Pai Fire Department, Duck Valley Indian Reservation Campground, a Community Health Facility, a Recreation Program, and the Shoshone-Paiute Tribe 101 Ranch (Sho-Pai, 2023). |
|  | Summit Lake Paiute Tribe | The major tribal enterprise includes the Natural Resource Department. The tribe also employs two fish and wildlife biologists, an environmental |

| State | Tribe(s) | Enterprises |
|-------|----------|-------------|
| | | specialist, and technicians to monitor and protect the tribe's natural resources (Summit Lake Paiute Tribe, n.d.). |
| **Oregon** | Fort McDermitt Paiute-Shoshone Tribes (also in Nevada) | Enterprises include the Say When Bar Café and Casino which recently reopened and the Fort McDermitt Wellness Center (Fort McDermitt Paiute-Shoshone Tribe, 2023). |
| | Burns Paiute Tribe | Enterprises include Tu-Wa-Kii Nobi (a safe environment for tribal youth), Old Camp RV Park, a Natural Resources Department, and the Tribal Transit Service (Burns Paiute Tribe, 2023). |
| **Arizona** | San Juan Southern Paiute Tribe | The Tribe leases its gaming device allocation rights to other tribes which enables the Tribe to provide services and carry out governmental functions (San Juan Southern Paiute Tribe, 2019). |
| **Utah** | Paiute Indian Tribe of Utah (5 Bands) | Enterprises include an Annual Powwow, the Native Goods Marketplace, Four Points Health, and the Economic Development Department (Paiute Indian Tribe of Utah, 2021). |

## Health & Healing Then

The Paiute had an unusual permanent cure for warts. Using fish bones placed through the wart at different angles would make the wart fall off and never return (Cabeen, 2021). Desert Princeplume was used as a tonic and the boiled root cured weakness after an illness. A mashed poultice of the root could be applied for throat pain (Train, Henrichs, & Archer, 1941).

## Health & Healing Now

The Paiute Indian Tribe of Utah has numerous health programs and services to promote tribal wellness. These include a diabetes education course, monthly nutrition education for adults and youth, and healthy shopping information. Exercise programs and fitness trackers are available and family services for vulnerable children and adults (Paiute Indian Tribe of Utah, 2021). The San Juan Southern Paiute Tribe provides Emergency Assistance and Elder and Disabled Assistance based on funds available in the Program Budget unless the Tribe lacks the financial resources to safely and adequately provide assistance (San Juan Southern Paiute Tribe, 2019). The Lovelock Paiute Tribe of Nevada has programs for elders and youth. The Tribal Elders Program includes congregate meals and a caregiver support program. The Johnson-O'Malley Program includes students from Head Start to three county high schools by providing supplemental services, such as school supplies, book fees, academic incentives, recognition for students, help with sports footwear, educational advocacy, and Elders in the classroom. The Indian Education Committee also provides tutoring and cultural classes and field trips when funding is available (Lovelock Paiute Tribe, n.d.). The Bishop Paiute Tribe of California uses the Comprehensive Opioid Stimulant and Substance Abuse Program to assist with an open resource lounge, transitional housing, case management, job search, clothing, and well-being services (Bishop Paiute Tribe, 2022). The Las Vegas Tribe of Paiute Indians provides services for out-patient health, pharmacy, behavioral health, optometry, dentistry, and diabetes prevention and treatment (Las Vegas Paiute Tribe, n.d.).

## Impact on Health of Interaction with White Culture Then

A treaty in 1869 awarded the Burns Paiute Tribe 1.8 million acres in Oregon, but in the Bannock War, they fled the reservation to avoid conflict and were force marched over 300 miles in knee-deep snow to Washington State. After five years, they were able to return, but found that the reservation was public domain, and they had no land. Their children weren't allowed in public schools. Until the 1920s they were forgotten. When Indian agents did come to their remote encampment to take children to boarding schools, many parents successfully hid their children. By the 1940s more children were sent to boarding schools and finally were admitted to public schools (Burns Paiute Tribe, 2023). From 1884 to 1911 a boarding school operated on the Duck Valley Reservation and high school students were sent away to boarding schools until 1946 when high school classes came to the reservation (Sho-Pai, 2023). The Paiute Indian Tribe of Utah was displaced by Mormon settlements in the 1800s. The new settlements were on Paiute gathering and hunting grounds and many plants that were a staple of their diet were destroyed. Access to land near water sources was denied and the land that was left was mostly impossible to farm. Poverty reduced the tribe to begging for survival. After 25 years of interaction with Mormon settlers, the Paiute population was reduced by 90% due to disease and loss of farmlands, water sources, and native plants (LaMore, 2021).

## Impact on Health of Interaction with White Culture Now

Today, mercury from mining operations has contaminated the Carson River and the Paiute-Shoshone Tribe of the Fallon Reservation and Colony has been advocating for clean-up since 1990. It is currently on the list for this to occur (Fallon Paiute-Shoshone Tribe, n.d.). The Summit Lake Paiute Tribe has a Natural Resource Department to manage water, air, soil, wildlife, fish, and plants on the Reservation and was recently awarded funds from the Bureau of Indian Affairs to address the effects of climate change in this area and produce a climate adaptation plan for the Tribe (Summit Lake Paiute Tribe, n.d.). The Bishop Paiute Tribe has a cooperative agreement with the USDA Agricultural Marketing Service to obtain fresh fruit and vegetables from local farmers and producers. Besides economic opportunities for growers, the produce will be distributed twice a month for a year to elders and Tribal community members who need food (Bishop Paiute Tribe, 2022). The Fort Independence Indian Reservation's Air Quality Specialist uses EPA-approved measures for air quality monitoring and submits this data into the EPA Air Quality System national database so residents and workers are alerted if unsafe particulate dust levels occur. The dried Owens

Lakebed which is 21 miles from the Reservation is one of the largest sources of fine dust particles in the U.S. and winds from there can cause multiple adverse health outcomes on the Reservation. Disease affected by outdoor air pollution includes respiratory diseases, diabetes, hypertension, stroke, cardiovascular disease, and premature birth/decreased birthweight (Fort Independence Indian Reservation, 2020). The Fort McDermitt Paiute-Shoshone Tribes has joined since 2021 with the Burns Paiute Tribe and other tribes to protest a Nevada lithium mine at Thacker Pass, which is considered sacred by the Tribe Conservationists also oppose the mine, believing it will pollute groundwater and destroy habitat for grouse, antelope, and other species by violating environmental laws. The mine suit was subsequently sent to the 9th Circuit Court of Appeals. On July 20, 2023, the Court ruled in favor of allowing the mine to go forward although there is concern about adverse environmental impact from the project (Solis, 2023).

## *Shoshone*

There are nine federally recognized Shoshone tribes. The Shoshone-Paiute Tribe of the Duck Valley Reservation in Nevada was discussed under Paiute. The others will be discussed here. Shoshone were known as "Grass House People" (Wikipedia.org, 2023) in reference to their lodgings.

| State | Tribe(s) | Enterprises |
|---|---|---|
| **Wyoming** | Eastern Shoshone Tribe of the Wind River Reservation | The Eastern Shoshone Tribe seeks diversification of their economy by creating SITTA LLC (Shoshone Indian Tribe Tribal Acquisition). They are developing the Eastern Shoshone Business Park, a mixed-use development that is being developed in phases. They also have created a buffalo enclosure that contains pure Yellowstone buffalo and engage in |

| State | Tribe(s) | Enterprises |
|---|---|---|
| | | conservation efforts (Eastern Shoshone, 2023). |
| Idaho | Shoshone-Bannock Tribes of the Fort Hall Reservation | The Shoshone-Bannock Tribes' enterprises include the Shoshone-Bannock Casino & Hotel and retail businesses. They also lease agricultural lands (Shoshone-Bannock Tribe, 2023). |
| Utah | Northwestern Band of the Shoshone Nation | The major enterprise for the Northwestern Band is Tope Technology which provides information technology, engineering, translation, VoIP services, and instructional design training for customers (Northwestern Band of the Shoshone Nation, n.d.). |
| Nevada | Duckwater Shoshone Tribe | The Tribe is primarily agricultural and also has the Duckwater Economic Development Corporation which operates a small convenience store and trucks to haul lime and ore for mines in the area (Duckwater Shoshone Tribe, n.d.). |
| | Ely Shoshone Tribe | Tribal enterprises include the Silver Sage Travel Center and an RV Park, the Ely Shoshone Campgrounds. They also have a marijuana dispensary and an annual Powwow (Ely Shoshone Tribe, n.d.). |
| | Te-Moak Tribe of Western Shoshone | Enterprises include a gas station and convenience store and the Newe Cannabis Dispensary (Te-Moak Tribe |

| State | Tribe(s) | Enterprises |
|-------|----------|-------------|
| | | of Western Shoshone, 2004-2022). |
| | Yomba Shoshone Tribe | The Tribe lives off the land, raising cattle and farming. They focus on resource management of their land, including grazing permits (Yomba Shoshone Tribe, 2017). |
| California | Timbisha Shoshone Tribe | The Tribe lives in Death Valley and there are few opportunities for economic development in their remote area. They are working on constructing a community center and are planning a future casino project (Timbisha Shoshone Tribe, n.d.). |

## Health & Healing Then

Vision quests and dreams enabled Shoshone men to gain a spirit helper. Shamans had curing powers and hosted tribal ceremonies. There were three types of Shamans—those who cured specific ailments, those who used their powers to benefit themselves, and those with general curing ability. The Shoshone also used the Sun Dance ceremony to renew their relationship with the land by singing, dancing, drumming, and seeing visions. The Shoshone respected the land and believed that plants and animals possessed a living spirit. They treated diseases and physical illnesses with different herbal remedies. Shamans used sweat lodges to detoxify the sick and smudge sticks (dried herbs) to cleanse the body, mind, and spirit of the afflicted person. Medicine wheels also aided in the healing process (Arnold, Bennett, Christensen, Harmon, Hatch, Reid, 2010).

## Health & Healing Now

Eastern Shoshone Tribal Health uses the Zone to promote health and disease prevention through wellness and fitness programs (eastern Shoshone, 2023). Today, the Western Shoshone face higher cancer rates which may be the result of nuclear testing done upwind of their communities. Fallout effects tainted wild game and the vegetation consumed by their livestock. This resulted in contamination of their primary food sources (Arnold, Bennett, Christensen, Harmon, Hatch, & Reid, 2010). The Yomba Shoshone Tribe's Human Services Department focuses on improving the quality of life and  protecting the elderly, disabled, and children from neglect and abuse. They serve as the contact point for social service agencies related to children's protection. placement, and adoption (Yomba Shoshone Tribe, 2017).

## Impact on Health of Interaction with White Culture Then

The Shoshone suffered from the introduction of diseases and their interactions with fur trappers and White settlers resulted in loss of natural resources and homelands. Mining companies obtained water rights depriving the tribes of their traditional water supply. The Timbisha Tribe had its adobe homes washed away with high power fire hoses in the 1960s to evict them from their home in Death Valley. They had no homeland until 2000 and water diversion has caused the mesquite trees that they harvest to decline (Feller, n.d.).  The Northwestern Band found their land plundered by Mormon farmers and emigrants heading to California. Their food supplies were depleted, and some hungry tribes ate stolen cattle to survive. This resulted in the Bear River Massacre which decimated the tribe and resulted in further loss of tribal lands (Northwestern Band of the Shoshone Nation, n.d.).

## Impact on Health of Interaction with White Culture Now

The Duckwater Shoshone Tribe has mitigated the Big Warm Spring to save a threatened species of fish (Duckwater Shoshone Tribe, n.d.). The Ely Tribe has used a grant to clean up a landfill that was unregulated from the early 1900s to the late 1950s. This area remains unsuitable for development (Ely Shoshone Tribe, n.d.). The Eastern Shoshone Tribe collaborates with the Wyoming Department of Health to decrease cancer rates through screening, early detection, education, referrals, patient navigation, and advocacy (Eastern Shoshone, 2023). The Northwestern Band is working with the Utah Conservation Corps to tear down thousands of invasive Russian olive trees, which are absorbing water that depletes the land. One tree can use 75 gallons of water daily and rehabilitating the site is a priority of the Tribe and the conservationists who want to restore the land (Anderson, 2022). The Timbisha Shoshone have always used mesquite harvesting and the trees are now unhealthy due to competition for water in the area and invasion of salt cedar trees in the mesquite groves. The Tribe is conducting the Mesquite Traditional Use Pilot Project to use traditional care for the mesquites. The project on two half-acre plots co-managed by the Timbisha and the National Park Service has also removed the salt cedar trees from the area. Restoring this land in traditional ways gives the mesquite trees an opportunity to thrive in the future (Timbisha Shoshone Tribe, n.d.).

## Confederated Salish and Kootenai Tribes

The Kootenai Tribe and its tribal history was addressed above. The Confederated Salish and Kootenai Tribes of the Flathead Reservation are also federally recognized and located in Montana. The Salish were also known as Flatheads. Their major enterprise is S&K Technologies, Inc. This company is a global small business in technology and aerospace for commercial customers and federal agencies. They also operate the Big Arm Resort and own Eagle Bank which especially focuses on increasing tribal home ownership (Confederated Salish & Kootenai Tribes, 2022).

Note: A small Kalispel Tribe also lives on the Reservation. Since their federal recognized tribe lives in the State of Washington, they will be discussed in West Coast tribes.

### Health & Healing Then

The Salish Sacred Medicine Tree was the story of a great medicine man who traveled the land to prepare for human beings by destroying evil monsters. He confronted a giant, evil bighorn sheep and asked it to use his horns to destroy a small pine tree. The bighorn sheep crashed into the tree and one of his horns was stuck through the tree. The medicine man cut off the ram's head and made the tree a sacred place for people to leave offerings, give thanks, and pray for well-being, health and good fortune. Insincere petitions would result in misfortune and death. The sacred Medicine Tree became a towering Ponderosa pine. When it was blown down in a storm in 2001, pine cone seeds were planted to grow a new tree and a 16-foot snag of the tree stands today for people to pray and leave offerings at the sacred site (Montana Cowboy Hall of Fame, 2021). Medicines came from roots, such as bitterroot. Spirituality was part of life and they believed that all things deserved respect and were interconnected (Flathead Watershed Sourcebook, 2010-2023).

## Health & Healing Now

The Tribes have several health services available for their members. Since diabetes is a health issue for them, the Tribal Health Network offers screening, education, and management for diabetes. Podiatry clinics are held monthly at both health centers along with lifestyle coaching, nutrition services, medication management, and diabetic eye care. The Safe On All Roads program from the Montana Department of Transportation works to reduce tribal traffic fatalities and incidence of impaired driving along with promoting seat belt use. The program also provides infant care seats and education on installation and use. The Reason to Live Native Program targets youth from 10 to 24 years to provide suicide screening, prevention, interventions, support groups, therapy, and healthy and cultural activities. Tribal Health fitness centers have equipment, health information, and classes with certified personal trainers to help participants achieve fitness goals (Confederated Salish & Kootenai Tribes, 2022).

## Impact on Health of Interaction with White Culture Then

During the 18th century the Salish encountered disease epidemics that wiped out half  the tribe. The fur traders killed animals that the Salish depended on for food and they tried to maintain their traditional lifestyle. They welcomed the Jesuits in the 1820s-1830s without realizing that the priests were bent on religious conversion and eliminating spiritual and traditional hunting practices  In 1904 the Flathead Allotment Act resulted in homesteading by non-Natives on the best agricultural lands. The Jesuits and boarding schools made children learn a new language (English) and lose their cultural traditions. When they rebelled, they were punished and some surviving elders remember abusive experiences (Flathead Watershed Source Book, 2010-2023).

## Impact on Health of Interaction with White Culture Now

The Natural Resource Department works to protect and preserve the environment in multiple areas. The Wildlife staff worked with big game hunters to help control chronic Wasting Disease in deer, elk, and moose. The Fisheries Program focused on protecting Bull Trout and Tribal Fish and Game Wardens improved compliance for licensed recreationists and boaters. The Information and Education Program helped with Mussel Walk events for students in area schools. Native Fish Keepers, Inc. exists to remove non-Native Lake Trout in the Flathead Lake-River System. It removes Lake Trout population and offsets the costs by processing removed fish for sale and donating all funds received to the hydropower mitigation funding sources for Lake Trout suppression. They also distribute over 3,000 pounds of fish to Tribal Health Centers and area food banks (Confederated Salish & Kootenai Tribes, 2022).

## *Ute*

There are three federally recognized Ute tribes. The Southern Ute Indian Tribe and the Ute Mountain Ute Tribe are in Colorado. The Ute Indian Tribe of the Uintah & Ouray Reservation  is in Utah. Ute means "the people" (native-languages.org, 1998-2020). The Ute Mountain Ute Tribe's enterprises include commercial construction services, a tribal farm and ranch with a 700 head cow/calf operation, a retail travel center with fuel islands and a convenience store, and the Ute Mountain Ute Casino and Hotel (Ute Mountain Ute Tribe, 2020). The Southern Ute Indian Tribe's enterprises include oil and gas production, real estate development, housing construction, and the Sky Ute Casino and Resort (Southern Ute Indian Tribe, 2023). The Ute Indian Tribe of the Uintah & Ouray Reservation's enterprises include managing land containing oil and gas deposits, retail businesses (grocery, gas stations, bowling alley, and coffee house), and Uinta River Technologies for Information Technology support (Ute Indian Tribe, 2023).

## Health & Healing Then

The Ute Tribe had traditions for health and to stay in harmony with nature. The Sun Dance lasted four days and focused on individual or community welfare where people hoped for cures for the sick or visions. The Bear Dance welcomed spring and focused on harmony with nature and leaving troubles behind. Shamans were both men and women who healed through songs and dances learned in dreams. They cured diseases of the body and spirit using fetish bags, eagle bones, eagle feathers, and medicinal plants (Bennett, 2010).

## Health & Healing Now

The Ute Indian Tribe of the Uintah & Ouray Reservation holds a monthly gathering for Ute elders who have been impacted by opioid misuse and stigma. To combat isolation, the group uses Talking Circles and creating art to engage members and build relationships. This is affiliated with the Tribal & Rural Opioid Resource Center. The Center provides support and evidence-based education and uses traditional and contemporary arts with talking circles in a program called Promote Art + Heal + Create. Monthly gatherings are open to the public and free for participants (Ute Indian Tribe, 2023).

## Impact on Health of Interaction with White Culture Then

Children's education was important to the Ute Tribe and was traditionally provided by a grandparent. After interaction with White culture, Ute children were sent to an Indian boarding school at Fort Lewis, Colorado beginning in 1891. They learned the basics of reading, writing, and arithmetic, but it was an industrial training school. Ute children could not wear tribal clothes and their names were changed for them to assimilate into White culture. They also were required to cultivate land and grow crops. By 1901, the students cultivated 200 acres of land for the school. The buildings were in poor condition and presented a fire hazard from stoves and oil lamps that were used for heat and light. By 1903, disease was rampant in this and other boarding schools and the government determined to support schools on reservations. The Ute Tribe built a school in Ignacio, Colorado for their children. In 1969, the Southern Ute Tribe began one of the first tribal Head Start programs in the country (Bennett, 2010).

## Impact on Health of Interaction with White Culture Now

The Ute Mountain Ute Tribe has health services for the community as well as tribal members. The Community Health Program promotes and enhances the well-being and health of everyone in two local communities. The Substance Abuse Program provides support, health, and nutrition services to elders 55 years or older. Ute Mountain W.I.C. provides nutrition/health screening and assessment to improve outcomes for pregnant, postpartum, and breastfeeding women and infants/children. The Sleeping Ute Diabetes Prevention Program provides education and support to encourage positive lifestyle changes that reduce the risk of type 2 diabetes. The Ute Mountain Public Safety Department provides quality emergency services to residents and visitors (Ute Mountain Ute Tribe, 2020).

# Tribal Government-What does Federal or State Recognition Mean?

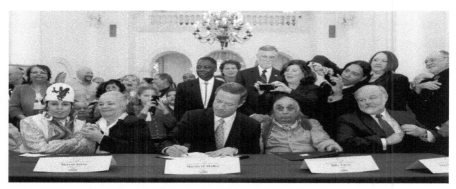

## Historic & Legal Perspective

Currently, there are 574 federally recognized Native American tribes in the United States (Congressional Research Service, 2023). Other tribes are either state recognized or not recognized at all. The United States Constitution in Article 1, Section 8 "To regulate Commerce with foreign Nations, and among the several States, and with the Indian tribes" (Cato Institute, 2013). Congress and the Executive and Judicial branches were authorized to negotiate with the tribes. In 1832 Chief Justice John Marshall stated in Worcester v. Georgia the principle that has guided how federal Indian law has evolved from then to today that Native tribes "had always been considered as distinct, independent political communities, retaining their original natural rights, as the undisputed possessors of the soil from time immemorial" (Bill of Rights Institute, 2023).

However, a year before in Cherokee Nation v. Georgia, the Supreme Court decision was that tribes were "domestic dependent nations" (Bill of Rights Institute, 2023). This established the trust doctrine as an important principle in federal Indian law. The trust doctrine was in other Supreme Court cases culminating in Seminole Nation v. United States in 1942. The Court opinion stated "the fiduciary duty of the Government to its Indian wards" and "recognized the distinctive obligation of trust incumbent upon the Government in its dealings with these dependent and sometimes exploited people" (Justice Murphy for the U.S. Supreme Court, 1942).

This reinforced the federal Indian trust responsibility toward Indian tribes which is also a legal obligation to protect assets, lands, treaty rights, and resources of the tribes. Language from Supreme Court cases suggest that the Government has legal responsibilities, moral obligations, and should fulfill the understandings and expectations of the relationship between the federally recognized tribes and the United States (Bureau of Indian Affairs, n.d.).

## Federal Recognition & Tribal Sovereignty

A federally recognized Native American or Alaska Native tribe has a government-to-government relationship with the United States and possesses tribal sovereignty or certain self-government rights. When Europeans first encountered Native tribes, the tribes were powerful and controlled the natural resources within their homelands. The European practice of establishing relations with other countries and recognition of tribal property rights made tribes seen as sovereign nations and the Europeans treated them as such. In the years since, the United States grew in power and size, while tribal populations decreased, and tribal sovereignty eroded. Today, tribal sovereignty is limited by treaties, executive orders, acts of Congress, court decisions, and federal administrative agreements. However, remaining tribal sovereignty of federally recognized tribes is protected from encroachment by states. This ensures that the participation and consent of these tribes is required for any decisions about their property and citizens (Bureau of Indian Affairs, n.d.).

## How tribes receive recognition

Most federally recognized tribes received that status one of the following ways: treaties, presidential executive orders, acts of Congress, other federal administrative actions, or federal court decisions. The Interior Department issued regulations for the Federal Acknowledgement Process (FAP) in 1978 to uniformly address requests for federal recognition by Indian groups. These regulations (25 C.F.R. Part 83) were revised in 1994 and are still in effect. Congress also enacted Public Law 103-454 in 1994 called the Federally Recognized Indian Tribe List Act (108 Stat. 4792, 4792). This Act formally established how a tribe could become federally recognized:

- "By Act of Congress,
- "By the administrative procedures under 25 C.F.R. Part 83, or
- "By decision of a United States court" (Bureau of Indian Affairs, n.d.).

In 2015, the Secretary of the Interior released a final rule for Part 83 with a consistent, more flexible process to account for unique tribal histories with input from tribal leaders. The new rule promotes transparency by posting publicly available petition materials online and uses a uniform evaluation period of 1900 to the present to satisfy seven mandatory criteria. These applications are reviewed by federal experts in anthropology, genealogy, and history to ensure the criteria are met and a decision is then made by the Assistant Secretary-Indian Affairs (US Department of  the Interior, 2021).

## Termination & Restoration

Some tribes had been previously recognized and terminated by Congress and were not allowed to use the Federal Acknowledgement Process. Only Congress can restore federal recognition to a tribe that has had their recognition terminated.

Today, some tribes are attempting to gain or regain federal recognition. The best example of a tribe regaining federal recognition after termination is the Menominee. In the 1950s, the federal government tried to terminate federal recognition for all tribes and chose the Menominee as one of the first tribes to be terminated in 1961. They lost their trust relationship with the federal government and their sovereign powers as a domestic dependent nation. This enabled non-Indians to buy Menominee lands and the tribe fought to regain trust status and federal recognition. They finally succeeded in 1973. Other tribes saw the negative consequences of termination for the Menominee and refused to accept termination causing the program to end (Milwaukee Public Museum, 2022).

## The Advantages of Federal Recognition

Sovereignty enables tribes to be self-governing, allowing tribal governments to regulate their own internal activities, and entering agreements with the United States and individual states. The trust relationship protects tribal lands from being purchased or taken by non-Indians. The federal authorities must protect sovereign status, tribal lands and property, and the rights of tribal citizens (Milwaukee Public Museum, 2022). Federally recognized tribes are eligible for funding from the Bureau of Indian Affairs and receive federal benefits, protections, and services that are not available to non-recognized tribes. Tribal governments make and enforce their own civil and criminal laws; levy taxes; determine and establish tribal citizenship; license and regulate activities in their jurisdiction; establish zones; and exclude people from tribal lands. Their limitations are also those applicable to individual states, such as inability to engage in war or foreign relations, or printing and issuing currency (Bureau of Indian Affairs, n.d.).

Although some states under Public Law 83-280 have civil and criminal jurisdiction over Indian victims and offenders in state courts, the states don't have regulatory power over lands held in trust by the United States for tribes. Federally recognized tribes are guaranteed fishing, hunting, and trapping rights; tribal government functions like domestic relations and enrollment; and freedom from state taxes. States cannot regulate land use, environmental control, licenses, and gaming on federal Indian reservations. Today, these tribes have strengthened their jurisdiction over criminal and civil actions on reservations based on subsequent state actions, court decisions and acts of Congress (Bureau of Indian Affairs, n.d.).

## Tribal Self-Government

Historically, Native tribes governed themselves with cultural traditions, tribal laws, religious customs, and kinship structures like clans and societies. Modern tribal governments mainly use elected leaders and a democratic process to govern. Although they are not subordinate to states, they often cooperate and collaborate with states via agreements or compacts on matters of mutual interest like law enforcement and environmental protection. Their laws may be more lenient or stricter than states around them and they regulate activities on their lands independently from state control. They determine inheritance rules for property not in trust status, regulate their property, use tribal ordinances to control conduct of tribal citizens, and use their traditional self-government systems whenever possible (Bureau of Indian Affairs, n.d.).

Many tribes have constitutions or articles of association. Some use documents approved by the Secretary of the Interior and usually their governments are similar to the federal branches:  legislative, executive, and judicial. There are numerous names for the tribal chief executive: chairman, chairwoman, chairperson, governor, mayor, principal chief, president, spokesperson, or representative. The chief executive chairs the tribal council or legislative body and the executive branch. Usually, the chief executive and tribal council are elected by eligible tribal voters. They have authority to act and speak for the tribe by representing it in negotiations with local, state, and federal governments. The council or tribal business committee creates laws, appropriates funds, authorizes expenditures, and conducts oversight of activities by tribal government employees and the chief executive (Bureau of Indian Affairs, n.d.).

Many tribes also have tribal courts to administer justice and interpret tribal laws.  These tribal courts usually have civil jurisdiction over tribal residents and non-Natives residing or doing business on reservations. They also have criminal jurisdiction over tribal members residing or conducting business on the reservation who violate tribal laws. Tribal courts use 25 C.F.R. Part 115 to determine competency, appoint guardians, determine paternity, authorize adoptions, marriages, and divorces, award child support, and resolve claims about trust assets. Of 574 federally recognized tribes, about 225 tribes compact or contract with the Bureau of Indian Affairs to perform the Secretary's adjudicatory function and 23 Courts of Indian Offenses that exercise federal authority. Tribal courts are supported by the Indian Tribal Justice Act of 1993 (P.L. 103-176, 107 Stat. 2005) to dispense justice in Indian Country (Bureau of Indian Affairs, n.d.).

## Tribal Self-determination & Self-Governance Laws

Congress enacted two major pieces of legislation to recognize that tribes must have input in the development and implementation of federal programs and policies directly impacting tribal members. The Indian Self-determination and Education Assistance Act of 1975, as amended (25 U.S.C. 450 et seq.) and the Tribal Self-Governance Act of 1994 (25 U.S.C. 458aa et seq.) give tribal governments authority to administer programs and services usually administered by the Bureau of Indian Affairs for their members. This legislation also upholds the principle of tribal consultation, and the federal government must consult with tribes on federal policies, actions, rules, or regulations that directly affects the tribes (Bureau of Indian Affairs, n.d.).

## State Tribal Recognition

Tribes seek state recognition to acknowledge their cultural and historical contributions. State recognition is usually authorized by state legislatures. Formal state recognition can build tribal-state collaboration and in some cases the tribe may qualify for federal and state support. The Department of Housing and Urban Development, Labor, Health and Human Services, and Education have authority to provide funding for state recognized tribes. State recognition  doesn't guarantee funding from the state or federal government. State recognized tribes may not be federally recognized and don't receive the same benefits for housing, health care, nutrition, or education. Some states include tribal participation on state commissions for policy decisions that affect Native Americans. Some states provide education and technical support for state recognized tribes although appropriations are not provided (National Conference of State Legislatures, 2016).

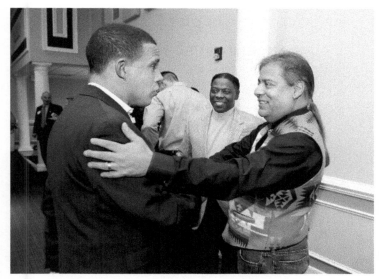

The benefits of federal recognition outweigh those of state recognition although some tribes are dually recognized, and others continue to seek federal recognition.

# Chapter 7
# Southwest Tribes

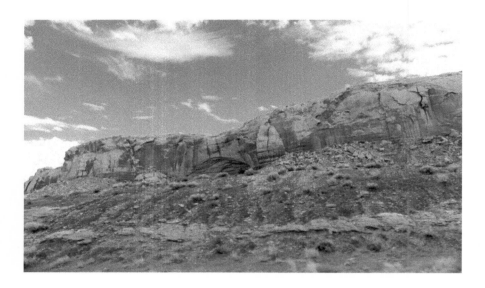

Tribes living in the Southwest included the Apache: Chiricahua (Western Apache), Jicarilla, Mescalero, San Carlos Reservation, Tonto, White Mountain, and the Yavapai-Apache Nation; Hopi, Hualapai, Havasupai, Maricopa, Navajo, O'odham, Pima, Pueblo, Quechan, Yaqui, Yavapai, and Zuni tribes.

## *Apache*

The Apache Tribe of Oklahoma (Plains or Kiowa Apache) was described in chapter 5. There are seven other Apache tribes in the Southwest. All are federally recognized. The name 'Apache' means "enemy" (native-languages.org, 1998-2020).

| State | Tribe(s) | Enterprises |
|---|---|---|
| **Oklahoma** | Chiricahua Apache (Fort Sill Apache Tribe) | Fort Sill Apache tribal enterprises include the Apache Casino Hotel, 3 Apache Markets (convenience |

| State | Tribe(s) | Enterprises |
|-------|----------|-------------|
| | | stores and fuel stops), and Fort Sill Apache Industries which provides government and commercial clients with diverse products and services (Fort Sill Apache Tribe, 2020). |
| **New Mexico** | Jicarilla Apache Nation | The Jicarilla Apache Nation has moved from tourism and recreation to oil and gas production as the chief enterprise (Ten Tribes Partnership, 2023). |
| **New Mexico** | Mescalero Apache | Major Enterprises of the Mescalero Apache Tribe are the Inn of the Mountain Gods Resort and Casino and Ski Apache Ski Resort (Mescalero Apache Tribe, 2023). |
| **Arizona** | San Carlos Apache Reservation | The San Carlos Apache Tribe's enterprises include the Apache Gold Casino as well as recreation activities and cattle ranching (Inter-Tribal Council of Arizona, 2011-2023). |
| **Arizona** | Tonto Apache | Tonto Apache enterprises include the Mazatzal Casino & Restaurant and outstanding basketry and beadwork for purchase (Inter-Tribal Council of Arizona, 2011-2023). |
| **Arizona** | White Mountain Apache (Fort Apache Reservation) | The White Mountain Apache Tribe's enterprises include the Hon-Dah Casino, Sunrise Park Resort, and Trophy Elk hunting (White Mountain Apache Tribe, 2022). |

| State | Tribe(s) | Enterprises |
|-------|----------|-------------|
| **Arizona** | Yavapai-Apache Nation | The Yavapai-Apache Nation's enterprises include the Cliff Castle Casino, Distant Drums RV Resort, YAN Transit bus service, a concrete supplier, and a convenience store & fuel stop (Yavapai-Apache Nation, 2023). |

## Health & Healing Then

Cattail pollen was sacred to the Mescalero Apache, was used in ceremonies, and was a symbol of fertility and well-being (Sanchez, 2018). According to tradition, White Painted Woman gave birth to two sons on White Mountain who grew up to kill all monsters and make peace on earth. Apache women were skillful at gathering and harvesting wild plants, using the Yucca for shampoo and the Mescal plant for food. Pollen was used by a medicine man and medicine woman in the puberty rite ceremony for a young girl to transition from childhood to womanhood. The ceremony was created by White Painted Woman and was a major commitment for the girl's family (Mescalero Apache Tribe, 2023). The Jicarilla Apache Tribe considered water sacred and used it in their religious ceremonies and rituals (Ten Tribes Partnership, 2023).

## Health & Healing Now

The Fort Sill Apache Family Violence Program supports services and emergency shelter for domestic violence victims and their dependents. Staff find temporary shelter, conduct local group counseling, and even pay for individual counseling. They collaborate with community resource agencies and provide Life Skills classes. The Program provides community education about all types of violence:  domestic violence, dating violence, school violence, and sexual assault. Staff offers training for schools, workplace staff, civic/religious organizations, law enforcement, and medical staff (Fort Sill Apache Tribe, 2020).

## Impact on Health of Interaction with White Culture Then

The Apache had a nutritious and diversified diet before being placed on the San Carlos Reservation in the mid-19th century. Restricted to the Reservation, they were prevented from obtaining their original diet and waited in lines for government rations of processed foods high in sugar, salt, saturated fat, and cholesterol (National Congress of American Indians, 2021).

## Impact on Health of Interaction with White Culture Now

The Traditional Western Apache Diet Project was created in 2011 to support the physical, social, cultural, and mental health of the Apache people. Staff of tribal health and wellness programs work together with educational resources to educate youth in community gardening projects. Project staff researched the traditional Apache diet and guided tribal members to increase consumption of traditional, healthy foods. All generations have benefitted from the programs about traditional foods and medicines (National Congress of American Indians, 2021).

## *Hopi*

The Hopi Tribe is federally recognized and located in Arizona. The word 'Hopi' means "peaceful or civilized person" (native-languages.org, 1998-2020). The Hopi Tribe owns the Hopi Tribe Economic Development Corporation (HTEDC) that consists of six entities including:

- the Hopi Cultural Center with lodging, restaurant and gift shop;
- the Muyawki Inn;
- Walpi Housing- a 74-unit apartment complex;
- Heritage Square- a rentable 15,000 sq. ft. property with an underground parking garage;
- Continental Plaza- four buildings with nearly 61,000 sq. ft. rental space and Corporation Headquarters; and
- Kachina Square with 56,000 sq. ft. rental space.

Plans are underway for a two-story, 44-unit hotel in 2024 called the Taawaki Inn (Hopi Tribe Economic Development Corporation, n.d.).

## Health & Healing Then

Hopi medicine men dispersed evil and used crystal gazing to determine the spirits or people responsible for an illness. They chewed the root of the jimson weed to induce visions and used herbs in treatment. They received fees for their services like jewelry, blankets and buckskin. Bonesetters received no compensation and used their knowledge of anatomy to set bones. They also gave massages and used herbs. Kachinas were kindly beings who came for six months to bring clouds and rain before returning to their mountain home in July. Ceremonies included ritual emetics (white aster), ritual smoking of tobacco mixed with herbs, white beans, and ears of corn. Several plants were used as symbols of water, including cottonwood, rushes, sedge, willows, and cattail. Multiple plants cured various illnesses. Gristle from globe mallow treated broken bones. Fleabane cured headaches. Holly grape healed sore gums. Dwarf lupine was used for eye trouble. Blue gilia relieved stomach aches and sand sagebrush aided indigestion. Yucca and thistle were laxatives and globe mallow cured diarrhea. Canaigre treated colds and Mormon tea was used for syphilis. People suffering from epileptic fits used sage as a treatment and jimson weed cured meanness. Painted cup prevented pregnancy and juniper was used to induce pregnancy (Whiting, 1978).

## Health & Healing Now

Hopi residents have suffered from high unemployment due to the reservation's remote location. The tribe has lacked infrastructure and funding. Some homes lack running water and the water they use has high levels of arsenic and drinking this water over time increases risk of diabetes, cancer, heart disease, and kidney disease. Tribal members have had increased cases of cancer. Climate change is increasing temperatures and drought posing a threat to water security According to Hopi Tribe Chairman Timothy Nuvangyaoma, "We all know water is life. If you're threatened with your water running out, it's definitely a concern for us out here on Hopi" (James, 2020).

## Impact on Health of Interaction with White Culture Then

The Spanish in the 1600s and later the Europeans gave the Hopi smallpox epidemics which decimated their population. When the Hopi homeland became part of the United States, the tribe was forced on the reservation. For many years afterward, the Hopi were pushed to assimilate by placing children in boarding schools, forcing men and boys to cut their hair, and pushing tribal members to convert to Christianity (Legends of America, 2023).

## Impact on Health of Interaction with White Culture Now

After a four-decade fight to secure water rights, the Hopi Tribe in 2020 faced having to justify its use of every drop of water to the Arizona Superior Court. Although the U.S. Supreme Court in 1908 ruled that reservations have a right to water, Arizona did not grant water based on the amount of arable land as other states do. In court, experts argued about how many Hopi lived in the area for centuries and how much water they had used for livestock and crops. The fertility rate of Hopi women and the viability of the tribe's economic projects were debated. The court examined lists of secret sacred springs to see how much water they could provide for religious ceremonies. In May 2022, the court awarded less than a third of the water requested. The court only included Hopi who live on the reservation fulltime. It also recommended water from the same contaminated, depleted aquifer and streams the Hopi already use. Water for subsistence and ceremonial gardens was denied. Even accessing the allotted water will require funding for pipes, dams, and other infrastructure through congressional action and negotiation with other tribes using the same groundwater. The Tribe is appealing the decision, but their dreams of farms, cattle ranching., and economic health benefits from additional water will not be realized from this court decision (grist.org, 2023).

## *Hualapai*

The Hualapai Tribe lives in Arizona and is federally recognized. The name 'Hualapai' means "people of the pine trees" (native-languages.org, 1998-2020). Major enterprises of the Hualapai Tribe are tourism, cattle ranching, and arts and crafts with the majority of employment in public schools, administration, and state/federal government. The tribe sells big game hunting permits and owns and operates the Hualapai River Runners offering rafting trips on the Colorado River. They also operate Grand Canyon West with a skywalk, helicopter, and boat tours (Hualapai-nsn.gov, n.d.).

## Health & Healing Then

For the Hualapai Tribe the canyons where people were created were sacred and the sun was the symbol of life (Hualapai-nsn.gov, n.d.). Traditional Hualapai ceremonies included the "Maturity" and "Mourning" Ceremony. The souls of the dead were thought to go northwestward to a beautiful land seen only by Hualapai spirits where plentiful harvests grew (Johnson, n.d.).

## Health & Healing Now

The modern Sobriety Festival is celebrated annually in June (Johnson, n.d.). The 2023 Hualapai Sobriety Campout included multiple activities for all ages. Activities included pottery and soap making skills, equine skills, a sweat lodge, and chair volleyball. The Hualapai Green Reentry Program involves youth in programs to learn different skills while detained in the Hualapai Juvenile Detention & Rehabilitation Center. Elders are involved to teach skills about the Hualapai language, traditions, and culture with the goal to develop self-confidence and leadership skills among these youth. After an intake assessment to understand each youth's needs, they are referred to appropriate services and a reentry plan is developed with the youth, family, and support individuals to establish goals and identify needs and strengths. After release, the youth can continue participating in community programs that include the Boys & Girls Club, the Agriculture Extension Office, and Youth Council (Hualapai-nsn.gov, n.d.).

## Impact on Health of Interaction with White Culture Then

The Appropriations Act of 1892 made education mandatory for Native tribes. In 1901, assimilation efforts began with an Indian boarding school on the reservation. The Hualapai children attended the Truxton Canon boarding school from 1901 to 1937. They were forced to lose their heritage and culture and their language was forbidden. In the fall of 1975, Hualapai children finally learned about their language and culture at the Peach Springs Bilingual/Bicultural School. For the next 25 years, they regained knowledge of zoology, ethnobotany, and ethnogeography (Cannon, 2018).

## Impact on Health of Interaction with White Culture Now

The sacred Cofer Hot Springs in the Big Sandy River Valley also has large deposits of lithium that is essential to manufacturing of electric vehicles. In 2018, the Australian Company Hawkstone Mining began exploratory drilling in the area with no notice to the Hualapai Tribe. The company eventually drilled nearly 50 test wells more than 300 feet deep in the sacred land. Now, they plan to create an open-pit mine and dig an underground slurry to pipe the ore to a plant in Kingman, Arizona about 50 miles away. Court actions have not favored the tribes by creating public lands for development. The Bureau of Land Management has rejected the Hualapai Tribe's request to be a coordinating agency on the project or allow a tribal elder walk to educate the agency about cultural resource sites imperiled by the drilling. Other sacred sites have been adversely impacted by gold mines, wind turbines, and other private interests and the tribe continues to pursue legal action for the sacred Springs (Kapoor, 2021). One positive development is the right of the Hualapai tribe to obtain water from the Colorado River. This legislation was signed by President Biden on January 5, 2023 and the tribe will perform an  environmental analysis for  a proposed water line, pumping station, and water treatment plant to bring water from the Colorado River to the reservation (Hualapai-nsn.gov, n.d.).

## *Havasupai*

The Havasupai Tribe is federally recognized and lives in Arizona. The name 'Havasupai' means "people of the blue-green water" (native-languages.org, 1998-2020). The Havasupai Reservation is eight miles below the Grand Canyon and can only be reached by foot, mule, or horseback. This isolated location has a hidden limestone aquifer whose blue-green waters nourish crops of beans, corn, and squash. The tribe creates beautiful arts and crafts and operates the Havasupai Lodge where reservations are required, and permits are issued for hiking. The trail is open 24 hours a day, but hikers are urged to be cautious. The store and café sell hamburgers, tacos, fries, water, soda, and Gatorade. Travel size toiletries, fruit, and canned goods are also available.  The tribe also makes reservations for pack mule trips and there is a rustic campground where reservations for camping can be made (Havasupai Tribe, 2017-2020).

## Health & Healing Then

The Havasupai Tribe was primarily vegetarian eating the crops they grew in the Grand Canyon. The land was sacred and on the South Rim the bands would tell their origin stories (Hobson, 2019).

## Health & Healing Now

Today, the Supai Health Station is open 5 days a week and is accessible only by helicopter, mule, or on foot. It is staffed by one physician on an appointment and walk-in basis. Transportation and communication continue to be issues for the Havasupai Tribe because of the isolation of the area. Services include behavioral health, limited laboratory, optometry, pharmacy, podiatry, primary care, public health education, public health nursing, and substance abuse counseling (ihs.gov, n.d.).

## Impact on Health of Interaction with White Culture Then

The Grand Canyon Railway and subsequent creation of Grand Canyon National Park disrupted the Havasupai Tribe whose small reservation in Supai didn't include the Tribe's Havasu waterfalls, which became part of the National Park. Older residents resented the incursion on their land and the Park tried to push the tribe out of the area (Hobson, 2019). In 1989, the Havasupai Tribe asked an Arizona State University anthropology professor to investigate why diabetes was increasing in their community. They provided blood samples for testing and no genetic link was found. However, other researchers used the samples to research medical disorders without the tribe's consent. These published papers reflected inbreeding and alcoholism. A subsequent lawsuit resulted in payment of $700,000 return of the samples, scholarships, and help obtaining federal funding for a health clinic (Sterling, 2011).

## Impact on Health of Interaction with White Culture Now

Today, the Havasupai Tribe partners with the Park and have regained some of their land. Their major concerns today are uranium mining, regaining as much land as possible, and establishing water rights to protect their aquifer (Hobson, 2019).

## *Maricopa*

The Maricopa Tribe is federally recognized and resides on two Arizona reservations at Gila river and Salt River. The word 'Maricopa' means "people who live toward the water" (Inter Tribal Council of Arizona, 2011-2023). They share the Gila River Indian Community  and Salt River Indian Community with the Pima Tribe. Enterprises in the Gila River Indian Community include large farming operations, restaurants, the Gila River Resorts & Casinos,  the Sheraton Wildhorse Pass Resort & Spa, two golf courses, and an equestrian center (Gila River Indian Community, n.d.). Enterprises in the Salt River Indian Community include leasing tribal land for development of the Pavilions, the largest retail development on Indian lands, and operating a landfill that has won national awards for environmental excellence and design. The Salt River Indian Community also operates two Casino Arizona locations near Scottsdale, Arizona (Inter Tribal Council of Arizona, 2011-2023).

## Health & Healing Then

The Pima and Maricopa Tribes believed in a Great Spirit and future rewards and punishments. They also believed in witches and would sacrifice property to find and destroy the evil one usually in the form of a stone or stick. They worked hard to find and destroy the object. If one of their family was considered bewitched, the person's life might be taken. When the family head died, all personal property was eaten, destroyed, or burned. The destroyed property was to be placed in the unknown world to benefit the deceased (Estes, 2013). The Man in Maze of the Salt River Reservation showed children that when negative events happen, they could find a physical, social, mental, and spiritual balance. The center of the maze was a person's goals and dreams where each person was met by the Sun God who passed them to the next world (Inter Tribal Council of Arizona, 2011-2023).

## Health & Healing Now

The Gila River Indian Community has a Community Services Department and a Tribal Health Department. The Community Services Department provides social and short-term financial support for tribal members. They meet with clients to discuss available services during intake and outreach. They also respond in crisis situations to meet immediate needs and make necessary referrals. Their Elderly Services Division serves as liaison with other agencies to support elderly and disabled residents. The Tribal Health Department's Animal Control Program's goal is to prevent spread of the rabies virus from dogs and cats to humans. It also provides diabetes prevention services, community nutrition services, health education and information, health surveillance monitoring, communicable disease control, environmental health services, and health system information and data (Gila River Indian Community, n.d.).

## Impact on Health of Interaction with White Culture Then

In the 1870s-1880s, Gila River water was cut-off because of construction of upstream dams by non-Native farmers and the tribe lost the ability to farm. From then until 1920, they faced starvation and famine. The federal government then distributed canned, processed food. This dietary change led to high rates of obesity and diabetes. The tribes were poor, and this poverty led to alcoholism and loss of rituals and traditions. This marginal existence lasted until the Coolidge Dam and San Carlos Reservoir were created in the 1930s. Some of the water restored part of the traditional farming practices (Gila River Indian Community, n.d.).

## Impact on Health of Interaction with White Culture Now

Today, the Gila River tribes are planning an irrigation project to deliver water from the Blackwater area to the Maricopa area. Both tribes must be involved and needs of community members must be addressed. Although this irrigation system will take years to accomplish, they are actively working toward this goal (Gila River Indian Community, n.d.).

## Navajo

The Navajo Nation is federally recognized and is located in Arizona, New Mexico, and Utah.

The word 'Navajo' means "farm fields in the valley" (Crow Canyon Archeological Center, 2023). The Navajo Nation has 12 enterprises and is the largest employer on the reservation (The Navajo Nation, 2023).

### Health & Healing Then

The Navajo always attached healing to a higher power and their culture embraced balance and spirit between the body, mind and nature. Herbal therapies could restore health and medicinal plants could maintain wellness. Evening primrose was used for dry skin and to heal sores. Burning sage and other herbs were used for smudging before ceremonies to clear negative or bad energy. Sage also was used to clean the inner ear, treat respiratory issues, and erase negative inner thoughts. Greenthread tea was sometimes called Navajo tea and soothed sore throats, treating stomach issues, calming nerves, preventing inflammation, and purifying the blood. A pinch or handful of an herb was used, and the remaining liquid was rubbed on the body after drinking a potion (Murphy, 2017).

### Health & Healing Now

Navajo Nation residents experience health problems from oil drilling, uranium and vanadium processing, water and air contamination. Methane, hydrogen sulfide, and oil leaks from abandoned wells increase pollution where people live. The irony is that many homes are above a natural gas line or residents worked for years for energy projects and still don't have water or lights in their homes. About 25% don't have an electrical connection and some don't have running water. During the Pandemic, the Navajo Nation had significant deaths because they lacked basic services of water and electricity. Even residents who have both services in their homes may use coal for heating in the winter because of odor from the gas line. Other residents use a garden hose to get water and an extension cord to connect an outside outlet to an interior outlet. Respiratory illnesses also impact tribal members (Redfren, 2023).

## Impact on Health of Interaction with White Culture Then

In 1863-1866, The Navajo or Diné as they call themselves were forcibly removed to New Mexico 370 miles away. Before they could return to the current Navajo Nation in 1868 almost one/fourth of the people died. Soon after that, the Nation fought outsiders who wanted to develop oil, coal, and other mineral deposits on their land. In 1921 the U.S. government collaborated with some of the younger tribal members who wanted the funds that could be made from development. They became a new Navajo Nation Council and agreed to the first oil leases in 1923. After that, large companies like Peabody, ARCO, General Electric, and BHP Billiton got wealthy from the reservation's oil, gas, uranium and other minerals. The Navajo Nation didn't fare as well. As oil wells were abandoned after the 1950s second oil boom, some were not plugged and methane leaks and contaminated water occurred (Redfern, 2023).

## Impact on Health of Interaction with White Culture Now

The Navajo Nation did not achieve financial independence from the oil booms. Those with oil reserves on their land get monthly royalty checks from the Department of the Interior averaging $20,000/year. Some tribal members only receive $7-$9/month. Sometimes, more than 100 people share a 100-acre allotment that has oil wells on the property. Old wells continue to leak, and health problems are prevalent. In July 2023, the young Navajo Nation President testified to the Energy and Mineral Resources Subcommittee of the House Committee on Natural Resources. He spoke in favor of lifting the Bureau of Land Management's 20-year, 10-mile ban on drilling around Chaco. The Navajo Nation Council had two reasons for recommending this action:

1. The Bureau of Land Management did not properly consult with the Nation about the buffer and

2. The oil money—any money—is needed to live on the reservation (median annual income-$ 27,000) where residents live in poverty (Redfern, 2023).

## O'odham

The O'odham tribes are federally recognized, and some members live on the Gila River, Salt River, and Ak-Chin Indian Communities. The Tohono O'odham Nation will be discussed here. Tohono O'odham means "desert people" (Encyclopedia.com, 2019). The O'odham Nation's lands include Sells, San Xavier, San Lucy District, and Florence Village in Arizona. The Nation's enterprises include the Desert Diamond Casinos, the Tohono O'odham Utility Authority which provides water and electric service, and the Tohono O'odham Economic Development Authority which acquires, owns, and manages business enterprises to create diversified revenue streams for the Nation. The Nation also has Tohono O'odham Community College, a two-year accredited school that prepares graduates for four-year universities and provides apprenticeships and a Building & Construction Trades Vocational Program (Tohono O'odham Nation, 2016).

### Health & Healing Then

The Tohono O'odham harvested the fruit of the saguaro cactus annually for their religion and reaffirmation of their relationship with their environment. The Nation believed the saguaro was once human. They used the syrup to make saguaro fruit wine and drank it at the fruit harvest ceremony on the O'odham New Year's celebration in June or early July to bring the summer monsoon. The saguaro served as food and in ceremonies. An experienced harvester could collect 12 to 20 pounds of pulp in 2-3 hours, and it took 20-30 pounds of fruit to produce a gallon of syrup (Cultural Resources, 2015). The Tohono O'odham respected and feared their shamans who could cause and cure illness. According to shamans, disease was either "wandering" or "staying". "Wandering" sicknesses were infectious diseases brought by others and were cured by Western medicine. "Staying" sicknesses were only in the Tohono O'odham tribe and never spread to outsiders or could be completely eliminated. They resulted from not respecting nature and the person could die if untreated too long. The shaman diagnosed the sickness and specialists in ritual used songs to treat it (Encyclopedia.com, 2019).

## Health & Healing Now

The Tohono O'odham Division of Behavioral Health addresses the needs of individuals with mental, behavioral, alcohol, drug, emotional, and relational issues. It provides services for youth and adults in community-based, in-home, and clinic settings. Therapy is individual, group, or family and there is an outpatient treatment program based on the 12-step Alcoholics Anonymous model since alcoholism is a concern in the Nation. Acupuncture Wellness uses the National Acupuncture Detoxification Association Model to help individuals cope with stress resulting from substance abuse. There is a suicide prevention program (the Good Road of Life), a domestic and sexual violence prevention program (Komckud Ki), and a psychosocial day treatment program for individuals with developmental disability or serious mental illness (Tas Tonlik Ki), Community workshops address suicide prevention, substance and crystal methamphetamine recovery, and conflict resolution (Tohono O'odham Nation, 2016).

## Impact on Health of Interaction with White Culture Then

From the 1800s to the 1960s, children were placed in boarding schools and did not learn the practical work and the cultural aspects of farming. Intergenerational knowledge was lost, and the traditional food system suffered. For example, the Tohono O'odham Nation produced approximately 1.6 million pounds of tepary beans annually on 20,000 acres of traditional crops in the 1930s. By 2000, only one elder grew traditional crops on about two acres and struggled to get 100 pounds of tepary beans a year. The loss of traditional farming was a loss to the Nation's culture and way of life (Himdag). Prayers, songs, and stories with traditional farming nearly disappeared. The arrival of non-Native commercial farms impacted tribal farming (Perez, 2022).

## Impact on Health of Interaction with White Culture Now

Obesity and diabetes are prevalent in the Tohono O'odham community (Encyclopedia.com, 2019). Today, the San Xavier Co-Op Farm has combined some lands to benefit the entire community by sustaining healthy farming and growing traditional crops. The traditional tepary beans and squash are connected to the Tohono O'odham culture and the Farmers Market is showing youth about traditional foods. The Ajo Center for Sustainable Agriculture shows how dryland farming techniques can use rainwater to cultivate traditional crops and distributes seeds to farmers, Youth are learning farming's role in food sovereignty (Perez, 2022).

## Pima

The Pima Tribe is federally recognized and lives on three Arizona reservations: the Gila River Indian Community, the Salt River Indian Community, and the Ak-Chin Indian Community. The first two Indian communities were discussed in the section on Maricopa. The word 'Pima' means "river people" (Gila River Indian Community, n.d.). The Ak-Chin Indian Community is comprised of Pima (also known as Akimel O'odham) and Tohono O'odham. Ak-Chin means "mouth of the wash" referring to the type of farming practiced there. Agriculture is the main industry, and the Community has invested in other enterprises to support their tribal members and the community. These enterprises include management relationships with Harrah's Ak-Chin Casino and Troon Golf in the Ak-Chin Southern Dunes Golf Club. They also own and operate the Ak-Chin Regional Airport (Ak-Chin Indian Community, 2021).

### Health & Healing Then

The Pima Tribe used plants to treat various health conditions. Mormon tea was a treatment for syphilis, screwbean mesquite was used for wound dressings, and banana yucca was a cathartic. Chaparral was an anti-dysenteric. Mesquite had multiple medicinal uses:  treating severe sunburn, eye ailments, sore throat, respiratory infection, disinfectant for open wounds, treating diarrhea, an emetic, and treating stomach disorders (SpottedBird, 2000).

(See also Maricopa)

## Health & Healing Now

The Elder Center in 2023 introduced soap making to create oatmeal soap that assists in controlling eczema, psoriasis, relieving irritation and itching, and moisturizing the skin. An annual caretaker seminar provides tools to empower and support caregivers. The Ak-Chin Indian Community is talking with Indian Health Services about infrastructure needed to enhance community healthcare services. Spiritual and cultural health are also addressed in the Ak-Chin Eco-Museum, which is a living museum in the land where residents act as curators and share their knowledge with visitors (Ak-Chin Indian Community, 2021).

## Impact on Health of Interaction with White Culture Then

(See also Maricopa) The Gila River cut-off also created a health crisis, and the Pima Tribe has the highest rate of Type II diabetes in the world (Scott, 2023).

## Impact on Health of Interaction with White Culture Now

The Ak-Chin Indian Community participated in an injury prevention program from 2015-2020 with Indian Health Service to prevent fall injuries and motor vehicle injuries. During that time, 86 homes were checked for fall hazards and changes were implemented for safety. Six to twelve elders participate regularly in weekly exercise classes to improve their balance and strength. Three events have been hosted annually to provide safety seat education and correct safety seat use. 230 car safety seats were provided to caregivers and parents. Regular safety observations occur to check adult seat belt use and proper child safety restraint use (his.gov, 2020).

## *Pueblo*

There are 19 Pueblo tribes in New Mexico, and all are federally recognized. The word 'Pueblo' means "town/village" or "nation/people" (The Free Dictionary, n.d.). Their enterprises are below.

| State | Tribe(s) | Enterprises |
|-------|----------|-------------|
| **New Mexico** | Pueblo of Acoma | Pueblo of Acoma enterprises include the Sky City Casino and Hotel, Sky City Cultural Center, and Big Game Trophy Hunts (Pueblo of Acoma, n.d.). |
| **New Mexico** | Pueblo de Cochiti | The Pueblo de Cochiti has a convenience store and fuel stop along with recreational areas on Cochiti Lake (Krasnow, 2016). |
| **New Mexico** | Pueblo of Isleta | Pueblo of Isleta owns and operates the Isleta Casino and Resort and Isleta Lakes & RV Park (Pueblo of Isleta, n.d.). |
| **New Mexico** | Pueblo of Jemez | Pueblo of Jemez enterprises include a convenience store, tourism and artisans, a visitor center, and timber harvesting (Pueblo of Jemez, 2023). |
| **New Mexico** | Pueblo of Laguna | The Laguna Development Corporation operates three casinos: the Route 66 Casino Hotel, Dancing Eagle Casino, and Casino Express. The Corporation also operates two travel centers, food and beverage venues, a grocery store, and an RV resort (Pueblo of Laguna, n.d.). |
| **New Mexico** | Nambé Pueblo | Nambé Pueblo enterprises include agriculture, the Nambé Falls Travel Center and tourism that includes recreational areas, textiles, and pottery production as well as ceremonials that are open to the public (Nambé Pueblo, 2014). |
| **New Mexico** | Ohkay Owingeh | Ohkay Owingeh's enterprises are the Ohkay Hotel & Casino, recreation, and tourism (Ohkay Owingeh, 2018). |
| **New Mexico** | Picuris Pueblo | Picuris Pueblo enterprises are the Picuris Smoke Shop, recreation, and tourism (Picuris Pueblo, n.d.). |

| State | Tribe(s) | Enterprises |
|---|---|---|
| **New Mexico** | Pueblo of Pojoaque | Pueblo of Pojoaque enterprises include Buffalo Thunder Resort & Casino, Cities of Gold Casino, Red Sage dining, and the Poeh Cultural Center & Museum (Pueblo of Pojoaque, n.d.). |
| **New Mexico** | Pueblo of Sandia | Pueblo of Sandia enterprises are the Sandia Resort & Casino, Bien Mur Indian Market, recreation at Sandia Lakes, and hunting at Bobcat Ranch (Pueblo of Sandia, n.d.). |
| **New Mexico** | San Felipe Pueblo | San Felipe Pueblo's major enterprise is the Black Mesa Casino (San Felipe Pueblo, 2023). |
| **New Mexico** | Pueblo de San Ildefonso | The San Ildefonso Pueblo's major enterprise is tourism and tribal artists have pottery available for purchase (San Ildefonso Pueblo, 2023). |
| **New Mexico** | Santa Ana Pueblo | Santa Ana Pueblo enterprises include the Santa Ana Star Casino & Hotel, golf courses, and a nursery (Santa Ana Pueblo, 2023). |
| **New Mexico** | Santa Clara Pueblo | Santa Clara Pueblo enterprises include the Santa Claran Hotel & Casino, the Black Mesa Golf Club, and recreation. Recreation has improved since wildfires occurred in the past 20 years due to collaboration with multiple agencies and mitigation assistance (New Mexico Tourism Department, 2023). |
| **New Mexico** | Santo Domingo Pueblo | Santo Domingo Pueblo enterprises are a gas station and convenience store and crafts that include beadwork, turquoise jewelry, and pottery (Santo Domingo Pueblo, n.d.). |

| State | Tribe(s) | Enterprises |
|---|---|---|
| New Mexico | Taos Pueblo | Taos Pueblo enterprises focus on tourism, including traditional crafts, arts, and concessions. Some members are employed in the town of Taos (Taos Pueblo, 2023). |
| New Mexico | Tesuque Pueblo | Tesuque Pueblo enterprises are the Tesuque Casino and the Santa Fe Suites. Many Tesuque artists also sell pottery sculpture, paintings, traditional clothing, and silverwork (New Mexico Tourism Department, 2023). |
| Nes Mexico | Pueblo of Zia | Pueblo of Zia enterprises are agriculture and livestock raising. They also have artists who produce pottery and traditional works of art (New Mexico Tourism Department, 2023). |
| New Mexico | Pueblo of Zuni | Pueblo of Zuni enterprises are agriculture growing wheat and maize, jewelry making, pottery, painting, and fetish carving (Pueblo of Zuni, 2016). |

## Health & Healing Then

The Pueblos shared common spiritual and religious beliefs. The Kachina religion believed that hundreds of these ancestral spirits communicated and lived with each tribe for half the year. These spirits included Earth Father, Earth Mother, and a serpent god who controlled rain. The Pueblo respected nature and their prayers and dance rituals requested renewal, large harvests, fertility, and successful hunts. Spirituality was integrated throughout their lives and beliefs showed harmony with nature. Ceremonies were often held in underground locations called kivas. Some religious rituals were practiced to cure diseases, protect their welfare, and seek rain. Kinship determined eligibility to govern or perform religious ceremonies. When the Spanish came, some Pueblo incorporated Christian beliefs with their traditional customs (Ketchum, 2017).

## Health & Healing Now

Pueblo de Cochiti youth are returning to farming through the Cochiti Youth Experience which teaches traditional farming techniques and the importance of food to community health, the land, and spirituality. The organization reaches youth at risk for alcohol use or truancy and helps them make better lifestyle choices. Most food at the Pueblo is manufactured and growing food helps tribal members improve their nutrition, diet, and exercise for better health. Youth are able to learn from elders and growing quality food is empowering. Since 2012, the program has served more than 2,311 meals to community residents, the number of mentors has nearly doubled, and youth participants have increased from 6 to 26. The Cochiti Youth Experience is benefitting the community and is replicable to other Native communities (Jakober, 2023).

## Impact on Health of Interaction with White Culture Then

The Spanish in the 1600s attempted to destroy the Pueblo tribes by making them pay taxes, bringing Catholic missionaries to threaten their religious beliefs, renaming pueblos with saints' names, and trying to eradicate the Pueblos culture. When protestant evangelical missions came in the early 1900s, the Bureau of Indian Affairs forced children to attend boarding schools. After the 1960s, Pueblos were exposed to anthropologists and seekers of Native spirituality as they clung to their traditional customs and religion (Nambé Pueblo, 2014).

## Impact on Health of Interaction with White Culture Now

The Pueblo of Isleta Resort and Casino implemented a no smoking policy inside the Casino when reopening after the Pandemic. They are continuing this policy today and have found benefits for patrons and staff that are also improving the bottom line. The smoking ban is accepted, and patrons don't complain about the smell in their rooms and on their clothing after a visit there. Revenue is increasing and business is up. Casino staff are surveyed on hire and at three months and results show that 95% of them appreciate working in a nonsmoking workplace. A bill to ban smoking in New Mexico was tabled in the 2023 legislative session, but the Casino's positive outcomes and health benefits may be used by the Tobacco Settlement Oversight Committee to reintroduce this legislative proposal (Jones, 2023).

## Quechan

The Fort Yuma Quechan Tribe's reservation is located within Arizona and California. The Tribe is federally recognized, and the name 'Quechan' means "those who descended" (encyclopedia.com, 2019). Agriculture is a major industry with lands leased to both tribal and non-tribal farmers. Other enterprises include tourism, the Quechan Casino Resort, the Paradise Casino, trailer and RV parks, and a grocery store (Fort Yuma Quechan Tribe, n.d.).

### Health & Healing Then

Dream power was a spiritual power found in special dreams and from ongoing interaction with souls of the dead. Dream power was used by leaders, warriors, ritual specialists, and healers. Smoking and abstinence produced results and many people had guardian spirits who lived on sacred mountains. Some singers and speakers knew rituals and some men had unusual dream power. Religious ceremonies honored deceased tribal members, and some were like large feasts. The Quechan believed soul loss or accidentally eating a poisonous substance caused disease. Either could be caused by violating a taboo or by a hostile sorcerer. Curers or healers used dream power by blowing smoke on the patient, massaging him or her, and by sucking out the substance. After death, the soul passed through four layers into the afterlife and the body and possessions were cremated. Some spirits returned to receive burned offerings (encyclopedia.com, 2019).

### Health & Healing Now

The Quechan Indian Tribe has a Social Services Victim Advocate who supports victims of domestic violence, sexual assault, dating violence, or stalking. Services include transitional housing support, emergency assistance, case management, crisis intervention, referrals to outside agencies, and help completing orders of protection/report filing. On May 4th, the Quechan Tribe President proclaimed that day "The Fort Yuma

Quechan Indian Nation MMIW Medicine Wheel Ride Day" and the Tribe hosted the Medicine Wheel Riders, a female biking group. Their mission statement is: "We are Indigenous Women Motorcyclists and Allies who create awareness events and fundraise for issues affecting Our Indigenous Women and Relatives as well as issues in our communities." They and male Rez Riders support advocates and groups who search for Missing and Murdered Indigenous Relatives (MMIR) and provide support to women and their families. Many ride for awareness of MMIW because members of their families or close friends have been victims (Fort Yuma Quechan Tribe, n.d.).

## Impact on Health of Interaction with White Culture Then

The Spanish attempted to make the Quechan people leave their religion for Catholicism and to use European farming methods. When the Americans came, the government forcibly relocated the Quechan and other tribes to reservations away from their homelands. The new land was not suitable for farming and their food systems were disrupted because they could no longer hunt, fish, and use their traditional farming practices. Mining practices also degraded tribal lands and caused environmental pollution (Cassar, 2023).

## Impact on Health of Interaction with White Culture Now

In 2022, the Quechan Indian Tribe and Earthworks successfully stopped gold drilling at Indian Pass. This area is important spiritually to the Tribe and drilling could be detrimental to the health of residents. While the mining company wants to continue exploration at nearby sites, another project concerns the Quechan in 2023. The new project wants to do gold exploration in the Cargo Muchacho Mountains. The project would build 8 miles of roads, drill down to 800 feet in 65 holes, use 2,000 gallons of water daily, and disturb the habitat of desert tortoises. After this, the company would build large mines to extract gold from rocks using cyanide. Cyanide is toxic to animals, the environment, and people. These areas are sacred to the Quechan, and they have fought 20 years to prevent projects like these that could damage the environment, water supplies, and fellow residents in two counties. The Bureau of Land Management has conducted an environmental assessment and has approved the new project despite strenuous objections by the Quechan Tribe and Earthworks who believe the assessment did not analyze direct, indirect, and cumulative impacts of gold extraction in this area. The Tribe and its allies are meeting with the Imperial County Planning Commission which must give final permission for the project to proceed. As a Quechan elder stated: "These mountains were created like, like we were created and they shouldn't be destroyed" (Stargazer, 2023).

## *Yaqui*

The Pascua Yaqui Tribe is federally recognized and lives in Arizona. The word 'Yaqui' means "person" (New World Encyclopedia, 2023). The Tribe has two casinos, Casino Del Sol and Casino of the Sun, and plans to build a third on land north of downtown Tucson (Duren, 2023). They also are employed in agriculture and ranching. The Tribe's Economic Development Department continues to diversify the tribal economy and generate additional revenue (Pascua Yaqui Tribe, 2023). There is also a Texas Tribe of Yaqui Indians who are state recognized and live in Lubbock, Texas. Their purpose is to preserve Yaqui culture, language, and traditions. They have tribal artisans who do beadwork, jewelry, and write books (Texas Band of Yaqui Indians, 2021).

### Health & Healing Then

Deer were central to Yaqui culture and the Deer served as a guide in death and on the Yaqui journey to heaven. A Yaqui deer dancer or Pascola learned the dance in a dream vision from a trained individual and performed the dance at ceremonies as part of a Yaqui cultural society. Another cultural society was the Coyote Bow Authority which provided security for ceremonies and still protects tribal leaders. Their ritual dance was performed only by men in cultural ceremonies, although women could serve as soldiers and leaders (Pascua Yaqui Tribe, 2023). Deer song rituals and the deer dance paid tribute to the balance between man and nature, the harmony of the forest, and the deer's spirit as well as giving thanks (New World Encyclopedia, 2023).

## Health & Healing Now

Although today's Yaqui religion is a combination of traditional beliefs and Catholicism, the Pascua Yaqui Tribe has a Traditional Healing program which is highly utilized. The program administrator supports transporting Traditional Healers to and from Mexico, ensures they have required supplies, and assists them as needed. The program uses Traditional Yoeme Practices to heal body, mind, and spirit. Therapies and services include counseling and emotional/spiritual consultations; smudging; limpia (cleansing); massage; and traditional healing rituals. Traditional Healing is based on cultural and spiritual values by developing trust between the person and the Healer. The Pascua Yaqui Behavioral Health Centered Spirit Program also provides substance abuse and mental health services to individuals and groups using a team approach to improve tribal members' health and well-being (Pascua Yaqui Tribe, 2023).

## Impact on Health of Interaction with White Culture Then

The Yaqui originated in Mexico and a significant number still live there. The earliest interactions with White culture involved Mexicans who invaded the tribe's homeland in the 1800s. Hundreds of Yaqui of all ages were forced to work as slaves in southeastern Mexico. Rich Yaqui lands were opened to commercial development and outside investors. Some Mexicans intermarried with Yaquis and began taking control of some Yaqui lands. Some Yaqui sought refuge in the United States to avoid this attempted genocide (Texas Band of Yaqui Indians, 2021).,

## Impact on Health of Interaction with White Culture Now

The Pascua Yaqui Tribe has a Charitable Organization that gives back to the Tribe and the community. They partner with the Community Food Bank of southern Arizona to establish a food pantry on the reservation where hundreds of residents in Pima County receive healthy foods they could not get otherwise. Food Security and Nutritional Support fights food insecurity and focuses on the long term goal of community food sovereignty. Another project of the Pascua Yaqui Tribe Charitable Organization is humanitarian aid for Yaqui villages in Mexico who are culturally and spiritually related to the Tribe. This humanitarian aid includes potable water services which the diversion of the Yaqui River by dams has resulted in lack of potable water for these Yaqui in Mexico (Pascua Yaqui Tribe, 2023).

## *Yavapai*

The Yavapai-Apache Nation of the Camp Verde Reservation was discussed earlier in this chapter. The Yavapai-Prescott Indian Tribe and Fort McDowell Yavapai Nation are also federally recognized and live in Arizona. The word 'Yavapai' means "people of the sun" (native-languages.org, 1998-2020). The Fort McDowell Yavapai Nation's enterprises include the Fort McDowell Farm, Fort McDowell Casino, the Poco Diablo Resort, the We-Ko-Pa Resort and Conference Center, the We-Ko-PA Golf Club, and the Eagle View RV Resort (Fort McDowell Yavapai Nation, 2013-2020). The Yavapai-Prescott Indian Tribe's enterprises include Bucky's Casino, the Yavapai Casino, and the Frontier Village Shopping Center (Yavapai-Prescott Indian Tribe, n.d.).

### Health & Healing Then

The Yavapai used various plants for health. These included:

1. arenaria or sandwort which was used for gastrointestinal disturbances and as a cathartic;
2. cyperus or sedge which treated colds and skin conditions;
3. euphorbia or spurg which treated venereal diseases;
4. chaparral which was an antirheumatic and treated sore throat and venereal disease;
5. lobeleaf groundsel which was a cold remedy and nose medicine;
6. curly dock which treated coughs, sore throats, and toothaches; and
7. jojoba which treated skin conditions and also was used as a cathartic (Gifford, 1936).

## Health & Healing Now

In 2021, the Hman Shawa Early Childhood Development Center created a community garden at Fort McDermott which helps children develop healthy eating habits. The community garden involves collaboration between the Tribal Farm, the Healthy Futures Program (funded by the Special Diabetes Program for Indians) and the Fountain Hills Community Garden. Children learn that vegetables and fruits are healthy and good for them. These vegetables mitigate and prevent obesity, diabetes, hypertension, kidney disease, coronary artery disease, and chronic constipation. The goal is to have a 'garden to table' concept to offset chronic diseases. Harvested fruits and vegetables are put in the school cafeteria, used in classroom education, donated to needy community families, and used in the diabetes classes of Healthy Futures (Fort McDowell Yavapai Nation, 2013-2020).

## Impact on Health of Interaction with White Culture Then

In the 1970s, a dam was proposed at the convergence of the Salt and Verde rivers that would have flooded much of the Fort McDowell reservation. The Yavapai Nation would have lost its ancestral lands. With limited financial resources, the Nation rallied other Native tribes and non-Native groups to oppose the Orme Dam Project. In 1976, they voted not to sell their land for the dam site and finally succeeded in 1981 when the Interior Secretary announced that the dam would not be built (Fort McDowell Yavapai Nation, 2013-2020). In 1990, the Yavapai Nation made a water settlement with the U.S. government to receive 36,000 acre-feet of water annually. With a $13 million low-interest loan from the Bureau of Reclamation, they were able to expand their farm and lease some of this water allocation to other communities. The Yavapai Nation also demanded that the Salt River Project on the Verde River maintain river water level to support bald eagles and other wildlife there (Kraker, 2004).

## Impact on Health of Interaction with White Culture Now

The Fort McDowell Yavapai Nation today farms 2,000 acres containing pecan trees, citrus trees, and alfalfa. Since navel oranges are no longer profitable due to competition from California orchards, they are increasing growth of lemons and grapefruit. Their citrus is available in local markets and shipped worldwide. The Nation realizes that good community relations is essential for successful farming operations and limits chemical use in areas bordering residential development. They have also met with the homeowners' association in Rio Verde to discuss their operation (Growing Magazine, 2018).

# Reservations & the Bureau of Indian Affairs

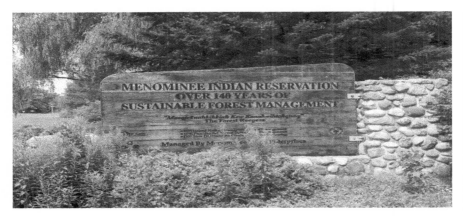

## History of Reservations

All Native Americans do not live on reservations, but reservations have impacted Native tribes since the mid-19th century. The Indian Appropriations Act of 1851 created the first reservations in Oklahoma with the stated goal of protecting Native tribes from encroachment by White people. However, the reservations' size decreased with White expansion. President Grant (1869-1877) intensified the reservation process by relocating numerous tribes and putting religious groups and officials in charge of the reservations to "civilize" tribes by converting them to Christianity. Their methods were described earlier and included boarding schools to teach children English and prohibit cultural traditions.

Many reservations had soil that could not support crops and attempts to use traditional farming practices were unsuccessful. This led to malnutrition and starvation for many tribes because government support was often late or inadequate. When tribes resisted, the government began to reduce the size of the reservations and forcibly relocated many tribes. The U.S. Army was sent to control the tribes and Grant's successor, Rutherford B. Hayes, began phasing out his Indian policies. Other legislation affected the reservations negatively and positively. The Dawes Act of 1887 created a policy of awarding parcels of land to tribal individuals instead of entire tribes. This resulted in further loss for the tribes when "excess" reservation land was given to Whites. In 1934, the Indian Reorganization Act returned ownership of the land to the tribes. This law increased reservation sizes and included government investment in health care, education, and infrastructure on reservations. The Act also relocated some tribes, and 61 tribal nations were terminated according to the government (Foster, 2023).

## Reservations Today

Today, there are three kinds of reserved federal lands: public, military, and Indian. On federal Indian reservations, the government holds the land's title in trust for the tribe. These reservations have been designated as permanent homelands for tribes based on treaty, federal law or administrative action, or executive order. Areas held in trust account for approximately 56.2 million acres and there are about 326 federal Indian reservations in the U.S. The largest is the Navajo Nation of Arizona, Utah, and New Mexico that has 16 million acres. Many smaller reservations are under 1,000 acres and the smallest reservation is a 1.32-acre cemetery belonging to the Pit River Tribe of California (Bureau of Indian Affairs, n.d.).

Not all reservations are on tribal homelands. Some were created by the government to resettle Native tribes relocated away from their homelands. All federally recognized tribes don't have reservations. Those that have reservations are considered sovereign nations and are usually exempt from state taxation and jurisdiction. There are also state reservations where a state holds lands in trust for a tribe. These lands are protected from state property tax, but are subject to the laws of that state. State trusts result from agreements or treaties between the state or earlier colonial government and the tribe. Other tribal members may live in non-native locations where they are employed, have businesses, and/or own property. They must comply with state and local laws and regulations and pay state/local taxes as state citizens (Bureau of Indian Affairs, n.d.).

## Eligibility Requirements & Trust Responsibilities

The federal government provides services to enrolled tribal members. These services from federal programs can include health, welfare, education, and social service programs to eligible individuals. Each federally recognized tribe determines the eligibility criteria for membership or enrollment differs for each tribe. Not all of these benefits are available to state recognized tribes and eligibility requirements also differ for federal programs. The Department of the Interior and the Secretary of the Interior are responsible for fulfilling trust responsibilities to federally recognized tribes. The Assistant Secretary-Indian Affairs, a representative from a Native American tribe, has been charged since 1977 with promoting economic well-being and self-determination of tribes by supporting their

government-to-government relationship with the United States through
the Bureau of Indian Affairs (Bureau of Indian Affairs, n.d.).

## History of the Bureau of Indian Affairs

Here is the chronology of the Bureau of Indian Affairs:

| Date | Participant(s) | Action |
|---|---|---|
| 1775 | Continental Congress | Committee on Indian Affairs established under Benjamin Franklin to handle tribal trade matters |
| August 20, 1789 | Congress & Secretary of War | Responsibility for managing tribal trade matters given to Secretary of War by Congress |
| April 21, 1806 | Secretary of War and War Department | Office of Indian Trade created to handle trade matters with tribes |
| May 6, 1822 | Congress & Secretary of War | Office of Indian Trade eliminated and responsibility for Indian matters back to Secretary of War |
| March 11, 1824 | Secretary of War | Bureau of Indian Affairs (BIA) established within War Department by Secretary as the Office of Indian Affairs |
| July 9, 1832 | Congress | BIA and Commissioner on Indian Affairs position legislatively established |
| 1849 | Congress | Interior Department created and BIA transferred there |
| September 17, 1947 | Interior Department | Bureau of Indian Affairs name formally adopted |

There have been 45 Commissioners of Indian Affairs since 1824 and six
have been Native Americans. The Bureau of Indian Affairs began by
seeking to suppress native tribes and has evolved to respect their self-
determination (Bureau of Indian Affairs, n.d.). The journey was difficult.
The Office of Indian Affairs as it was known banned ceremonial dances
and placed Indian children in boarding schools to assimilate them into

White society. They were considered hostile by many tribal members. The Bureau also controlled "Individual Indian Money" accounts and denied access to some tribal members. Initially, most office personnel were non-Native White administrators even though the government in 1834 officially gave Native people preference for hiring. This lasted until the 1970s, when Native hiring increased. By 2010, 95% of the Bureau of Indian Affairs employees were Native Americans and the relationship between the agency and the tribes improved (Gershon, 2021).

## The Bureau of Indian Affairs Today

The Bureau's Mission Statement describes today's relationship between the tribes and the Bureau:

"The BIA's mission is to enhance the quality of life, to promote economic opportunity, and to carry out responsibility to protect and improve the trust assets of American Indians, Indian tribes and Alaska Natives. We will accomplish this through the delivery of quality services, maintaining government-to-government relationships within the spirit of self-determination" (Bureau of Indian Affairs, n.d.).

Besides providing services and programs to tribes. The Bureau maintains criteria to determine which tribes are federally recognized. Since tribal recognition provides access to the services listed earlier, some people (particularly non-Natives) believe tribal recognition is not an appropriate role for the government. However, federally recognized tribes see reduced criteria and undermining the government's recognition authority as eroding the political standing of tribes as sovereign nations (Gershon, 2021).

Land and water rights continue to be areas of contention, but Bureau employees across the United States collaborate with tribal governments to address job training, employment assistance, agriculture and economic development, managing natural resources, justice and law enforcement, and governance with the goal of improving tribal communities' quality of life. Examples of the role of the Bureau of Indian Affairs are varied and include:

1. funding and administering program services for federally recognized tribes;
2. collaborating with tribes to administer trust land and its natural resources;
3. maintaining nationwide district law enforcement offices in Indian Country to conduct investigations and protect all residents there;

4. building roads, dams, bridges, and infrastructure in Indian Country;
5. assisting with fires or natural disasters;
6. administering the Guaranteed Indian Loan Program to increase business development and entrepreneurship by tribes;
7. administering federal employment/training and economic development programs for tribes;
8. administering Bureau programs if tribes are unable or unwilling to do so; and
9. performing fiduciary duties for leases and probate of Indian trust estates for individual beneficiaries (Bureau of Indian Affairs, n.d.).

Although relationships between the Bureau of Indian Affairs and the tribes have sometimes been strained, tribes have learned how to work with the agency. As one tribal leader stated "The BIA is a great resource if you know how to use it" (Gershon, 2021).

The Bureau provided health care services until 1955 when that responsibility transferred to the Department of Health and Human Services as the Indian Health Service (Bureau of Indian Affairs, n.d.). Tribal health services will be discussed at the end of the following chapter.

## History of Native American Education

The chronology of Native American education is applicable here as it has evolved over many years.

| Date | Native American Education | Outcome |
|------|---------------------------|---------|
| 1819 | Indian Civilization Act | Up to $10,000/year to support religious groups who would teach Indians with mission schools; directly funded until end of 19th century; some exist today |
| 1879 | Government & Boarding Schools | Schools established to provide industrial/vocational education with the goal of cultural assimilation; regimented used student labor to maintain the schools |
| 1891 | Contracts | Federal officials required to negotiate individual contracts with school districts |
| 1921 | Snyder Act | Authorized the Bureau of Indian Affairs to financially support Native education |

| Date | Native American Education | Outcome |
|---|---|---|
| 1928 | Meriam Report | Brookings Institute independently investigated the Indian Office. The report was critical of vocational government-run programs and called for more child-centered progressive education. |
| 1934 | New Indian Deal-Johnson O'Malley Act | Secretary of the Interior could contract with territories and states to pay to educate Indian students |
| 1934 | Indian Reorganization Act | Introduced teaching of Indian history and culture in Bureau of Indian Affairs schools |
| 1940 | Bilingual texts | Secretary of the Interior and Commissioner of Indian Affairs endorsed using Native languages in textbooks to increase learning English |
| 1966 | Rough Rock Demonstration School | First Indian-controlled school established in the Navajo Nation |
| 1968 | Bilingual Education Act | Legislation to help Native Americans use their own languages |
| 1968 | Navajo Community College | First tribal college to improve high college drop-out rate for Native students |
| 1970s | Survival Schools | The American Indian Movement opens some small schools to promote Indian culture and focus on basic living and learning skills |
| 1972 & 1975 | Indian Education Act (1972) & Indian Self Determination and Education Assistance Act (1975) | Congress passes legislation to improve federal efforts to provide quality education to Native Americans since past approaches have had dismal results. Tribes could contract with the Bureau of Indian Affairs to determine suitable programs for their children. |
| 1978 | Tribally Controlled Community College Assistance Act | Legislation providing funding for Native students attending tribal colleges |
| 1978 | Education Amendments Act | Provided funds directly to tribally operated schools, permitted local hiring of teachers and staff, and created a direct line between the Education Director and the Assistant Secretary-Indian Affairs |

| Date | Native American Education | Outcome |
|------|---------------------------|---------|
| 1990 | Native American Languages Act | Legislation to promote freedom by Native Americans to develop, practice, and use their Native languages |
| 2001 | No Child Left Behind Act | Revision of Elementary & Secondary Education Act to raise academic achievement of minority students |
| 2006 | Esther Martinez Native American Language Preservation Act | Legislation using Native languages as the instruction language in Indian immersion schools |
| 2006 | Bureau of Indian Education | Office of Indian Education Programs renamed to reflect the purpose and organizational structure of other programs within the Office of the Assistant Secretary-Indian Affairs |
| 2013 | Education Trust Report | "The State of Education for Native Students" shows no improvement in achievement levels since 2005 |

(Reyhner, 2013 [updated 2019] & Bureau of Indian Education, n.d.)

Additional updated information based on the table:

1. The current Indian Education Act has funding for special programs for Native students both on and off the reservation.
2. There are 35 tribal colleges in 13 states.
3. Since adoption of the No Child Left Behind Act, Native students are the only group whose achievement has not risen.
4. Today, some Native groups use charter school funding to teach a curriculum for the culture and community (Reyhner, 2013 [updated 2019]).

## Role of the Bureau of Indian Education

The Assistant Secretary-Indian Affairs is responsible for the Bureau of Indian Education which is to manage and direct all education functions and funding expenditures. Its mission is:

"Provide students at BIE-funded schools with a culturally relevant, high-quality education that prepares students with the knowledge, skills, and behaviors needed to flourish in the opportunities of tomorrow, become healthy and successful individuals, and lead their communities and sovereign nations to a thriving future that preserves their unique cultural identities" (Bureau of Indian Education, n.d.).

There are 183 Bureau of Indian Education (BIE) elementary and secondary schools in 23 states on 64 reservations which serve approximately 46,000 Native students. Of these schools, 128 are tribally controlled and 55 are BIE-operated. The BIE also operates or funds off-reservation boarding schools and dormitories near reservations for Native students attending public schools. The Bureau serves postsecondary students through scholarships and funding support for tribal colleges. It also operates two postsecondary institutions for Native students: the Southwest Indian Polytechnic Institute in Albuquerque, New Mexico and the Haskell Indian Nations University in Lawrence, Kansas (Bureau of Indian Education, n.d.).

The Bureau administers the Replacement School Construction program that replaces all or portions of existing facilities when upgrading existing facilities is not feasible. The Bureau uses an Education Facilities Replacement Construction Priority List in funding to determine which schools need replacement (Bureau of Indian Education, n.d.).

There continue to be issues impacting the Native education system. Currently, Native students fail to achieve proficiency or graduate at a higher rate than other students. The Government Accountability Office (GAO) added the Bureau of Indian Education to their High-Risk List in 2017 as a government agency in need of transformation and vulnerable to mismanagement. The Bureau remains on this list because the agency needs to improve its monitoring and capacity as well as demonstrating progress in school administration (Government Accountability Office, 2022).

Many BIE-funded schools have struggled in several areas for the following reasons:

1. Leadership-Organizational realignments and leadership turnover in the Bureau of Indian Affairs resulted in fragmentation and inadequate communication between Indian Affairs offices. The Government Accountability Office (GAO) recommended in 2015 that a strategic plan be developed for BIE and that the Bureau have a strategy for communicating with schools. A strategic plan was developed for 2018-2023 that has a communication strategy (Bureau of Indian Education, n.d.).

2. Curriculum-Academic standards vary from state to state and standardized exams don't capture all that communities value in education. Test scores are also lower in poorer districts because

those students lack time or resources for learning outside school. The Bureau does not provide pre-K programs and Head Start programs lack resources for pre-K ones. School Family and Child Education Programs (FACE) by the Bureau use integrated learning for parents and children successfully, but they are not in all BIE schools. There were only 49 of these programs in the 2018-2019 academic year. The Bureau has not had a statistically valid method to evaluate schools because standardized education and assessments are based on multiple state standards (Woods & Philip, 2021)

3.  Staffing-In May 2022, the Bureau had a staff vacancy rate of almost 33% and the School Operations Division had a vacancy rate of about 45%. This significantly reduces the Bureau's ability to oversee and support schools (Government Accountability Office, 2022). Attracting skilled principals and teachers is also difficult in Native as well as other rural schools(The Red Road, 2023).

4.  Funding-According to the GAO, the Bureau of Indian Education "has not fully implemented its program for risk-based monitoring schools' use of federal education funds" (Government Accountability Office, 2022).

5.  Technology-The Bureau of Indian Education does not have a program to routinely assess and monitor technology needs and assets at schools. The GAO found this led to major delays in giving distance learning devices to students during the Pandemic school closures (Government Accountability Office, 2022).

6.  School Safety/Construction-The Bureau of Indian Education developed a long- term capital asset plan in September 2021 to guide school construction. A plan was also developed in January 2022 to increase school building safety in areas like sprinkler systems and fire alarm maintenance (Government Accountability Office, 2022). Many of these schools are in disrepair with leaking roofs, mold, and asbestos (The Red Road, 2023).

The Bureau of Indian Education is planning to use its Strategic Transformation of Education Plan and an eLMS digital tool to improve educational outcomes. This program is in its first year and plans to use Blended Learning strategies and eLMS with an integrated curriculum to engage students and encourage real-time collaboration between leaders and support staff and teachers and students. Besides increasing IT infrastructure and digital connectivity for schools, it is designed to support professional development for teachers, leaders, and IT professionals (Bureau of Indian Education, n.d.). It will take time to see if this will truly transform education in BIE and tribal schools, but it is a start on the journey to the future.

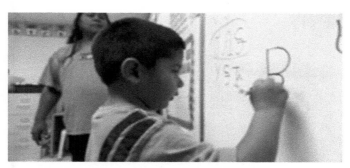

# Chapter 8
# West Coast Tribes

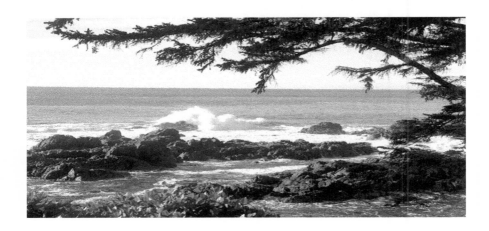

The West Coast, particularly California, has numerous small Native tribes who live in Rancherias or Missions. After listing them in alphabetical order, they will be discussed in their locations as several tribes are combined in either Rancherias or Missions. They are: Achomawi, Bear River, Cahuilla, Chasta, Chehalis, Chemehuevi, Chinook, Chukchansi, Chumash, Colville, Coos, Cupeno, Diegueno/Kumeyaay, Hupa, Kalapuya, Kalispel, Karuk, Klamath, Luiseno, Maidu, Mattole, Miwok (Me-Wuk), Modoc, Mojave, Molalla, Mono, Nomlaki, Pit River, Pomo, Samish, Serrano, Shasta, Siuslaw, Spokane, Stillaguamish, Tachi, Tillamook, Tolowa, Tulalip, Tule River, Umatilla, Umpqua, Wailaki, Washor, Washoe, Wiyot, Wintun. Yana, Yokuts, Yuki, and Yurok tribes.

## Achomawi

The Achomawi live on the Alturas Indian Rancheria in California and are federally recognized. The word 'Achomawi' means "river people" (encyclopedia.com, 2019). They operate the Desert Rose Casino and the Rose Café (500Nations.com, 1999-2023). The tribe did not exist until 1924 when the Office of Indian Affairs bought 20 acres for about 40 homeless Indians (Magagnini, 2015).

## Health & Healing Then

Since the tribe did not exist until 1924, there is no record of past health & healing practices.

## Health & Healing Now

There are only two tribal members who descended from the original 40 Native residents. The Achomawi have adopted non-Natives to increase federal health and education grants that are based on the number of enrolled tribal members. In 2015, the tribe had three to seven members (Magagnini, 2015).

## Impact on Health of Interaction with White Culture Then

Since the tribe did not exist until 1924, there is no record of health impact from interactions with White culture.

## Impact on Health of Interaction with White Culture Now

The economic health of the Achomawi tribe has been impacted by the adoption of two White men who have divided the small tribe in conflict over revenues. The Desert Rose Casino makes about $700,000 in revenue annually and receives $1.1 million in revenue sharing from California's large casino tribes. The tribe also receives several hundred thousand dollars in federal funds for tribal governments. Wanting to diversify their finances, the tribe adopted White men who said they could get a second casino. Neither achieved that goal, but they are now (as of 2015) being paid monthly. One, who is in prison for fraud, received $5,000/month and the other served as tribal administrator for $7,500/month and $400,000 in retroactive payments. The two descendants of original members, a brother and sister, quarreled over the direction of the tribe and the tribe has spent over $2 million on legal fees without resolution (Magagnini, 2015).

## *Bear River Band*

The Bear River Band of the Rohnerville Rancheria includes members of three tribes: Mattole, Bear River, and Wiyot. The tribe is federally recognized and resides in California. Mattole comprise many of the members and 'Mattole' means "member of the Athapaskan people". The Bear River Band's enterprises include the Bear River Casino Resort, Family Entertainment Center, and Recreation Center, a gas station, and a tobacco shop. The Tribe was established in 1910 as a home for homeless Native people (Bear River Band of the Rohnerville Rancheria, 2021).

## Health & Healing Then

The Mattole and Bear River group intermarried. Their land use pattern had them move within their territory to be where seasonal foods became available. Family groups shared a winter site. Small bands that were kinship-based collaborated together in hunting and fishing. Headmen were selected for their ability to resolve disputes and their wealth, but ruled by making suggestions within the small social structure. Small bands used plant resources in season. Acorns from the oak trees were processed for storage. They traded for obsidian which had ceremonial value. They also practiced annual burning to induce plant growth in the spring. This environmental manipulation reduced overgrowth and maintained wild grasses, shrubs, and clover on the prairies (Roscoe, 1985).

## Health & Healing Now

Since the Bear River Band was not federally recognized until 1983, services are limited. The Tribe is working to secure grants to develop and expand health, social services, education, housing, cultural renovation, and economic development. Social Services has several programs to support tribal residents:

1. Healthy Families Program has monthly classes for tribal families to develop life skills;
2. Elders Program provides support for elders, including home visits, referrals, social activities, cleaning, and utility assistance;
3. Lice Policy provides supplies to prevent lice infestations in homes;
4. Food for People provides food distributions monthly for families on and off the Rancheria;

5. Victim Services provides support, services, and advocacy to members affected by crime; and

6. Homeless Housing Assistance Program supports tribal households who are homeless or at risk for homelessness (Bear River Band of the Rohnerville Rancheria, 2021).

## Impact on Health of Interaction with White Culture Then

Although the Mattole had brief interactions with traders and trappers before the 1800s, the mid-nineteenth century brought an influx of White settlers who took over Native land for cattle ranching. Soon, they were living on the most suitable agricultural lands. By 1859, many traditional foods were depleted or kept from the Mattole by White settlers claiming the land. They also shot much of the game in the area and exterminated elk herds in the region along with reducing the number of deer. The Mattole killed and ate the settlers' cattle to keep from starving. Settlers engaged in genocide by offering bounties for killing Mattole people. Eventually, the tribe was placed on a reservation and descendants were discouraged from practicing their way of life, including religious rituals (Roscoe, 1985).

## Impact on Health of Interaction with White Culture Now

The Bear River Band is collaborating with California State Polytechnical University at Humboldt to have cultural classes including a weaving circle. They also have joined the Farmer's Market group with partners at Cal Poly Humboldt helping volunteer weekly and preparations are continuing with plantings for the Tribal Garden greenhouse (Bear River Band of the Rohnerville Rancheria, 2021).

## *Big Lagoon Rancheria*

Big Lagoon Rancheria is the home of the Tolowa and Yurok tribes in California. The Tribe has been federally recognized since 1918 and has 24 enrolled members and eight households in the 20-acre reservation (Unite Indian Health Services, 2022). Since Yurok will be discussed later, 'Tolowa' means "People of Lake Earl" (Everything Explained Today, 2009-2023). The Tribe partners with the Los Coyotes Band to operate the

Barstow Casino and Resort and also owns the Arcata Hotel (AAA Native Arts, 1999-2023).

## Health & Healing Then

Tolowa shamans could be men or women and they treated the sick with trances, dancing, magic formulas, and sucking sources of evil out of the sick persons. The Headman was usually the richest person in the village (Countries and Their Culture, 2023). The Tolowa used a variety of plants medicinally. California mugwort was used as a tea for pinworms. Wild ginger leaves were a poultice for infections. Western skunk cabbage was a treatment for lumbago, arthritis, or stroke. The roots of Oregon grape treated coughs and purified the blood. Cuts and boils were treated with a poultice from Mexican plantain or dwarf plantain (Baker, 1981).

## Health & Healing Now

United Indian Health Services incorporates traditional customs and values into health care services at the Potawot Health Village Clinic where the Blue Lagoon Rancheria tribe can obtain chronic and acute outpatient services, including obstetric services. Pediatric and well child care services are available along with referrals for mental health, infectious diseases, and cardiology (United Indian Health Services, 2022).

## Impact on Health of Interaction with White Culture Then

The Tolowa experienced epidemics of smallpox and other infectious diseases, like cholera and measles, in the 1800s resulting in high mortality (Countries and Their Cultures, 2023). Over 90% of their population was murdered by Whites in a series of massacres and attempted genocide in the mid-1800s. By 1910, their population dropped from 1,000 to 150 due to these attacks for which Gov. Gavin Newsom apologized in 2019 (Everything Explained Today, 2002-2023).

## Impact on Health of Interaction with White Culture Now

The Business, Consumer Services and Housing Agency has joined with the California Interagency Council on Homelessness to grant $20 million for the Big Lagoon Rancheria and 21 other tribes in the state to support projects addressing housing insecurity and homelessness in their communities. The Big Lagoon Rancheria will receive $1.5 million to develop facilities and a program supporting transitional-aged youth (CAL ICH, 2023).

## Blue Lake Rancheria

The Blue Lake Rancheria is home to Yurok, Wiyot, and Tolowa tribes in California. It was founded in 1908 for homeless Indians. After being terminated in 1958, it again received federal recognition in 1983 (Blue Lake Rancheria, 2023). Since Tolowa was previously discussed and Wiyot will be addressed later, the focus here will be on Yurok. 'Yurok' means "downriver" (encyclopedia.com, 2019). Blue Lake Rancheria has multiple enterprises, including the Blue Lake Casino & Hotel and Powers Creek Brewery (Blue Lake Rancheria, 2023).

### Health & Healing Then

The Yurok Tribe believed that redwood trees were sacred living beings, and they were respected and served as guardians over sacred places. Canoes were also essential to transport dancers and ceremonial people to the White Deerskin Dance. Dentalia shell necklaces were used in ceremonies, such as the White Deerskin Dance. Jump Dance, and Brush Dance (Yurok Tribe, 2023). Plants were also used medicinally. Prince's pine treated aches and pains and relaxed muscles. Mountain balm treated coughs and colds. Western skunk cabbage was used for stroke, arthritis, and lumbago. Broadleaf plantain was used as a poultice for boils and a giant trillium poultice treated burns (Baker, 1981).

### Health & Healing Now

The Blue Lake Rancheria focuses on food sovereignty by creating and managing multiple food programs to serve tribal members, children, K-12 students, and elders. Over 60,000 meals are prepared and delivered annually The Tribe also has a community garden which grows all natural foods for the meals programs and restaurants. The Tribe also is transitioning to a zero-carbon community for environmental, economic, health, and resilience benefits. Their goal is to achieve zero net carbon emissions by 2030 through public/private partnerships and collaboration with local, regional, state, and national agencies. (Blue Lake Rancheria, 2023).

## Impact on Health of Interaction with White Culture Then

In the mid-1800s, White settlers and gold miners moved into Yurok country and destroyed villages. Many Yurok were massacred, and disease killed many others. At least 75% of the Yurok tribe died by the end of the gold rush. When the tribe was relocated  to a reservation, there was pressure to learn English and eliminate tribal customs and traditions (Yurok Tribe, 2023).

## Impact on Health of Interaction with White Culture Now

The Blue Lake Rancheria Tribe supports education, public safety, transportation, and social service/community-building activities for the region as well as to support tribal members. They have provided funds for scholarships, the Blue Lake Unified School District, the Blue Lake Volunteer Fire Department, City of Blue Lake Parks and Recreation City of Blue Laske Wastewater Treatment Plant, local non-profits and advocates, and emergency preparedness strategies (Blue Lake Rancheria, 2023).

## *Cahuilla*

Several Cahuilla Bands are federally recognized in California. 'Cahuilla' means " the master," "the one who rules'" or "the powerful one" (Augustine Band of Cahuilla Indians, 2018). Here are the Bands and their enterprises:

| Cahuilla Band | Enterprises |
|---|---|
| Agua Caliente Band of Cahuilla Indians | The Agua Caliente Band's enterprises include Agua Caliente Casinos, Indian Canyons Golf Resort, Agua Caliente Fuel, Tahquitz Canyon, and the Spa at S'ec-he (Agua Caliente Band of Cahuilla Indians, 2023) |

| Cahuilla Band | Enterprises |
|---|---|
| Augustine Band of Cahuilla Indians | The Augustine Band has the Three7Nine Enterprises Management Corporation which oversees the Augustine Casino, Cahuilla Ranch, and Temalpakh Farm (Augustine Band of Cahuilla Indians, 2018). |
| Cabazon Band of Mission Indians | The Cabazon Band has a tribally-owned and operated electrical facility which provides water, wastewater, electrical, and fiber optic services on over 1,600 acres. It also provides electricity to the Events Center and the Fantasy Springs Resort and Casino (Cabazon, Tribal Utility Authority, 2023). |
| Cahuilla Band of Mission Indians | The Cahuilla Band of Indians' enterprises include the Cahuilla Casino Hotel and the Mountain Sky Travel Center (Cahuilla Band of Indians, 2023). |
| Los Coyotes Band of Cahuilla & Cupeño Indians | The Los Coyotes Band has the Los Coyotes Reservation Campground and issues hiking permits for Hot Springs Mountain (Los Coyotes Band of Cahuilla & Cupeño Indians, 2021). |
| Morongo Band of Mission Indians | The Morongo Band owns and operates the Morongo Casino, Resort and Spa (Morongo Band of Mission Indians, 2022). |
| Ramona Band of Cahuilla | The Ramona Band of Cahuilla has developed its reservation off-grid using wind and solar energy with propane as a back-up energy source. Their Red Hawks hand crew has been contracted for projects on federal lands and dispatched to incidents throughout California for fire suppression services, mop-up and assistance after incidents. The Band |

| Cahuilla Band | Enterprises |
|---|---|
|  | wants to further develop the Red Hawks for dispatch throughout the U.S. (Ramona Band of Cahuilla, 2021). |
| Santa Rosa Band of Cahuilla Indians | The Santa Rosa Band provides electricity to local, state, and federal agencies at Toro Peak under the Santa Rosa Cahuilla Corporation and owns and operates the Santa Rosa Pit Stop (Santa Rosa Band of Cahuilla Indians, 2023). |
| Torres Martinez Desert Cahuilla Indians | The Torres Martinez Desert Cahuilla Indians own and operate the Red Earth Casino and the Torres Martinez Travel Center (Torres Martinez Desert Cahuilla Indians, n.d.). |

## Health & Healing Then

The mesquite bean and other plants were carefully gathered to avoid damaging the plant. Snakeweed was used as a cure for toothaches and as a gargle for sore throats. Wild tobacco was considered sacred, and it was used for medicinal or ritual purposes by shamans (Spotted Bird, 2000). Cahuilla spiritual beliefs involved supernatural forces and beings. These were reflected in their rituals and ceremonies that included healing and renewal of the natural world (Cahuilla Band of Indians, 2023).

## Health & Healing Now

The Morongo Band is an example of a tribe with multiple programs to promote the health and well-being of their people. Morongo Child and Family Services provides crisis intervention and focuses on safeguarding the rights of families and children with support and professional personnel. The Victims Service Program has a Legal Advocate and Attorney to assist at-risk victims/survivors with access to services free of charge. Assistance is available for primary and secondary victims as well as related victims. Safety and confidentiality are paramount in their services. The Morongo Elder Program provides tribal elders with recreational activities and their annual Christmas party includes Elder Guests from other reservations. The Morongo Tribal TANF Program provides financial assistance, education, job training, and career development. Besides referrals for community services, this team provides education and activities for youth and promotes healthy families by demonstrating life skills (Morongo Band of Mission Indians, 2022).

## Impact on Health of Interaction with White Culture Then

Many Cahuilla people died in infectious disease epidemics after interaction with White people. In 1863, a smallpox epidemic decimated the tribe resulting in deaths of over 80% of the population (Augustine Band of Cahuilla Indians, 2018). After establishment of reservations, the Dawes Act of 1887 divided reservation land to individual members wanting to assimilate into White culture. Children were sent to government schools and traditional Native spiritual practices were banned (Agua Caliente Band of Cahuilla Indians, 2023).

## Impact on Health of Interaction with White Culture Now

The Temalpakh Farm uses sustainable, organic practices to protect the land and create healthy products certified by the California Certified Organic Farmers as USDA organic. Their produce is nutritious and wholesome for the community because produce is only treated with materials approved and certified by the Organic Material Review Institute (Augustine Band of Cahuilla Indians, 2018). The Cahuilla Band of Indians believes in the importance of philanthropy to address community and social needs, provide innovative solutions, become engaged and active in the community, promote collaboration, and fund neglected or underfunded areas. They provide funds for schools, sports programs, civic, and educational programs (Cahuilla Band of Indians, 2023). The Agua Caliente Band also provides funds to local food banks, schools, libraries, youth groups, healthcare organizations, and public service agencies to give back to the community (Agua Caliente Band of Cahuilla Indians, 2023). The Morongo Band also funds community outreach to support local and national nonprofit organizations (Morongo Band of Mission Indians, 2022).

## Diegueno/Kumeyaay

Numerous Diegueño/Kumeyaay Bands are federally recognized in California. The Kumeyaay were called Diegueño by the Spanish after the Mission of San Diego (Britannica.com, n.d.).

Here are the California Bands and their enterprises:

| Diegueno/Kumeyaay Bands | Enterprises |
| --- | --- |
| Barona Band of Mission Indians | The Barona Band of Mission Indians own and operate the Barona Valley Ranch Resort and Casino and the Barona Gas Station (Barona Band on Mission Indians, 2020). |
| Campo Band of the Kumeyaay Nation | The Campo Kumeyaay Nation's enterprises include Mut Hei (economic development), the Golden Acorn Casino & Travel Center, Campo Materials (construction materials), and Kumeyaay Wind farm (Campo Kumeyaay Nation, 2013). |
| Capitan Grande Indian Reservation | The reservation is uninhabited-See Barona Band of Mission Indians (Kumeyaay, 2023). |
| Ewiiaapaayp Band of Kumeyaay Indiana | The Ewiiaapaayp Band of the Cuyapaipe Reservation has seven enrolled members. Their enterprise Leaning Rock Water dissolved in 2020. No other enterprise is found, except an annual three-day Powwow in July with native arts, a barbeque, and camping (Wikiwand.com, n.d.). |
| Inaja-Cosmit Band of Indians | The Inaja Band of the Inaja & Cosmit Reservation had 21 enrolled members in 1973 and none lived on the reservation. No enterprises are found (Wikipedia.com, 2023). |
| Jamul Indian Village | The Jamul Indian Village owns and operates the Jamul Casino and Jamul Indian Village Development Corporation (Jamul Indian Village, 2021). |

| Diegueno/Kumeyaay Bands | Enterprises |
|---|---|
| La Posta Indian Reservation | La Posta owned and operated the La Posta Casino and Marie's Restaurant which closed in 2021 (Everything Explained Today, 2009-2023). Their website does not list any current enterprises (La Posta Band of Mission Indians, n.d.). |
| Manzanita Band of the Kumeyaay Nation | Manzanita Band does not list any businesses or enterprises. They were awarded funding for solar PV energy in 2020 (tribalsolar.org, 2020). |
| Mesa Grande Band of Diegueño Indians | The Mesa Grande Band farms, raises livestock, or works in neighboring towns (Mesa Grande, 2023). |
| San Pasqual Band of Mission Indians | The San Pasqual Band's enterprises include the Valley View Casino & Hotel, Native Oaks Golf Club, Shawii Kitchen, the Pit Stop Market, and the Horizon Fuel Center (San Pasqual Band of Mission Indians, 2018). |
| Santa Ysabel Band of Diegueño Indians | Iipay Nation of Santa Ysabel's enterprises include the Santa Ysabel Botanical Facility (cannabis), and Biostar Solar. They are also groundbreaking for the Santa Ysabel Roadside Store in October 2023 (Iipay Nation of Santa Ysabel, n.d.). |
| Sycuan Band of the Kumeyaay Nation | The Sycuan Band operates the Sycuan Casino Resort, the Marina Gateway Hotel and Conference Center, the Sycuan Market and convenience store, and are part-owner of a Major League Soccer team (Sycuan Casino Resort, n.d.). |
| Viejas Band of Kumeyaay Indians | The Viejas Band owns and operates the Viejas Casino and Resort, Viejas Outlets, and Ma-Tar-Awa RV Park (Viejas Band of Kumeyaay, 2022). |

## Health & Healing Then

The Kumeyaay used herbs and plants for medicinal purposes. Aloe Vera pulp was spread on sores to heal and for any skin conditions. Angel hair (growing on buckwheat) was used for spider and insect bites when applied as pulp. Oak apple could be chewed for a sore throat or boiled as a disinfectant. Banana skin and cucumber relieved itch and stings of burns or insect bites. Black walnut could relieve stomach ailments. Buckwheat as a tea could relieve diarrhea in babies. Young cactus leaves could help heal gum problems. Cat tails soothed burns and poison ivy. Elderberry stems could heal diabetic sores and blossoms reduced fevers. A fern poultice was used to heal difficult wounds. Horsetail stems as a tea were used to control blood pressure. Juniper berries could freshen bad breath if chewed and tea from berries or leaves was used for kidney or liver problems. Watermelon seeds in tea treated urinary infections. Yerba Santa treated colds and congestion and the blossoms treated asthma (Kumeyaay, 2023).

## Health & Healing Now

The Manzanita Band was exposed to electrical pollution from wind turbines on a neighboring reservation in 2012. 'Stray voltage' caused levels of transient voltage 1,000 times above normal. This can increase risk of diabetes, cancer, leukemia, heart disease, and attention deficit disorder. This issue was debated, and a Manzanita tribal consultant stated that children there had higher rates of attention deficit disorder and sleep disorders and cancer are also present (Jannen, 2012). In 2020, a project began to provide solar PV energy to Manzanita tribal homes and community buildings to address this issue (tribalsolar.org, 2020).

## Impact on Health of Interaction with White Culture Then

Between 1850-1875, settlers came and took over tribal lands. According to an article in 1869, 22,000 Natives in California died of deprivation and disease (mesa Grande, 2023).The Barona Band was removed from the Capitan Grande Reservation in 1932 when the city bought the reservation to build a reservoir. Some federal funds from the sale enabled the Band to buy the current reservation. Until the early 1990s, the Tribe lived in poverty without electricity or other services and struggled to exist by ranching and farming (Barona Band of Mission Indians, 2020).

## Impact on Health of Interaction with White Culture Now

The Barona Band has rebounded from poverty through gaming and has given back to their people and their community. They provide 100% of vision, dental, and medical coverage to all tribal members, including non-tribal spouses and dependents. They also have created over 3,500 jobs and 97% are held by non-Natives. The Band donates to multiple charitable organizations and has created infrastructure, including housing, wastewater treatment, and education expansion (Barona Band of Mission Indians, 2020). The Sycuan Band also donates to charitable and nonprofit organizations (Sycuan Casino Resort, n.d.). In 2021, the Manzanita tribal police chief admitted selling fake badges to outside wealthy individuals to become "members' of the Manzanita Tribal Police Department for large payments by receiving a badge supposedly letting the holder carry a concealed weapon. He admitted he stole over $300,000 in this scam and has been prosecuted (East county News Service, 2021).

## *Chemehuevi*

The Chemehuevi Indian Tribe is federally recognized and located in California. The word 'Chemehuevi' for themselves means "people" (Feller, n.d.). Tribal enterprises include the Havasu Landing Resort & Casino, a campground, and a marina (Chemehuevi Indian Tribe, 2023).

## Health & Healing Then

The Chemehuevi had a spiritual connection to the land. Their cultural practices encompassed ceremonies and rituals (Stamper, 2023). The Mountain Sheep Song and Deer Song were inherited, and Chemehuevi could only hunt in those areas if the man owned the song. Only a song owner could sing it ritually. A High Chief taught his people a moral code and led them in peace. The High Chiefs' Talking Song was only sung at Mourning ceremonies and funerals (Feller, n.d.).

## Health & Healing Now

The Wellness Center has a variety of programs to ensure tribal health and wellness. The Community Health Representative provides case management and assessment to help clients with short and long-term goals. The Community Health Representative (CHR) conducts group and individual education/prevention services and assists with home management skills. Traditional Native approaches are incorporated in multiple settings to provide primary care services. The Wellness Center also provides diabetes services, an alcohol/substance abuse program, child abuse services, and domestic violence programs (Chemehuevi Indian Tribe, 2023).

## Impact on Health of Interaction with White Culture Then

In 1908, the Supreme Court ruled that Native water rights would have priority over other locations. In the twentieth century the Bureau of Reclamation began a canal to send waters on Chemehuevi land to Tucson and Phoenix from the Colorado River. The creation of the Parker Dam and Lake Havasu reservoir washed away homes and flooded covered productive farmland, leaving the Tribe with desert they were unable to farm. In the 1960s, the Tribe was not federally recognized and didn't receive infrastructure funding to access the water via canals, pipes, and pumps. The government allotted them about 3.7 billion gallons of water annually, but they could not transport the water to expand farming (Olade & Smith, 2023).

## Impact on Health of Interaction with White Culture Now

The Chemehuevi Environmental Department is encouraging neighboring cities to collaborate to protect the environment. Small changes in precipitation and temperature may seriously impact plants and animals in the area. Drought and wildfires have increased which destroy plants and wildlife. Planting non-Native plants and irrigation of crop fields leads to increased salt levels in soil that won't support indigenous plants. The Environmental Department is developing innovative, cost-effective methods to slow or stop abuse of the land. They are focusing on promoting community awareness, education, action, and participation by everyone who impacts the environment (Chemehuevi Indian Tribe, 2023).

## Cher-Ae-Heights Indian Community of Trinidad Rancheria

The Trinidad Rancheria is home to Wiyot, Tolowa, and Yurok people in California. The Tribe is federally recognized and, since Yurok and Tolowa tribes have been previously discussed, the Wiyot tribe will be examined here. 'Wiyot' is the name of a river in their homeland (native-languages.org, 1998-2020). Enterprises in the Trinidad Rancheria include the Sunset Restaurant, the Seascape Restaurant and Pier, Seascape Home Rental, and the Heights Casino Trinidad Rancheria, 2023).

### Health & Healing Then

The Wiyot population declined between the 1800s and 1910 from physical genocide, European diseases, forced removal, starvation, and exposure (Wiyot Tribe, n.d.).

### Health & Healing Now

The Social Services Department provides services to tribal families in the Child Welfare System. The Department delivers case management, school and court advocacy, home visits, and referrals for children when placement is indicated. Care providers and guardians who foster eligible children receive support and advocacy. The Department staff facilitate reconnecting families to traditional cultural practices. Substance Use Disorder Services conducts assessments, education, case management, counseling sessions (individual and group), referrals, aftercare and cultural activities. Victim Services provides emergency services, advocacy, referrals, emotional support, and safety planning. Behavioral Health offers assessment, referrals, individual counseling sessions, Neuro-Feedback Intervention, and therapeutic groups for crime victims (Trinidad Rancheria, 2023).

## Impact on Health of Interaction with White Culture Then

The Trinidad Rancheria began in 1906 when Congress permitted the government to purchase small land tracts to house homeless California Indians. The Rancheria was originally Yurok lands and residents were Yurok, Tolowa, and Wiyot who shared similar cultures. For years, they required permits to access and gather native plants and medicines on their lands and could not access spiritual and sacred places in state parks (California Department of Parks and Recreation, 2023).

## Impact on Health of Interaction with White Culture Now

The Trinidad Rancheria Environmental Program's mission is to protect land, air, water, wildlife, and cultural resources. They have monitored water quality for over two decades and their data is accessible to the public online via the Water Quality Portal. They work with the community to maintain and improve watersheds and coastal waters for everyone's benefit as active participants in the Trinidad Bay Watershed Council. Since non-point source pollution (pollution from a large area instead of a single source) threatens the Rancheria's water supply, they identify potential sources and implement practices and projects to minimize the impact on local water quality. The Rancheria also protects Trinidad Bay by identifying, preventing, and eliminating sources of contamination. The Environmental Program has increased their capacity to respond to oil spills in the harbor and its surrounding waters. Their Invasive Weed Management Program manages invasive plants on tribal land. In 2022, they successfully removed over 8,000 pounds of invasive plants from local watersheds (Trinidad Rancheria, 2023).

## *Confederated Tribes of Siletz*

The Confederated Tribes of Siletz Indians are multiple tribes in Oregon who are federally recognized. These tribes are Clatsop, Chinook, Klickitat, Molala, Kalapuya, Tillamook, Alesa, Siuslaw/Lower Umpqua, Coos, Coquelle, Upper Umpqua, Tututni, Chetco, Tolowa, Takelma, Galice/Applegate, and Shasta. 'Siletz' means "crooked river" (encyclopedia.com, 2019). Tribal enterprises include the Siletz Tribal

Business Corporation for economic development, the Chinook Winds Casino Resort, and RV parks (Confederated Tribes of Siletz Indians, 2023).

## Health & Healing Then

Shamans learned from guardian spirits in dreams. Special sweathouses were used to cure illnesses. Some sickness was believed to be caused by objects inside the patient's body. The shaman waved a carved wand and pierced the person's skin. Then, he sucked out the object which he often brought with him. Shamans also used potions for fertility, luck in hunting, and longevity. If a shaman couldn't heal successfully, he could be killed. The tribes had many ceremonies, including the naming ceremony for children, celebration of puberty, and powwows where feather dances and fiddle dances occurred. The Siletz believed that after death bad people went to land below the earth and good people went to the land in the sky. The Ghost Dance religion was practiced from the 1870s and the Indian Shaker Church in 1923 combined elements of traditional practices with elements of Christianity (encyclopedia.com, 2019).

## Health & Healing Now

The Siletz have an extensive behavioral health program. Their Prevention Program is based on four healing principles:

1.  "Healing from problems associated with alcohol, tobacco, and other drugs comes from within ourselves, our Tribe, and our community."
2.  "Our journey is linked to the past. We will use traditions, cultural values, and knowledge to strengthen ourselves and our community."
3.  "Positive messaging to our children and families about the harmful effects of alcohol, tobacco, and other drugs."
4.  "The healing of the individual, the community, and the tribe go hand in hand and are inseparable" (Confederated Tribes of Siletz Indians, 2023).

Substance use treatment includes assessment, evaluation, referral to resources, education, counseling, and recreational therapy. Transitional living centers provide housing, life skills, referrals, education for parents, prevention of domestic violence, Talking Circles, and support for recovery. CEDARR (Community Efforts Demonstrating the Ability to Rebuild and Restore) began as a Meth Task Force and uses community education to achieve its goals (Confederated Tribes of Siletz Indians, 2023).

## Impact on Health of Interaction with White Culture Then

Pandemics involving nearly the total population resulted in 75% to 90% of deaths from smallpox and other diseases beginning in the 1770s. Trappers engaged in economic warfare in the 1800s. When White settlers arrived, about 2.5 million acres were claimed by settlers and Native people were killed to acquire the best locations. The reservation was established in late 1855 and the tribes were removed to there. This period was marked by violence, disease, starvation, poverty, and depression. The tribes were taught faming and worked long hours for little results. Allotment in the late 1800s had the effect of reducing tribal lands and the traditional way of life (Confederated Tribes of Siletz Indians, 2023).

## Impact on Health of Interaction with White Culture Now

The Siletz Charitable Contribution Fund uses part of gaming revenues for distribution to charitable organizations. In 2022, the Tribal Council approved 134 awards for $909,235. Their charitable donations focused on health, education. public safety, and food security. These grants support local nonprofits and governments in neighboring counties. Recipients include schools, libraries, cultural organizations, alcohol and drug treatment groups, environmental and natural resources groups, the Oregon Council on Problem Gambling, historical preservation, housing organizations, fire and emergency responders, and arts organizations (Confederated Tribes of Siletz Indians, 2023).

## *Elk Valley Rancheria*

Elk Valley Rancheria was a piece of land in California reserved for homeless Indians after the Landless California Indians Act of 1906. Tribes comprising the Rancheria include Tolowa and Yurok people and the

Rancheria is federally recognized. The Rancheria owns and operates the Elk Valley Casino with plans to create a world-class destination and resort (Elk Valley Rancheria, 2023).

## Health & Healing Then

Tolowa-See Big Lagoon Rancheria

Yurok-See Blue Lake Rancheria

## Health & Healing Now

The Elk Valley Rancheria invests in education, both in college education for tribal members and by supporting early childhood education programs at Elk Valley Head Start (United Indian Health Service, 2022).

## Impact on Health of Interaction with White Culture Then

Tolowa-See Big Lagoon Rancheria

Yurok-See Blue Lake Rancheria

## Impact on Health of Interaction with White Culture Now

California's Proposition 64 has required tribes to give up sovereignty if opening a cannabis business. The Proposition legalized recreational cannabis, but required tribes to cede authority to the state government. The Elk Valley Rancheria established a regulatory framework and authorized an independent marijuana business to set up a cultivation facility on tribal land. When the company was refused a state license, the tribe entered into an agreement with the Del Norte County government to allow the Rancheria to lease land to cannabis tenants that would be regulated by the tribe. The tribe and state both license the facility. In 2019, the tenant business achieved a license by the California Department of Food and Agriculture. The economic impact for the Rancheria, the tenant company, and the County has validated the tribe's efforts to use cannabis as an additional economic engine (Herrington, 2020).

## *Hoopa Valley Tribe*

The Hoopa Valley Tribe is comprised of Hupa Indians and is federally recognized. 'Hupa' means "people of the place where the trails return" (Wikipedia, 2023). Their economic enterprises include the Hoopa Mini Mart, Hoopa Shopping Center, Lucky Bear Casino, the Tsewenaldin Inn Motel, and a cement company (Hoopa Valley Tribe, 2003-2020).

### Health & Healing Then

The Hupa Tribe used six annual ceremonies to express their spirituality. These ceremonies were:

1. New Year's Festival to connect tribal members to the natural world;
2. Planting Festival to pray to the creator and bless seeds for a good harvest;
3. Make-the-World Ceremony to honor all living things;
4. Two Solstice Celebrations to thank the creator for life and pray for longevity for all;
5. Home Dance/Tree Dance to invoke peace; and
6. Harvest Festival to thank the creator for the harvest (Cassar, 2023).

They used music to share stories and traditions between generations and used plants like yarrow leaves and wild ginger root for medicinal purposes (Cassar, 2023).

### Health & Healing Now

In 2021, the Tribal Council declared a state of emergency about the local opioid epidemic. The Tribe has developed several actions since then to address this concern. These actions include:

1. CPR education and weekly Narcan training;
2. Visits to grades 3-12 by behavioral health experts to educate about dangers of drugs;
3. Increasing youth job opportunities;

4. Posting anti-drug abuse signs;
5. Grief talking circles;
6. Increasing focus on data collection to attract funding for this issue;
7. Lobbying at State and Federal levels for additional resources;
8. Increasing community awareness about the crisis; and
9. Partnering with the Humboldt County Drug Task Force and the Klamath-Trinity Joint Unified School District (Hoopa Valley Tribe, 2023).

## Impact on Health of Interaction with White Culture Then

The Hoopa Valley Tribe leased land by the Copper Bluff Mine in 1958 to Celtor Chemical Works. The company extracted zinc and copper from the mine for four years, but didn't pay the royalty payments to the tribe from 1960. The company also was cited for polluting the Trinity River and left tailings (waste materials left after processing ore) at the river and mill site. This Superfund site was cleaned up between 1983 and1988, but additional contamination was discovered in 2016 (Hoopa Valley Tribe, 2023).

## Impact on Health of Interaction with White Culture Now

The San Mateo High School Interact Club in coordination with the Rotary Club has installed a playground at the Tish Tang Campground and is working with the Hoopa Valley Tribe to install additional play structures in the tribal community (Hoopa Valley Tribe, 2023). As follow-up to the previous section, the EPA and the Hoopa Valley Tribe plan a second major clean-up of the Celtor Chemical Works site. This process will involve excavation of sites to remove contaminants and remove mine tailings so people won't be exposed to this contaminated waste. The EPA has also consulted with the Hoopa Valley Tribal Fisheries and the National Marine Fisheries Service about the project. The main exposure concern is ingestion of wind-blown particles in this recreation area and closure of river access during the clean-up period is essential for health of users (Hoopa Valley Tribe, 2023).

## *Indians of the Santa Ynez Reservation*

The Santa Ynez Band of Chumash Indians is federally recognized. 'Chumash' originally meant "the first people" and today's elders say "bead maker" or "seashell people" (encytclopedia.com, 2019). The Band's enterprises include the Chumash Casino, Chumash Capital Investments LLC (economic development), the Corque Hotel, Chumash Gas Stations, and real estate investments (Santa Ynez Reservation, n.d.).

### Health & Healing Then

Shaman priests were also astronomers and women could become chiefs and priests. Caves were used for religious ceremonies and Chumash drawings illustrated their bond with the environment (Santa Ynez Reservation, n.d.). The Chumash priest-astrologers could find meaning in the position of heavenly bodies. They also took toloache from jimsonweed which caused them to go into trances and see visions. Then, they painted pictographs of their visions in sacred caves (encyclopedia.com, 2019).

### Health & Healing Now

The Santa Ynez Tribal Health Clinic provides multiple services to all residents of the Santa Ynez Valley and Santa Barbara communities. These services include:

1.  Medical primary care for all age groups (immunizations, examinations, podiatry, chiropractic care, same-day care, and minor surgical procedures);
2.  Dental services;
3.  Behavioral health services (psychotherapy, drug and alcohol counseling, psychiatric evaluation and medication management, suicide prevention, and mental health education); and
4.  Community and Social Services Programs (elder services, injury prevention services, child welfare services, and transportation for Chumash community members for health care appointments and 'essential errands') (Santa Ynez Reservation, n.d.).

## Impact on Health of Interaction with White Culture Then

After the Spanish arrived in 1769, they established five missions on Chumash lands and introduced European diseases that nearly decimated the tribe. In 1834, the Mexican authorities broke their promise to distribute remaining land among the Chumash which further reduced the Chumash population. By 1870, Americans became dominant, and the region prospered for everyone except the Chumash. Those who stayed in the area performed menial work on area ranches and farms to survive. Many tribal members left the reservation and those who remained had no running water or electricity (Santa Ynez Reservation, n.d.). During the Spanish period, children who were five or six years old were removed from their homes and put in dirty, disease-prone barracks where they were trained in occupations the Mexicans considered useful, performed labor without pay, and were made to attend religious services. If their parents protested, they were beaten, imprisoned, and sentenced to hard labor for disobedience (encyclopedia.com, 2019).

## Impact on Health of Interaction with White Culture Now

The Chumash Casino has become the largest employer in the Santa Ynez Valley and has increased tourism to the area. Besides improving the economic health of the Tribe, the Santa Ynez Band of Chumash Indians Foundation contributes to the Santa Barbara community. In September 2023, their Charity Golf Classic raised funds for Savie Health in Lompoc, the Sansum Diabetes Research Institute in Santa Barbara, and the California Central Coast Alzheimer's Association Chapter. Savie Health will use Foundation funds to provide patient care services to low-income and uninsured residents. Sansum will use Foundation funds to improve the lives of people impacted by diabetes and the Alzheimer's Chapter will provide support groups and education for local families (Santa Ynez Reservation, n.d.).

## *Kalispel Indian Community*

The Kalispel Tribe of Indians is federally recognized and located in the State of Washington. 'Kalispel' means "ear pendants" in French describing tribal adornments (native-languages.org, 1998-2020). The Tribe has several diverse enterprises operated by the Kalispel Tribal Economic Authority. These include the Kalispel Casino, Kalispel Market & Fuel, Kalispel Auto Sales, and Kalispel Storage (Kalispel Tribe of Indians, 2023).

## Health & Healing Then

The Kalispel Tribe believed in spiritual forces and used traditional practices for spiritual guidance, connection to nature, and living in harmony with all creatures. They used dance and music in ceremonies to connect with the spirit world. Regalia represented tribal traditions and identity. Elders had an essential role in guiding tribal decisions and each clan had specific duties and responsibilities. They believed they were responsible for protecting the environment and that every creature had a spirit to be honored and respected. Traditional medicine used natural plants and herbs to treat sickness and promote wellness. Storytelling was used to hand down traditions and customs from one generation to another (Justo, 2023).

## Health & Healing Now

Kalispel Tribe Victim Assistance Services seeks to empower tribal citizens to end violence. Their advocacy services support:

1. Crime victims;
2. Victims of domestic violence, sexual assault, stalking and dating violence;
3. Legal and medical services;
4. Counseling and referral services;
5. Community outreach and education;
6. Support groups; and
7. Emergency assistance (Kalispel Tribe of Indians, 2023).

They also collaborate with other tribal communities to acknowledge the impact of crime on the reservations, its traumatic impact on families, and awareness of support and services available locally (Kalispel Tribe of Indians, 2023).

## Impact on Health of Interaction with White Culture Then

From 1880 to 1910, the Tribe lost much of its land to White settlers who claimed it under the Homestead Act. As the tribal population decreased, the Whites introduced alcohol which broke down the Kalispel family unit. The Tribe subsisted for many generations with unemployment, substandard housing, limited economic opportunities and prejudice and discrimination. In 1965, the Tribe had one telephone and only a couple of reservation homes had running water. Tribal members lived in poverty on land that was not suitable for development (Kalispel Tribe of Indians, 2023).

## Impact on Health of Interaction with White Culture Now

The Kalispel Tribe's Kalispel Charitable Fund supports numerous non-profit organizations in the area to improve everyone's lives. Funds are distributed in alignment with tribal goals in health care, education, environmental conservation, social services, and arts and cultural activities (Kalispel Tribe of Indians, 2023).

## *Karuk*

The Karuk Tribe is federally recognized. 'Karuk' means "upriver" (native-languages.org, 1998-2020). The Tribe owns and operates the Rain Rock Casino, the Klamath River RV Park, and Áan Chúuphan high-speed internet (Kurak Tribe, 2015).

## Health & Healing Then

The Karuk Tribe used the California mugwort as a poultice for rheumatism and arthritis. Little prince's pine leaves were drunk to treat kidney, bladder, and women's issues. Naked buckwheat roots prepared a medicine for abdominal ailments. Coastal manroot poultices could draw boils and heal bruises (Baker, 1981). The Karuk believed that a disease object lodged in the body or supernatural pain caused severe illness. Wrongdoing by a family member could also make children ill and the shaman forced a public confession to cure the child. Shamans received their fees in advance, but the fee had to be refunded if the patient died (encyclopedia.com, 2019).

## Health & Healing Now

In 1922, a groundbreaking was held for a new medical and dental office building to increase space and technology support. The Karuk Tribe Division of Victim Assistance increased educational outreach in 2022 to share information about human trafficking, sexual assault awareness, missing and murdered indigenous persons, elder abuse, domestic violence awareness, and identity theft prevention and awareness. The Tribe is also focusing on housing projects and college and vocational educational training (Karuk Tribe, 2015).

## Impact on Health of Interaction with White Culture Then

After interaction with White culture, the Karuk Tribe contracted diseases for which they had no immunity. They were also displaced and not recognized as a tribe until the 1970s (encyclopedia.com, 2019).

## Impact on Health of Interaction with White Culture Now

The Karuk Tribe joined with the Pacific Coast Federation of Fisherman's Associations and Environmental Law Foundation in 2023 to enforce a minimum waterflow standard for the Scott River, which supports most of the Southern Oregon-Northern California Coho remaining in the world. The California Department of Fish & Wildlife also urged this action for the Shasta River, an adjacent watershed, which is an important spawning area for Chinook salmon. The California Water Control Board endorsed these requests and is beginning to work on a permanent waterflow solution (Kurok Tribe, 2015).

## *Luiseño*

There are six federally recognized Luiseño tribes in California. An additional Luiseño tribe is not recognized. 'Luiseño' means "People of the West" (Bacich, 2023). Here is information about each federally recognized band's enterprises:

| Luiseño Bands | Enterprises |
|---|---|
| La Jolla Band of Luiseño Indians | The Band's enterprises include the La Jolla Trading Post and Casino, La Jolla Zip Zoom, and the La Jolla Indian Campground (CasinosAvenue, 2023). |
| Pala Band of Mission Indians | Pala Band enterprises include the Pala Casino, Fox Raceway, Pala SkatePark, Pala Fitness Center, and Pala Shooting Range (Pala Band of Mission Indians, 2023). |
| Pauma Band of Luiseño Mission Indians | The Pauma Band's enterprises include Casino Pauma and a thriving agricultural program (Pauma Band of Luiseño Indians, n.d.). |
| Pechanga Band of Indians | The Pechanga Band's enterprises include the Pechanga Resort and Casino, the RV Resort, and Pechanga Gas Station Plaza (Pechanga Band of Indians, 2023). |
| Rincon Band of Luiseño Indians | The Rincon Band's enterprises include the Rincon Economic Development Corporation and ownership of Harrah's Resort Southern California (Rincon Band of Luiseño Indians, 2023). |
| Soboba Band of Luiseño Indians | The Soboba Band's enterprises include Soboba Resort Casino, Soboba Roadrunner Express, Soboba Pharmacy, and the Soboba Economic Development Corporation (Soboba Band of Luiseño Indians, n.d.). |

## Health & Healing Then

People with religious knowledge had power because many beliefs were kept secret and those who received this knowledge were required to understand and use it correctly. Many animals, including ravens and rattlesnakes, had spiritual meaning. Rituals led by chiefs and shamans were part of everyone's life. These included birth, coming of age, marriage, and death ceremonies. Ceremonies for boys contained ordeals, visions, and dancing; while ceremonies for girls contained essential knowledge and advice for marriage. Music was part of the most important ceremonies (Bacich, 2023).

## Health & Healing Now

The Pauma Band and other Native bands developed a consortium in the 1970s called the Indian Health Council (IHC) and opened a modern clinic with expanded services in 2000. The culturally-appropriate health care resulted in multi-generational services. These services include prenatal care, well-child care, diabetes clinics, adult fitness classes, domestic violence prevention and treatment, prevention of youth substance abuse, orthodontics, eye clinics, mammograms, and podiatry. The IHC also provides outreach for youth programs, health fairs, environmental health, and rabies clinics for surrounding communities (Pauma Band of Luiseño Indians, n.d.). The Soboba Band is focusing on implementing clean energy solutions and installed a solar microgrid to combat power outages in their high-fire risk region. The microgrid provides critical services by powering the fire station and emergency operations center via mutual aid agreements with the Band and surrounding community (Soboba Band of Luiseño Indians, n.d.). The Rincon Band has a unique Equine-Assisted Experiential Health Therapy Program called Pegasus Rising. It is geared to returning military personnel with PTSD or Traumatic Brain Injury and their families using rescued horses (Rincon Band of Luiseño Indians, n.d.).

## Impact on Health of Interaction with White Culture Then

After the Rincon Reservation was created in 1875, the Luiseño people were forced to give up most of their ancestral lands and natural resources. They had to rely on the federal government for financial support to provide for tribal members. This support was meager and progress toward basic services often didn't exist at all or was very slow until 2002 when gaming arrived (Rincon Band of Luiseño Indians, 2023). The Pauma Band's treatment in the early twentieth century by Indian Health Service was indifferent. Local agencies used government directives to round-up native children who had their tonsils removed even if the hadn't been diagnosed with tonsilitis (Pauma Band of Luiseño Indians, n.d.).

## Impact on Health of Interaction with White Culture Now

The Pauma Band of Luiseño Indians uses gaming and economic resources to support health, education, welfare, and environmental services to meet tribal members' needs. Based on their social and cultural tradition to help the needy, the Band also partners with other organizations in the area by supporting schools, museums, universities, and cultural organizations. They purchased a certified organic farm and provide the Tierra Miguel Foundation with a long-term lease to ensure that the non-profit organization can preserve the farm for agricultural use (Pauma Band of Luiseño Indians, n.d.). The Pechanga Band of Indians issued a grant in 2019 to support the City of Lake Elsinore with traffic control during the "super bloom" in flower-covered hills. Traffic became a public safety issue and the Band and the city joined together to conserve and protect the natural resources as well as those enjoying the area (Pechanga Band of Indians, 2023).

## *Maidu*

There are six federally recognized Maidu tribes in California. Seven other tribes are not federally recognized. 'Maidu' means "man" (Alexander, 2023). Their enterprises are listed below.

| Maidu | Enterprises |
| --- | --- |
| Berry Creek Rancheria of Maidu Indians | The Berry Creek Rancheria's enterprises include the Gold Country Casino and Hotel, a smoke shop, Coffee Tyme coffee shop, a gas station, a mini-mart, and an RV Park (Berry Creek Rancheria of Maidu Indians, n.d.). |
| Enterprise Rancheria of Maidu Indians | The Enterprise Rancheria owns the Hard Rock Hotel & Casino Sacramento at Fire Mountain and the Rocktane Gas and Smoke Shop (Hard Rock Hotel & Casino Sacramento at Fire Mountain, 2023). |
| Greenville Rancheria of Maidu Indians | The Greenville Rancheria provides medical and dental services to the |

| Maidu | Enterprises |
|-------|-------------|
|  | community and its Environmental Protection Agency protects natural resources and addresses environmental health and safety issues (Greenville Rancheria, 2023). |
| Mechoopda Indian Tribe of Chico Rancheria | The Mechoopda Indian Tribe uses the Mechoopda Business Development as an economic engine. Other businesses include pest control, a coffee shop, a law office, a wedding and event videography company, and an auto repair company (Mechoopda Indian Tribe, 2023). |
| Mooretown Rancheria of Maidu Indians | Mooretown Rancheria's enterprises include Feather Falls Casino, Feather Falls Casino Brewing Company, The Lodge at Feather Falls Casino, and KOA RV Park (Mooretown Rancheria of Maidu Indians, 2022-2023). |
| Susanville Indian Rancheria | Susanville Indian Rancheria owns the Diamond Mountain Casino & Hotel (Diamond Mountain Casino & Hotel, 2023). It also is founder and owner of SIRCO Holdings to diversify tribal businesses. SIRCO has several construction companies that contract with the federal government, housing duplexes, a mini-mart and coffee/cigarette shop, and an environmental services firm (Susanville Indian Rancheria, 2023). |

## Health & Healing Then

The Maidu people lived in small villages and the main village had a ceremonial lodge where the headman lived. He advised tribal members and spoke for them with others. Religious practices involved male secret societies who used masks, dances, and spiritual rites. The Maidu respected animals and an annual celebration was the Bear Dance which honored bears leaving hibernation in the spring. Other ceremonies were conducted to ward off disease and natural disasters (Alexander, 2023). Local plants were used for medicine and their religion promoted a peaceful lifestyle (Mooretown Rancheria of Maidu Indians, 2022-2023).

## Health & Healing Now

Enterprise Rancheria has several tribal assistance programs. These include:

1. the Tribal Nutrition Assistance Program of $150/month for adult tribal members;
2. LIHEAP for help with residential utility bills and emergency assistance with utility shut-offs and energy related emergencies;
3. the Food Voucher Program to assist with grocery cost annually; and
4. the Emergency & Human Services Assistance Program/Disability Program for tribal elders (55 and older) and disabled tribal members for emergency support of $1,500/year.

The Tribe also provides grants for members starting local businesses. They also started the kNow Tobacco NOW! Project in 2020 to educate and empower people to understand the difference between Commercial Tobacco and Sacred Tobacco and stop smoking practices introduced by non-Natives (Enterprise Rancheria, 2023). Berry Creek Rancheria also provides homeowners' assistance, housing assistance, and emergency rental assistance to tribal members. Their Wellness Department believes that medicine is seen "in many forms, a smile, a laugh, a hug, a sound, the forms and symbols are limitless. Wellness is having the understanding that We are the medicine, and our feelings, thoughts, and behaviors are meaningful" (Berry Creek Rancheria of Maidu Indians, n.d.).

## Impact on Health of Interaction with White Culture Then

The Concow-Maidu tribe contracted European diseases after contact with White culture which reduced the population White settlers appropriated Native lands and government treaties promised benefits that didn't come. The tribe was left homeless, and members were forcibly removed to reservations where many died or were killed in the journey. This was the "Maidu Trail of Tears". The Mooretown Rancheria began on 80 acres with only eight acres that were usable (Mooretown Rancheria of Maidu Indians, 2022-2023).

## Impact on Health of Interaction with White Culture Now

The Greenville Rancheria's Tribal Environmental Protection Agency protects natural resources by coordinating with other agencies for environmental preservation. Some examples include:

1. air quality coordination with the Plumas County Public Health Department;
2. water protection coordination with multiple agencies;
3. soil protection using information from the U.S. Forest Service and National Resources Conservation Service;
4. timber harvesting to protect spiritual and cultural sites and watersheds;
5. safety programs following standards of the Department of Homeland Security, Indian Health Service, State Indian Health Program, and FEMA; and
6. environmental health coordination with Tehama and Plumas counties, the State of California, the Bureau of Indian Affairs, and Indian Health Services (Greenville Rancheria, 2023).

## *Miwok (Me-Wuk)*

There are ten Miwok tribes that are federally recognized. There are also seven non-federally recognized tribes in California. 'Miwok' means "people" (Encyclopedia.com, 2019). Their enterprises are listed below.

| Miwok (Me-Wuk) | Enterprises |
|---|---|
| Buena Vista Rancheria of Me-Wuk Indians | Tribal enterprises include the BVR Smoke Shop, Harrah's Northern California Casino, and the Bryte and Broderick Community Center (Buena Vista Rancheria Me-Wuk Indians, 2023). |

| Miwok (Me-Wuk) | Enterprises |
|---|---|
| California Valley Miwok Tribe | The small California Valley Miwok Tribe is part of the monthly USDA Food Distribution Program to its citizens (California Valley Miwok Tribe 2003-2019) Additional information is under Impact on Health of Interaction with White Culture Now. |
| Chicken Ranch Rancheria of Me-Wuk Indians | Tribal enterprises include the Chicken Ranch Casino (with expansion planned for 2024), the Jamestown Hotel, and the Mathiesen Memorial Health Clinic (Chicken Ranch Rancheria of Me-Wuk Indians of California, n.d.). |
| Federated Indians of Graton Rancheria | The tribe owns and operates the Graton Resort and Casino (Federated Indians of Graton Rancheria, 2023). |
| Ione Band of Miwok Indians | The Ione Band has the Ione Band Development Corporation and is seeking to establish a gaming facility (Ione Band of Miwok Indians, n.d.). |
| Jackson Rancheria of Me-Wuk Indians | The tribe owns and operates the Jackson Rancheria Casino Resort, an RV Park, Lone Wolf Restaurant and Lounge, Pacific Grill, and Margaret's Café & Bakery (Jackson Rancheria Casino Resort, 2023). |
| Shingle Springs Band of Miwok Indians | The Shingle Springs Band's enterprises include the Development Corporation, the Red Hawk Resort Casino, Shingle Springs Health & Wellness Center, and Express Fuel & Mart (Shingle Springs Band of Miwok Indians, n.d.). |
| Tuolumne Band of Me-Wuk Indians | The Tuolumne Band's enterprises include the Tuolumne Economic Development Authority, the Black Oak Casino, and Four Seasons Native |

| Miwok (Me-Wuk) | Enterprises |
|---|---|
| | Plant Nursery (Tuolumne Tribal Council, n.d.). |
| United Auburn Indian Community | The United Auburn Indian Community is governing entity for Thunder Valley Casino Resort and Whitney Oaks Golf Club and an investor in Danny Wimmer Presents music festivals (United Auburn Indian Community, n.d.). |
| Wilton Rancheria Indian Tribe | The Wilton Rancheria Tribe owns and operates the Sky River Casino (Wilton Rancheria, 2023). |

## Health & Healing Then

The Miwok Tribe believed all things are interconnected and respected and loved the environment. They saw plants and animals as brothers and sisters. Their spiritual connection to nature was seen in their ceremonies and rituals. Each of these had a purpose and reflected gratitude, respect, and spirituality. Music and traditional dance with symbolic movements told stories to honor spirits and tell stories. Women were responsible for gathering and farming along with spiritual guidance and leadership (Justo, 2023).

## Health & Healing Now

The Federated Indians of Graton Rancheria Tribal Temporary Assistance for Needy Families of Sonoma and Marin counties focuses on four goals;

1. "Provide assistance to needy families so that children may be cared for in their own homes or in the home of relatives."
2. "End the dependence of needy parents on government benefits by promoting job preparation, work and marriage."
3. "Prevent and reduce out of wedlock pregnancies and establish goals to prevent pregnancies." and
4. "Encourage the formation and maintenance of two parent families." (Federated Indians of Graton Rancheria, 2023).

## Impact on Health of Interaction with White Culture Then

Early interaction with White culture was marked by disease and enslavement which decimated their population and destroyed much of their culture. Many Miwok lived in poverty and their homelands were taken by settlers. Although the government established Rancherias as permanent sites for Native people, these sites were not always permanent (Evans, 2023).

## Impact on Health of Interaction with White Culture Now

With assistance from a federal grant in 2022, the Graton Rancheria Tribe addressed housing assistance for low-income tribal families to reduce homelessness and help families move into safe, sanitary housing. Their Tenant Based Rental Assistance Program served 31 low-income tribal households in 2022. Two of these were disabled and four were elder households. The Tribe also assisted five elder moderate-income households with rental assistance (Federated Indians of Graton Rancheria, 2023). The California Valley Miwok Tribe is currently fighting disenrollment of tribal citizens by the Bureau of Indian Affairs and the Chairperson expressed concern that non-enrolled individuals have been allowed to vote in a Secretarial Election to adopt, amend, or revoke tribal governing documents (California Valley Miwok Tribe, 2003-2019).

## *Modoc/Klamath*

Two Modoc Tribes are federally recognized: the Modoc Nation of Oklahoma and the Klamath Tribes of Oregon. Since the Modoc originated on the California-Oregon border, both tribes will be discussed in this section. 'Modoc' means "southerner" (encyclopedia.com, 2019). The Modoc Nation has multiple enterprises including the Stables Casino, Eagle Technology Group, a construction company, the Bison Range, a marketing and advertising agency, a shredding service, a market, and a farm (Modoc Nation, 2023). 'Klamath' means "the people" (native-languages.org, 1998-2020). Klamath Tribe's businesses include the Kla-Mo-Ya-Casino, Kla-Mo-Ya-Hotel, Crater Oaks Junction Travel Center, and agriculture (The Klamath Tribes, 2023).

## Health & Healing Then

The Modoc believed spirits inhabited animals and used sweathouses to hold religious ceremonies where the body was purified by sweating to request health and good fortune. Shamans or healers could be men or women who fasted for five days alone to learn healing songs and dances from the spirits. They learned how to affect the weather, and some could inflict disease or death. Shamans sucked objects out of sick individuals and sang to make them well. They used herbs for minor illnesses. Sores and skin swelling were treated with puffball fungus and cough medicine was made from stems and rabbitbrush leaves. Headaches and rheumatism were treated with sagebrush leaves (encyclopedia.com, 2019). The Klamath believed the Creator provided everything needed to live and celebrated the spring fish runs with the Return of c'waam Ceremony (The Klamath Tribes, 2023).

## Health & Healing Now

The Klamath Tribal Health & Family Services provides medical, dental, behavioral health, and pharmacy services. Multiple specialty programs include:   Diabetes Management Program, Immunization Programs, Nutrition Services, Community Fitness Center, Car Seat Program, Juvenile Crime Prevention, Oral/Dental Health Prevention for Children, Native Youth Suicide Prevention, Tobacco Prevention and Education Program, and Substance Use Prevention & Education (The Klamath Tribes, 2023).

## Impact on Health of Interaction with White Culture Then

The Modoc experienced diseases after interacting with White settlers and their lands were taken to accommodate the settlers. In the second half of the nineteenth century, the Modoc were sent to live on the Klamath Reservation. The tribes historically were enemies, and the Klamath harassed the newcomers. The government agent failed to provide provisions specified in the Treaty of Council Grove.  In October 1873, 155 Modoc, including 59 women and 54 children, were loaded in train cars for transporting cattle to be sent to the Wyoming territory. Men and boys were shackled to the floor of the cars. When orders were changed, they arrived in Baxter Springs Kansas having traveled 2,000 miles in cattle cars. They were tired, cold, and hungry. The first years resulted sickness and death, especially of children and the elderly. The Quaker agent and his family swindled the Tribe and provided inferior goods. Bad food and inadequate medical care took a toll on the Tribe (Modoc Nation, 2023).

## Impact on Health of Interaction with White Culture Now

The Klamath Tribes contributes to the area economy via employment and donations  to local organizations for projects such as the Green Schoolyard Project. The Klamath collaborate with local government to government relationships and strive to improve the ecosystem and local environment. They provide economic opportunities for Tribal and non-Native residents (The Klamath Tribes, 2023).

## *Fort Mojave Indian Community*

The Fort Mojave Indian Community in California is federally recognized. 'Mojave' means " the people by the river" (Fort Mojave Indian Community, 2023). Their enterprises include the Avi Resort & Casino, Mojave Resort & Huukan Golf Club, Fort Mojave Tribal Utilities, Fort Mojave Telecommunications Inc., and Aha Macav Power Service [electric utility company] (Fort Mojave Indian Community, 2023).

## Health & Healing Then

Mojaves had a clan system named for areas above the earth (birds, clouds and sun), things on the earth, and things below the earth. Originally there were 22 clans ruled by a clan chief and leaders from three regional groups with their approval and support. Dreams were  the source of knowledge and visions were shared with the tribe. Learning to treat illness required fasting and other trials to be considered gifted. The river was the center of existence and, when Mojaves died, they were cremated to enter the spirit world. Their belongings and property were burned with the body and their names were never spoken again (National Park Service, 2023).

## Health & Healing Now

The Fort Mojave Indian Tribe Behavioral Health offers outpatient assessment and intervention to families and all age groups for alcohol/substance abuse, behavioral problems, and mental illnesses. Education, therapy, crisis intervention, consultation, and referrals are services provided. Behavioral Health conducts workshops and consults with local school personnel about mental health issues seen in local schools. They also coordinate multiple events during the year, such as the New Year's Eve Sobriety Gathering and the Child Abuse Awareness Event. The Tribe also has a Domestic Violence Program which promotes cultural and traditional values to nurture respect for women and prevent abuse in all forms-physical, sexual, verbal, emotional, psychological, and spiritual. The Program coordinates activities throughout the year to prevent violence, including February National Teen Dating Violence & Prevention Activities and April Sexual Assault Awareness Activities (Fort Mojave Indian Community, 2023).

## Impact on Health of Interaction with White Culture Then

In 1890, Fort Mojave became an industrial boarding school. A compulsory law was passed for Native education and children were forcibly sent to the school. If they ran away, they were often whipped and locked in an attic on bread and water for days. Children could not speak their language or follow cultural traditions. In 1905, they were made to use English surnames instead of their clan and individual names (National Park Service, 2023).

## Impact on Health of Interaction with White Culture Now

The Fort Mojave Tribal Band and Rez Life Bird Singers celebrate their culture and share it with others. The Tribal Band has performed across the United States for generations. The Rez Life Bird Singers perform traditional songs and dances that celebrate the desert and its people. Recently, they went to the Yale Campus to share their history and culture with Yale students. The Yale Alumni Service Corps is also planning a service trip to the Fort Mojave Indian Community in 2024 where they and the Tribe will collaborate on a series of cultural, educational, fitness, and sports-related projects (Yale University, 2023).

## Mono

There are five federally recognized Mono tribes in California. 'Mono' means "people" (Wikipedia, 2023). Their enterprises are listed below.

| Mono | Enterprises |
|---|---|
| Big Sandy Rancheria of Mono Indians | Big Sandy Rancheria's enterprises include BSR Distribution (provides products to other federally recognized California tribes). The Mono Wind Casino, and fuel distribution/general store (Big Sandy Rancheria, 2023). |
| Cold Springs Rancheria of Mono Indians | The Cold Springs Rancheria does not list businesses and focuses on administering an Indian Housing Block Grant (HUD, 2022). 2021 income was $15,648 with 46% below poverty line and 33 households/35 housing units (U.S. Census Bureau, 2021). |
| North Fork Rancheria of Mono Indians | The North Fork Rancheria does not list businesses and is seeking to build a casino and hotel off-reservation (Benjamin, 2023). See more details below in Impact on Health of Interaction with White Culture Now. |
| Table Mountain Rancheria | Table Mountain Rancheria has the following enterprises: Table Mountain Casino, Eagle Springs Golf Course, Eagle's Landing Restaurant, Mountain Feast Buffet, and the TM Café (Native-Americans.com, 2012). |
| Tule River Indian Tribe | The Tule River Tribe has an Economic Development Corporation with the following businesses: Eagle Mountain Casino, Stoney Creek Barbeque and Eagle Feather Trading Post 1 & 2 (Tule River Tribe, 2023). |

## Health & Healing Then

Every two to five years, the Mono burned grasslands to clear out dead material, recycle plant nutrients, eliminate insect pests, and thin shrubs that blocked the sunlight. Wild ginger had multiple uses. It was used as a poultice to bring boils to a head or relive toothaches. It was a sedative for insomnia or hysteria and tea from wild ginger roots treated colds, constipation and indigestion. Buckwheat treated headaches, stomach disorders, and menstrual problems. Gumplant was a remedy for poison oak (Reid, Wishingrad, & McCabe, 2009).

## Health & Healing Now

Access to safe drinking water has been an issue on the Cold Springs Rancheria. The Tribe has worked with a Rural Development Specialist to develop short- and long-term solutions for water disinfection. New equipment was required, and the Specialist provided training on usage. They also developed an interim plan to disinfect water until parts are available for repairs (RCAC, 2020). Big Sandy Rancheria's Community Services Department provides nutrition, fitness, educational, and cultural programs to the community throughout the year. Their motto is "Strong Families*Strong Community" (Big Sandy Rancheria, 2023).

## Impact on Health of Interaction with White Culture Then

The Mono and other tribes experienced a malaria epidemic in 1832 and in 1850, California passed the Act for the Government and Protection of Indians. This Act was called the California Slave Act and allowed for indenture of Native children and women considered "vagrant" adults. The North Fork Rancheria of eighty acres was put in trust for the Tribe in 1916, but was not suitable for farming and could support only a few families. The Tribe lost federal recognition in 1958 which was not restored until 1983 after a class action suit (North Fork Rancheria, 2020).

## Impact on Health of Interaction with White Culture Now

The Tule River Tribe has worked to secure its water rights since 1971. This resulted in the 2022 Tule River Water Settlement Act to confirm land for a water storage project. This reservoir project will mitigate decreasing river flows causing water scarcity. A reliable water supply will improve the economy and infrastructure and improving water access will also help fight wildfires and invest in climate change measures (Tule River Tribe, 2023). The North Fork Rancheria wants to improve the Tribe's economic health by building a casino and hotel project off the Rancheria. The compact covering this project was approved in 2022, but is opposed by Madera residents Stand Up For California who challenge "off reservation gaming". The site is 36 miles from the Rancheria and the compact occurred before the land was put in trust for the Tribe. The compact has been placed on hold until a November state referendum. Opponents believe that off reservation gaming is not legal, and the North Fork Rancheria's lawyers state the Tribe negotiated in good faith and the compact is in effect based on federal law. At the time this is written (October 2023), this situation has not been resolved (Benjamin, 2023).

## Picayune Rancheria of Chukchansi Indians

The Picayune Rancheria is federally recognized and is located in California. 'Chukchansi' refers to the regional language and the tribe is classified as Yokuts which means "people" (Wikipedia, 2023). Their enterprises include the Chukchansi Gold Resort & Casino, the Tribal Nation Flower Company (cannabis dispensary), and Willow Glen Smoke Shop (Picayune Rancheria of the Chukchansi Indians, 2023).

### Health & Healing Then

Chukchansi followed the custom of  pruning and burning the land to increase food production (Coarsegold Historic Museum, 2023).  They traditionally harvested plants and were good stewards of the land. They used roundhouses and sweat lodges in their cultural traditions (Picayune Rancheria of the Chukchansi Indians, 2023).

### Health & Healing Now

The Chukchansi people still have substandard housing even though they have received federal grants from HUD. Some families live in used mobile homes without services for water, sewer, and electricity. The Chukchansi

Indian Housing Authority is working to provide housing services by helping tribal members complete applications for housing services. They also provide elder services in their Administration on Aging Department. These services include a Hot Meal Program, the Elders Food Card Program to ensure money for healthy groceries, the Utility Assistance Program for elders, and the Arts & Crafts Program as part of congregate meal service (Picayune Rancheria of the Chukchansi Indians, 2023).

## Impact on Health of Interaction with White Culture Then

In the mid- to late-1800s, the Chukchansi people contracted diseases for which they had no immunity and were restricted to small allotments of land. Many young women were forced to marry outside the tribe and parents were strongly encouraged or forced to send their children to faraway boarding schools. Some of these children never returned further reducing the population (Coarsegold Historic Museum, 2023).

## Impact on Health of Interaction with White Culture Now

The Tribe believes in education and collaborates with multiple organizations in programs to assist adults and high school students gain skills and explore career/employment opportunities. Their Career Development and Adult Education Center partners with area agencies, such as Madera County Workforce Development Office, Oakhurst Chamber of Commerce, West Hills Community College, and Madera Adult School to help tribal members succeed in  education and employment. Career Pillar, an online program, has interactive video tutorials for those who need interview support.  There is also an after-school program for youth that includes tutors and cultural learning activities (Picayune Rancheria of the Chukchansi Indians, 2023).

## *Pit River Tribe*

The Pit River Tribe is located in several locations and is federally recognized. 'Pit River Indians' refers to their unique deer hunting technique of digging pits along the river for the deer to fall into. The Tribe's members are descendants of Achomawi (meaning river) and Atsugewi (referring to Hat Creek). It is comprised of eleven Bands at six rancherias: Big Bend Rancheria; Likely Rancheria; Lookout Rancheria; Montgomery Creek Rancheria; Roaring Creek Rancheria; and XL Ranch (encyclopedia.com, 2019). Enterprises include the Pit River Casino, XL Ranch, and state and federal government (Pit River Tribe, n.d.).

## Health & Healing Then

The Achomawi believed every person had a soul-shadow for good that spoke to them and that everything-rocks, trees, mountains, etc.-was alive. The Atsugewi believed in nature spirits and guardian spirits that guided them through life. The Pit River Tribe believed that illnesses were caused by evil spirits, bad blood or loss of the soul. There were three types of shaman:

1. Singing doctors who cured by singing to healing spirits;
2. Sucking shaman who sucked out the object causing the disease; and
3. Bear doctors (men or women) who could either cure or harm (encyclopedia.com, 2019).

Plants and herbs had healing properties. Wild parsley treated stomach aches, coughs, and colds. If a person rubbed their legs with chewed angelica roots, snakes were kept away (encyclopedia.com, 2019).

## Health & Healing Now

Two health clinics serve the Pit River Tribe today. They are the Burney Clinic and XL Clinic which provide ambulatory health services. The Behavioral Health Department provides substance abuse counseling, anger management, family and marriage therapy, and assists in locating alternative resources. It is available to all Native clients regardless of resources and to non-Natives with insurance. The Outreach Team focuses on health promotion and disease prevention for the Native community. They conduct home visits, diabetes and other education classes, and car seat checks as part of their role (Pit river Tribe, 2023).

## Impact on Health of Interaction with White Culture Then

The Pit River Tribe's interactions with White culture mirrored those of other tribes. They experienced attempts at genocide, government-supported massacres, forced relocation, boarding schools for their children, and assimilation efforts. In the early 1900s, Mt. Shasta Power purchased tribal lands that were of cultural importance to the Tribe which impacted the following section (International Indian Treaty Council, 2021).

## Impact on Health of Interaction with White Culture Now

In 2021, the Pit River Tribe celebrated victories that protected their sacred locations and reinstated their jurisdiction over traditional lands. In 2018, ConnectGen, a Houston energy corporation proposed installation of over 70 wind turbines on a mountain of cultural and ecological importance to the Pit River Tribe. The Tribe began efforts to oppose the Fountain Wind Project and their testimony convinced the Shasta County Planning Commissioners and the Shasta County Board of Supervisors to deny the application. The project would have endangered plant and animal habitats and the Tribe was concerned about protecting sensitive environments in the area. According to a Pit River leader "this mega wind project would have forever erased ancestral, sacred and ceremonial sites, decimated eagles, hawks, bats, and would have placed miles of electrical lines through forest lands already at extremely high fire risk. Our Nation stood together with our neighbors and allies to protect our homes, lands, and natural resources against powerful interests" (International Indian Treaty Council, 2021).

On November 5, 2021, 789 acres of land was returned to tribal stewardship by Pacific Gas & Electric Company. According to a Pit River Tribal member "Protection of our sacred lands and waterways cannot effectively happen without Tribal management and stewardship" (International Indian Treaty Council, 2021).

## Pomo

There are 20 Bands of Pomo Indians that are federally recognized. The Federated Indians of Graton Rancheria are also a Miwok tribe and were discussed there. 'Pomo' means "those who live at red earth hole" (Wikipedia, 2023). Their enterprises are listed below.

| Pomo | Enterprises |
|---|---|
| Big Valley Band of Pomo Indians | The Big Valley Band's enterprises include the Konocti Vista Resort, Konocti Harbor Resort, a marina, an RV Park, and a convenience store (Big Valley Band of Pomo Indians, n.d.). |
| Cloverdale Rancheria of Pomo Indians | The Cloverdale Rancheria plans to build a casino to increase their economic self-sufficiency. This is not completed as of October 2023 (Rancheria of Pomo Indians, 2008). |
| Coyote Valley Band of Pomo Indians | The Coyote Valley Band's enterprises include the Coyote Valley Casino, Coyote Valley Smoke Shop, a convenience store, a propane station, and diesel for RVs and trucks (Coyote Valley Band of Pomo Indians, 2021). |
| Dry Creek Rancheria of Pomo Indians | Dry Creek Rancheria's enterprises include River Rock Casino, Bellacana Vineyards, and DCR Fire Department (Dry Creek Rancheria, n.d.). |
| Elem Indian Colony of Pomo Indians | No business are listed on the website. The Tribe participates in HUD housing assistance and the California Indian Manpower Consortium (Elem Indian Colony, 2023). |
| Federated Indians of Graton Rancheria | Covered under Miwok tribes |
| Guidiville Rancheria | Guidiville Rancheria planned a casino project at Point Molate that has not happened. However, they and their |

| Pomo | Enterprises |
|---|---|
|  | developer, Upstream Point Molate LLC, can now acquire the land for $400. The future of the land is unclear (Lauer, 2022). |
| Habematolel Pomo of Upper Lake | Habematolel Pomo of Upper Lake's enterprises include the Running Creek Casino, and e-commerce ventures (Habematolel Pomo of Upper Lake, 2023). |
| Hopland Band of Pomo Indians | The Hopland Band's principal enterprise was the Sho-Ka-Wah Casino (closed due to wildfires). The Tribe manages nearly 40 grants (Hopland Band of Pomo Indians, 2023). |
| Kashia Band of Pomo Indians of the Stewart's Point Rancheria | The Kashia Band has acquired government grants and will now manage the Kashia Coastal Reserve lands (Kashia Band of Pomo Indians, n.d.). |
| Koi Nation of the Lower Lake Rancheria | The Koi Nation wants to build a casino in Sonoma County as the Lower Lake Rancheria is not habitable (The Koi Nation of Northern California, 2023). |
| Lytton Rancheria | Lytton Rancheria's enterprises include the San Pablo Lytton Casino and vineyards (Lytton Rancheria of California, 2022). |
| Manchester Point-Arena Band of Pomo Indians | The Manchester Band owns and operates the Garcia River Casino and the Black Pearl Grill (Manchester Point-Arena Band of Pomo Indians, 2023). |
| Middletown Rancheria of Pomo Indians | Middletown Rancheria's enterprises include the Twin Pine Casino & Hotel, Mount St. Helena Brewery, and Uncle Buddy's Pumps (Middletown Rancheria of Pomo Indians of California, 2021). |
| Pinoleville Pomo Nation | The Pinoleville Pomo Nation has |

| Pomo | Enterprises |
|---|---|
|  | grants assisting them with education services and watershed protection. They also have an active vocational rehab program (Pinoleville Pomo Nation 2020). |
| Potter Valley Tribe | The Potter Valley Tribe has Gram's Coffee House and has acquired 140,000 acres of watershed lands for forestry, agriculture, outdoor recreation, and natural resource protection (Potter Valley Tribe, 2023). |
| Redwood Valley Rancheria of Pomo Indians | The Redwood Valley Rancheria manages environmental, social, educational, and infrastructure programs (Redwood Valley Rancheria, 2023). |
| Robinson Rancheria of Pomo Indians | The Robinson Rancheria's enterprises include the Robinson Rancheria Resort & Casino, Pomo Pumps, the Recycle Center, and the Smoke Shop (Robinson Rancheria, 2020). |
| Round Valley Indian Tribes | Round Valley Indian Tribes' enterprises include the Hidden Oaks Casino, the Golden Oaks Motel, and the Hidden Oaks Convenience Store (Round Valley Indian Tribes, n.d.). |
| Scotts Valley Band of Pomo Indians | The Scotts Valley Band's enterprises include the Scotts Valley Energy Corporation, Biochar Production, and the Clean Carbon Corporation (Scotts Valley Band of Pomo Indians, n.d.). |
| Sherwood Valley Rancheria of Pomo Indians | The Sherwood Valley Band owns the Sherwood Valley Casino and a Smoke Shop (Sherwood Valley Band of Pomo Indians, n.d.). |

## Health & Healing Then

The Pomo were very spiritual, and the roundhouse was the center for ceremony and worship (Hopland Band of Pomo Indians, 2023). The Pomo used a variety of plants medicinally. Poison oak wood was used by sucking doctors to make objects they used in curing. Four painted poison oak pegs were put in the ground at the patient's feet to disperse poison or disease. The curing doctors used medicine arrows and bows made from poison oak to drive the illness toward the patient's feet for the pegs to work. A poultice of poison oak was also used to treat boils. Death camas also had multiple uses. Besides its use as a poultice for boils, the bulb was a poultice for pain relief of bruises and strains. It's bulb also was mashed and applied to painful joints twice daily for a month for rheumatism. Fendler's meadowrue (coyote angelica) was an emetic, a laxative, and a treatment for gonorrhea. This plant also had spiritual properties. Shooting star roots were crushed to relieve toothache. Yerba Santa was valued as medicine. It treated colds, coughs, bronchitis, asthma, flu, consumption (tuberculosis), fever, rheumatism and could purify the blood. Hound's tongue was used to treat sores and Durango root was a laxative and treated stomach pains. Jimsonweed was used by doctors for divination by altering states of consciousness. It could occasionally result in death. Red larkspur's powdered dried root was blown in a person's face to make him or her drowsy. Yarrow also had multiple uses. It treated nausea, diarrhea, and serious burns. California sagebrush was an analgesic, treated nosebleeds, fever, colic, sore eyes, and dermatitis. It also was used as a deodorant (Welch, 2013).

## Health & Healing Now

The Elem Indian Colony lives by an abandoned mercury mine which leached into Clear Lake for 35 years and contaminates it today with mercury, arsenic, and antimony. Tribal members had a high rate of health issues, including cancer, miscarriages, autism, and developmental disabilities. The EPA spent 25 years and $100 million in attempts to clean up the area. Now, they estimate it would take another 20 years to succeed. Many Elem have moved, but others are reluctant to leave their homes (Dolton-Thornton, 2019).

## Impact on Health of Interaction with White Culture Then

The Cloverdale Rancheria was federally recognized in 1921 and terminated in 1958. It was not reinstated until 1983 and in 1994 the Highway 101 bypass was opened through the center of the Rancheria after Tribal landowners were forced to sell their land by Cal-Trans for the freeway. The Rancheria was split by the freeway leaving little development value or future habitation (Rancheria of Pomo Indians, 2008). When new settlers arrived in Northern California, the Pomo lost valuable agricultural lands and the Rancheria shrunk to a small part of their ancestral land. Most of the tribe's former villages, gravesites, and sites of gathering sedge for basket weaving were flooded by the Warm Springs Dam and Lake Sonoma in 1983 (Dry Creek Rancheria, n.d.).

## Impact on Health of Interaction with White Culture Now

The Big Valley Band of Pomo Indians monitors cyanobacteria and cyanotoxin in Clear Lake with the Elem Indian Colony since 2014 when they began this work to protect the lake, Tribal citizens, residents and visitors. Since 2021, Big Valley has been solely responsible for this monitoring (Big Valley Band of Pomo Indians, n.d.). The Lytton Rancheria provides more than 50% of San Pablo's operating budget and sponsors an annual golf tournament to provide $100,000 a year to the Brookside Foundation for community healthcare. The Tribe also donates to the Boys and Girls Club of San Pablo and Friendship House in San Francisco for alcohol and drug rehabilitation. They also installed wind machines to save water use from the Russian River and use sustainable practices for its vineyards (Lytton Rancheria of California, 2022).

## *Quartz Valley Rancheria*

The Quartz Valley Indian Reservation population are members of the Klamath, Karuk, and Shasta tribes. 'Shasta' means "plain speakers (Alexander, 2019). The Tribal website connects to their LinkedIn site which states "Government Administration" is their industry (Quartz Valley Rancheria, n.d.).

## Health & Healing Then

The Klamath and Karuk were discussed elsewhere. The Shasta Tribe's religion included guardian spirits and shamans. Spirits were in mountains, animals, and rocks (Sage-Answers, 2023).

## Health & Healing Now

The Anav Tribal Health Clinic provides medical, dental, and behavioral health services to tribal members through prevention, education, and healthcare maintenance. They also participate in Purchase Referred Care, a program funded by Indian Health Services with some funding available for dental and medical care referred to another facility or provider. Community Health focuses on prevention and health education, including school-based, individual, and family therapy (Quartz Valley Indian Tribe, n.d.).

## Impact on Health of Interaction with White Culture Then

The Shasta Tribe was reduced by malaria in 1826 after interaction with trappers. From 1848, miners entered the Shasta homeland and Shasta lands were lost. Although Shasta reside today on the Quartz Valley Indian Reservation, some Shasta elsewhere are not recognized, and the Shasta Nation continues to pursue federal recognition (Alexander, 2023).

## Impact on Health of Interaction with White Culture Now

The Tribal Environmental Department uses multiple grants for environmental issues that can impact health or safety. The Department is also charged with protecting the natural environment, responding to environmental emergencies, serving as a resource to the community, and promoting coordination and cooperation between the Reservation and local and federal agencies (Quartz Valley Indian Tribe, n.d.).

## *Redding Rancheria*

The Redding Rancheria is home to Pit River, Wintu, and Yana tribes and is federally recognized. Pit River and Wintu are discussed elsewhere. 'Yana' means 'people' (encyclopedia.com, 2019. Redding Rancheria's enterprises include the Redding Rancheria Economic Development Corporation, Win-River Resort and Casino, and Win-River Mini Mart (Redding Rancheria, 2023).

## Health & Healing Then

Yana healers or shaman were usually men although women sometimes healed using herbs. The Yana believed foreign objects in the body caused pain and the shaman either sucked them out of the body or grabbed them out of the air around the patient. Then, he put the object in a container sealed with pitch to prevent the sickness from escaping (encyclopedia.com, 2019).

## Health & Healing Now

Redding Rancheria Trinity Health Center is an ambulatory care center for both Native and non-Native communities. Services include medical, behavioral health, diabetes care, physical therapy, and nutritional services. The Center offers events throughout the year for disease prevention and health promotion. The Redding Rancheria Tribal Health Center provides similar services in Shasta and Trinity County. These include talking circles, senior focus group, youth classes, smoking cessation, cooking classes, and a health fair. Churn Creek Healthcare is a family practice and urgent care center. The Rancheria also offers a Native American Head Start Program and full-day child care for pre-school children (Redding Rancheria, 2023).

## Impact on Health of Interaction with White Culture Then

In the 1840s, White settlers moved into Yana territory. Their cattle ate the Yana's food supply. In the 1860s, the Army began a campaign of genocide against the tribe and stealing food resulted in their forced relocation. Many of the Yana people were very ill and died on the way to their new reservation or were too ill to finish the journey. In 1908, surveyors took all of the Yahi's winter supplies. Soon, only one Yahi survived in the University of California's museum as a live exhibit. He was frequently ill because he had little resistance to the settlers' diseases and died of tuberculosis in 1916. No other Yahi were ever found, and the Yana joined the Redding Rancheria (encyclopedia.com, 2019). The Bureau of Indian Affairs only built a few substandard houses, and the Rancheria was terminated in 1959 letting non-Natives buy parcels of Rancheria land. This occurred until 1983 when 18 tribes, including those on the Rancheria, were restored as federally recognized (Redding Rancheria, 2023).

## Impact on Health of Interaction with White Culture Now

The Redding Rancheria shares grants for nonprofits from the Redding Rancheria Community Fund. In 2023, they donated to the Happy Valley Little League, Axion Repertory Theatre, and Riverfront Playhouse. They also support schools, 4-H, youth camping, and hold Powwows to share their culture with others (Redding Rancheria, 2023).

## *Resighini Rancheria*

The Resighini Rancheria is comprised of Yurok people and is federally recognized. Its business enterprises include the Cher'ere Campground and RV Park. The Tribe also hunts and fishes on the Rancheria (Resighini Rancheria, n.d.).

## Health & Healing Then

Resighini Rancheria ancestors were responsible for caring for the lands where they resided in the Klamath River Basin. Their traditional ceremonies included the Brush Dance, Jump Dance, Boat Dance, and White Deerskin Dance (Resighini Rancheria, n.d.).

## Health & Healing Now

The Tribal Historic Preservation Office began in 2021 and is charged with protecting, preserving, and managing sacred cultural and historic sites. The Office is a liaison between the Tribe and local, state, and federal agencies as well as private organizations to ensure that sacred places and indigenous knowledge are preserved for the future. The Natural Resources Department also plays a significant role for the health and safety of the residents. The Department is responsible for:

1.  safety of the Tribal Community Drinking Water System;

2. surface water monitoring of the Klamath River and adjacent streams;
3. assessment and management of nonpoint source pollution;
4. monitoring and conservation of wetlands;
5. protecting cultural resources;
6. solid waste management;
7. land management; and
8. emergency management (Resighini Rancheria, n.d.).

## Impact on Health of Interaction with White Culture Then

Tribal lands were lost with the influx of White settlers in the second half of the nineteenth century. The location of the Rancheria on the Klamath River floodplain resulted in floods in 1955 and 1964 that destroyed all structures there along with many towns on the river in the region (Resighini Rancheria, n.d.).

## Impact on Health of Interaction with White Culture Now

In May 2023, the Rancheria's Tribal Council signed a historic agreement with the National Park Service and California State Parks at Redwood National and State Parks (RNSP) to partner on projects to protect cultural and natural resources. The agreement is designed to protect cultural resources and sites. The Tribe will participate in RNSP cultural education programs, and the team will meet twice a year to collaborate on park management projects and economic development to benefit the Rancheria and RNSP. The Rancheria is also a partner in the Tribal Marine Stewards Network which works to return management and stewardship of coastal and ocean territories to California Tribes (Resighini Rancheria, n.d.).

## *Samish*

Samish Indian Nation is a federally recognized tribe living on the state of Washington. 'Samish' means "people who are there/who exist" (Wikipedia.org, 2023). The Nation's enterprise is Fidalgo Bay Resort, a cottage and waterfront RV resort offering outdoor activities (Samish Indian Nation, 2017).

## Health & Healing Then

The Samish people defined spiritual leadership as success at healing. Being respectful and acknowledging family connections, rights, and privileges denoted social status. There was a kinship network and people were respected for spiritual strength. They believed the natural and spiritual world could not be separated and used a prayer or song to give thanks for the gifts of food, air, roots, plants, and nature (Samish Indian Nation, 2017).

## Health & Healing Now

The Samish Health Department has an award winning Diabetes Project of ongoing support and case management outreach for Tribal citizens. The Samish Elders Department also provides congregate nutritional meals three days a week for Tribal elders. They also provide elder support services and caregiver support services in a four county area (Samish Indian Nation, 2017).

## Impact on Health of Interaction with White Culture Then

In the 1770s, many tribal members died of smallpox. By the 1840s, traders intermarried with Samish women. As settlers arrived, they discriminated against these women and mixed-race children. Smallpox epidemics continued to decimate the Samish. Whites were vaccinated, but not Natives. In 1879, nine White men were charged with being married to Native wives because territorial law prohibited such marriage. Mixed-race marriages were common, and some were legalized in civil ceremonies. Settlers also desecrated burial sites on Samish Island forcing the Samish to rebury their remains (Samish Indian Nation, 2017).

## Impact on Health of Interaction with White Culture Now

The Samish Indian Nation collaborates with federal and state agencies on grants for environmental protection and preservation of cultural resources. The Samish Department of Natural Resources uses traditional ecological knowledge for environmental monitoring and protection and restoration of freshwater, marine, and terrestrial environments. They study plant and animal populations and engage in restoration projects and debris removal on beaches and rivers. The Tribal Historic Preservation Office consults with private and public agencies to enhance interagency relationships that will preserve and protect Samish resources and heritage. In their role, they monitor archeological sites and conduct project site visits for artifacts (Samish Indian Nation, 2017).

## Santa Rosa Indian Community (Tachi Yokut Tribe)

The Santa Rosa Indian Community is the home of the Tachi Yokut Tribe in California. Santa Rosa is federally recognized. 'Yokut' means "people" and Tribal enterprises include the Tachi Palace Casino & Resort, the Sequoia Inn, and Yokut Gas (Tachi Yokut Tribe, n.d.).

### Health & Healing Then

The Yokut used different plants for medicinal purposes. Manzanita was sometimes drunk as cider to stimulate the appetite. To control the density of these shrubs and increase their production, the Yokut routinely burned these areas every two to three years in controlled burns. This also reduced the population of harmful insects within dead wood. The pitch of digger pine was used to treat arthritis (Woodrow, 2013).

### Health & Healing Now

The Tribe supports education in various ways. Education Health Nutritional and Social Services supports cognitive and social development of children and their families. The Tachi Yokut Early Education Center offers two early childhood programs, one for 3-year-olds and one for 4-5 year olds. The Department of Education has multiple services for youth:

1. academic tracking to monitor grades and attendance;
2. transportation if students miss their bus or don't have a ride to school;
3. WASP Program of after-school study sessions for homework assistance;

4.  School Clothing Allowance Reimbursement Program (SCARP) twice a year;
5.  school meal reimbursements;
6.  recognition dinners twice a year for families and students recognized for academic achievements;
7.  attendance trip for students with 90% attendance or less than nine days absent;
8.  graduation merits with funds based on diploma type and GPA; and
9.  higher education which fully funds higher education costs for any Tribal member based on full or part-time status (Tachi Yokut Tribe, 2017).

## Impact on Health of Interaction with White Culture Then

When the Santa Rosa Rancheria was established in 1921, the area was desolate farmland and the Tribal people lived below poverty level. Many of them lived in tin houses, huts, chicken coops and old cars. The average level of education was third grade, and the primary income source was as field laborers. Living conditions remained below poverty level for most residents until the 1980s. The average education level increased to eighth grade and government programs like Head Start and 638 funds from the Indian Self-Determination and Education Assistance Act were available along with an Alcoholics Anonymous program (Tachi Yokut Tribe, n.d.).

## Impact on Health of Interaction with White Culture Now

Gaming has provided a way out of poverty for the Tribe. The Indian Gaming Regulatory Act passed by Congress enabled the Tribe to pursue gaming from bingo to today's Tachi Palace Casino and Resort, which employs over 400 people. One-third of these are Native people and the average education level has risen to twelfth grade and college levels. Housing and living conditions have moved to wood housing, mobile homes, and wood frame houses. Youth employment opportunities have increased, and many former employees have successful positions in the community and serve as positive role models for youth. Unemployment is below 25% and the Tribe is moving toward economic self-sufficiency (Tachi Yokut Tribe, n.d.).

## Santa Ynez Band of Chumash Indians

The Santa Ynez Ban is federally recognized and located in California. 'Chumash' means "the first people". The Band's enterprises include Chumash Capital Investments LLC, the Hadsten and Corque Hotel, the Chumash Casino Resort, Azimuth Technology LLC, Chumash Gas Stations, and real estate and retail investments (Santa Ynez Band of Chumash Indians, n.d.).

### Health & Healing Then

In Chumash society, shaman priests also were astronomers and women could become priests and chiefs. They used caves for religious ceremonies and drew human and animal figures on cave walls to show the spiritual bond of the Tribe to the environment (Santa Ynez Band of Chumash Indians, n.d.).

### Health & Healing Now

The Santa Ynez Tribal Health Clinic provides medical, dental, behavioral health, community, and social services. Their behavioral health providers treat the entire family by providing a full range of services including:

1. drug and alcohol counseling;
2. psychotherapy for individuals;
3. family therapy;
4. couples therapy;
5. EMDR (Eye movement desensitization and reprocessing) psychotherapy; and
6. Psychiatric evaluation and medication management (Santa Ynez Band of Chumash Indians, n.d.).

The Community and Social Services Department focuses on those who have limited access to resources. This includes Elder Services, injury prevention services, case management/advocacy for children in foster care, and transportation for needed health services and necessary tasks (Santa Ynez Band of Chumash Indians, n.d.).

## Impact on Health of Interaction with White Culture Then

The Chumash population declined due to European diseases for which they had no immunity. After their lands were taken by Whites, they survived by menial work on local farms and ranches. Their children attended the Sherman Institute, a government boarding school where they experienced forced assimilation. Chumash students attended only two hours of class per day. The rest of the time, they worked and learned trades. They could not speak their own language, dress in Chumash clothes, and eat their Native diet (Santa Ynez Band of Chumash Indians, n.d.).

## Impact on Health of Interaction with White Culture Now

The Chumash Foundation was established in 2005 and has donated more than $25 million to the community since then via grants to community organizations. It's goal is to make the community better for all residents by focusing on opportunities for disadvantaged people, supporting youth, and protecting the environment. They provide grants for technology in schools and Team Chumash volunteers donate their time and talents to community causes. Since Team Chumash was formed in 2015, the volunteers have contributed over 7,800 hours in over 160 events, earning and awarding $160,000 in grants for causes they support (Santa Ynez Band of Chumash Indians, n.d.).

## *Spokane Tribe*

The Spokane Tribe of Indians is federally recognized and resides in the state of Washington. 'Spokane' means "children of the sun" (U-S-History.com, 2023). The Spokane Tribe owns and operates the Mistequa (formerly Chewelah) Casino Hotel, Spokane Casino, and Two Rivers Resort (Mistequa Casino Hotel, 2023). Other Tribal enterprises are Two Rivers Marina, Two Rivers RV Park, and Wellpinit Trading Post (Spokane Tribe, n.d.).

## Health & Healing Then

The Spokane believed in a Great Spirit along with other spirits, such as thunder, wind, and supportive animal spirits. Their spiritual life was part of the land and other living creatures and plants. They celebrated first salmon catches, and the first fruits, berries, and roots harvested each summer with firstling rites (U-S-History.com, 2023).

## Health & Healing Now

The Food Distribution Program is available for anyone on the reservation who does not receive food stamps and off-reservation members of federally recognized tribes. An emergency food bank and food vouchers are also available. The Air Quality Department offers radon checks for homes and air quality assessments. The Spokane Tribe also provides utility assistance, elder assistance, vocational rehabilitation services, diabetic services, and mental health/behavioral health services (Spokane Tribe, n.d.).

## Impact on Health of Interaction with White Culture Then

The Spokane experienced syphilis, smallpox, influenza, and other diseases after contact with White culture. After they were relocated to reservations, their native lands were taken, and ancient villages and burial grounds were frequently destroyed, and White settlers built houses. Tribal members were given English names and faced prejudice and discrimination. Alcoholism and other diseases were prevalent (U-S-History.com, 2023).

## Impact on Health of Interaction with White Culture Now

Within the Spokane Reservation, there is a former uranium mine-Midnite Mine-that has been designated as a superfund site. The mine operated from 1955-1965 and employed many Tribal members without adequate safety precautions. After closure, there remained pits of exposed radioactive ore, groundwater contaminated with heavy metals and acid, and a mill site with tailings. The government expressed concern about contaminated water in the open pit mine in 1988. The most recent clean-up began in 2016 and the current owner petitioned the EPA in 2018 to relax clean-up standards. Currently treated ground water is pumped into Blue Creek and residents are concerned about the quality of drinking water. Families living near the mill site have found radiation spikes in their well water. The Blue Creek area contained sweat lodges and the mouth of Blue Creek is an important traditional fishing area. The Tribe has the support of the Spokane Riverkeeper, a nonprofit organization, and the Upper Columbia United Tribes to maintain clean-up standards (Gebauer, 2020). There is also a Midnite Mine Community Liaison who collaborates with the EPA and the current owner to keep the Tribe informed about the remediation project and handle grievances and complaints for community members (Spokane Tribe, n.d.).

## Stillaguamish

The Stillaguamish Tribe of Indians is federally recognized and resides in the state of Washington. 'Stillaguamish' refers to the river where they lived, and they call themselves "the river people". Their enterprises include the Angel of the Winds Casino, River Rock Tobacco & Fuel, smoke shops and convenience stores, and a cannabis dispensary (Stillaguamish Tribe of Indians, 2020).

### Health & Healing Then

The Stillaguamish used cedar medicinally and in spiritual ceremonies. Many plants were resources for medicine. Indian plum when used as a tea was a tonic. Pacific ninebark was a laxative. Salmon berry had several uses. It was a pain killer and cleaned infected wounds and burns. Red elderberry leaves treated boils and sore joints. Devils club also had multiple uses, including treating arthritis, rubbing on sore feet, improving lung function, and for blood sugar imbalances and adult onset diabetes (Stillaguamish Tribe of Indians, 2020).

### Health & Healing Now

The Stillaguamish Tribe has several resources for health. The Behavioral Health Program has a Healing Center that provides drug and alcohol assessments, support groups, education for adult family members, drug and alcohol information/education, out-patient services, and treatment for smoking cessation and mental health issues. There is a Massage Therapy Clinic available to address individual needs in a safe, secure environment (Stillaguamish Tribe of Indians, 2020).

## Impact on Health of Interaction with White Culture Then

The Stillaguamish were part of the Treaty of Point Elliott in 1855 and were told a reservation would be provided for them when their land was ceded to the White population. This didn't happen and the majority of the tribe stayed in their original homeland without federal recognition until 1976 when their current reservation was granted to them (Stillaguamish Tribe of Indians, 2020).

## Impact on Health of Interaction with White Culture Now

The Water Resources Program focuses on both water quality and water quantity to support salmon by monitoring the Stillaguamish watershed and collaborating with local, state, and federal governments to identify and address threats. The Department collects evidence about water quality and takes measurements to ensure availability of adequate water supply. They also participate in regional programs to monitor and protect Port Susan's water and partner with the Washington Department of Health to ensure that shellfish are safe to eat. The area has had contaminants, and the Department collects water from sixteen sites monthly for fecal coliform analysis (Stillaguamish Tribe of Indians, 2020).

## *Tolowa Dee-ni' Nation*

The Tolowa Dee-ni' Nation is federally recognized and resides in California. 'Tolowa' means "People of Lake Earl" (Everything Explained Today, 2009-2023). 'Dee-ni' call themselves "human being". The Nation's enterprises include the Lucky 7 Casino, Howonquet Lodge, Lucky 7 Fuel Mart, and Xaa-wan'-k'-wvt Village & Resort (Tolowa Dee-ni' Nation, n.d.).

## Health & Healing Then

Tolowa shamans could be men or women and they treated the sick with trances, dancing, magic formulas, and sucking sources of evil out of the sick persons. The Headman was usually the richest person in the village (Countries and Their Culture, 2023). The Tolowa used a variety of plants medicinally. California mugwort was used as a tea for pinworms. Wild ginger leaves were a poultice for infections. Western skunk cabbage was a treatment for lumbago, arthritis, or stroke. The roots of Oregon grape treated coughs and purified the blood. Cuts and boils were treated with a poultice from Mexican plantain or dwarf plantain (Baker, 1981). The Dee-ni' believed after death they would live with their ancestors and knew that everything had a spirit and was sacred. They prayed every day at dawn before they bathed and again before going to sleep. They left an offering and sang for each animal, herb, and fruit used during the year (Tolowa Dee-ni' Nation, n.d.).

## Health & Healing Now

The Department of Community & Family Wellness Services has several programs to address the cultural, economic, and social needs of tribal citizens. It's goal is to help children, youth, and families to be healthy individuals. One of these programs is the Clothesline Project which was founded nationally in 1990. The Project helps women who have experienced sexual or domestic violence share feelings and thoughts anonymously and provides community education. T-shirts and polo shirts are color coded to signify the type of abuse and if the victim survived. The Department sought donation of t-shirts or polo shirts in all sizes in certain colors to create Clothesline Project workshops (Tolowa Dee-ni' Nation, n.d.). The shirts are turned inside out so only the color shows to signify:

1. white for women who died of violence;
2. yellow or beige for battered or assaulted women;
3. red, pink, and orange for survivors of rape and sexual assault; and
4. blue and green for survivors of incest and sexual abuse (The Clothesline Project, 2023).

## Impact on Health of Interaction with White Culture Then

The Tolowa experienced epidemics of smallpox and other infectious diseases, like cholera and measles, in the 1800s resulting in high mortality (Countries and Their Cultures, 2023). Over 90% of their population was murdered by Whites in a series of massacres and attempted genocide in the mid-1800s. Towns across California offered rewards for scalping and killing Dee-ni' from $0.25 per scalp to $5.00 for a severed head. Many Dee-ni' were forced to live in the Camp Gaston concentration camp in 1868. Removal to camps like Camp Gaston were called the Dee-ni' Holocaust. The Federal trust relationship with the Tolowa was terminated in 1960 and they lost all land except an offshore rock, a cemetery, and a church (Tolowa Dee-ni' Nation, n.d.).

## Impact on Health of Interaction with White Culture Now

When lightning strikes ignited several fires in August 2023, the Nation opened a comfort shelter for the entire Del Norte County community. Services included showers, water, coffee, charging stations, and light snacks. Food boxes and ice for cold drinks were also donated. The Dee-ni' also provides direct donations to the community from the profits of their enterprises (Tolowa Dee-ni' Nation, n.d.).

## *Tulalip Tribes*

The Tulalip Tribes is federally recognized and resides in the state of Washington. 'Tulalip' means "small-mouthed bay". Tribal enterprises include the Tulalip Resort Casino, Tulalip Bingo & Slots, Quil Ceda Creek Casino, Quil Ceda Village, Tulalip Liquor & Smoke Shop, and Salish Networks (Tulalip Tribes, 2016-2023).

## Health & Healing Then

Western Redcedar needles were used as tea to treat respiratory or urinary tract infections. The tree also had spiritual or healing powers. Douglas fir's pitch was a salve for wounds and skin irritations. The needle tips were also ingested as a source of Vitamin C. Red alder bark relieved pain and inflammation and it's properties were similar to aspirin (Elsworth, 2022).

## Health & Healing Now

The Legacy of Healing Program provides multiple services for abuse victims that include emergency housing, education, outreach, counseling, group therapy, and transitional housing. In-person crisis intervention is available, and they also focus on children from violent homes who are also primary victims of violence. Their goal is a community where violence is not hidden or tolerated. The Tulalip Tribes Village of Hope Tiny Homes Project is a housing development for homeless adults that provides case manager services to address recovery solutions for the homeless (Tulalip Tribes, 2016-2023).

## Impact on Health of Interaction with White Culture Then

The Tulalip Boarding School was required for students through eighth grade from 1857-1932. Children were removed from their families to become assimilated into White culture. Students were forbidden to use their Native language, dress, or cultural heritage. One half of a day was spent in class learning English, geography, mathematics, and penmanship. The other half of the day was spent in manual labor. This labor kept the school running. It included clearing land for crops, farming, fishing, chopping wood, and caring for farm animals. Girls cooked, cleaned, served meals, did laundry, sewed, and mended. Every student participated in this school/work cycle six days a week. On Sunday, there was church and religious teaching. Saturday evenings were set aside for entertainments and socials. Discipline for infractions included extra work and sometimes students were beaten with a strap. Most students didn't finish eighth grade and few boys graduated. They left to work in logging as young at 13-14 years old. Younger students were frequently homesick and had to be comforted by older ones (Tulalip Tribes, 2016-2023).

## Impact on Health of Interaction with White Culture Now

Casino revenues have funded a new health clinic and many new and expanded community programs. The Tulalip Tribes support education and provide financial aid for students pursuing higher education. They also provide a Higher Education Resources Handbook with information about scholarships, internships, training opportunities, and fellowships. It contains data about developing a higher education financial plan, study assistance, and reference letter tips. Their Higher Education Department assists students with their educational goals by matching their goals to opportunities (Tulalip Tribes, 2016-2023).

## Washoe

There are two federally recognized Washoe tribes-the Reno-Sparks Indian Colony and the Washoe Tribe of Nevada & California. 'Washoe' means "the people" (Reno-Sparks Indian Colony, 2019). The Washoe Tribe of Nevada and California has the Washoe Development Corporation to oversee economic development. The Corporation has leased 37.2 acres to Tahor Forest Products to develop a saw mill that will create 30+ jobs, generate sustainable income, and sustain a healthy forest. (Washoe Tribe of Nevada and California, 2020). The Reno-Sparks Indian Colony's businesses include government services, economic development, finance, housing, recreation, human services, public works, and utilities (Reno-Sparks Indian Colony, 2019).

### Health & Healing Then

The Washoe people were part of their environment, and they were responsible for maintaining it. The animals provided information about creation and guidance about how to live. Each band served as a social and economic unit that was efficient and dependent on nature (Reno-Sparks Indian Colony, 2019). Plants were gathered for food and medicinal use (Washoe Tribe of Nevada and California, 2020).

### Health & Healing Now

The Washoe Tribal Health Center has an injury prevention program to reduce fall risk for Tribal members 50 years or older or disabled. Their services include home safety and risk assessments, education for injury prevention, group exercise, assessments for ramps and grab bars, and referrals for medical and vision issues. Diabetes management is also a priority. This program encourages healthy lifestyles through nutrition, education, exercise, and weight loss. Individual counseling is available for obesity, diabetes, heart disease, chronic kidney disease, and hypertension (Washoe Tribe of Nevada and California, 2020).

## Impact on Health of Interaction with White Culture Then

By the 1880s, settlers were taking so much of the Tribe's land that the Washoe had trouble finding food. After the Dawes Act created allotments, the Washoe could not continue communal land use and poverty, poor health, inadequate housing, and unemployment affected the Tribe and others (Reno-Sparks Indian Colony, 2019). In California, the gold rush depleted natural resources and the mining industry and logging scarred the mountains. Fisheries were significantly reduced, and livestock replaced the forest animals the Washoe needed (Washoe Tribe of Nevada and California, 2020).

## Impact on Health of Interaction with White Culture Now

Lake Tahoe is sacred to the Washoe people. To begin Tribal conservation efforts under the surface, a member of the Washoe Environmental Protection Department (WEPD) and two other Tribal members obtained their open water diving certification with a non-profit environmental dive center named Clean Up The Lake. Environmental scuba diving can ensure clean water and healthy ecosystems for future generations. This enables monitoring and documenting this environment to address littering and aquatic invasive species. The Washoe Tribe also assists US Fish and Wildlife Service's Senior Fishery Biologist to track five released Lahontan cutthroat trout released in Lake Tahoe with tracking devices. They were able to determine if the trout were in the same location as released and if they had been eaten by a predator. Results showed that four of the five trout were still in the same location. The survey took 6 days of 24-hour shifts to complete (Washoe Tribe of Nevada and California, 2020).

## *Wiyot*

The Wiyot Tribe is federally recognized and resides in California. 'Wiyot' is the name of a river in their homeland (native-languages.org, 1998-2020).

The Wiyot Tribe has developed a strategic plan that includes expanding and protecting land resources. They have relied on grants for funding and are seeking business opportunities and alliances to develop a gas station and convenience store (Wiyot Tribe, n.d.).

## Health & Healing Then

Most ceremonial leaders and healers of the Wiyot Tribe were women who journeyed to mountaintops at night to receive powers. The Tribe held an annual World Renewal Ceremony at the beginning of each year. There was a ceremonial dance that lasted 7 to 10 days using ceremonial masks (Wikipedia.org, 2023). There was also a coming of age ceremony for young women (Wiyot Tribe, n.d.).

## Health & Healing Now

There are extended foster care programs for children turning 18 and apartment assistance. However, waiting lists are long and many do not have a job or income to rent an apartment. Some youth are sleeping in cars and others don't want to leave the community to obtain services. A Jaroujiji case manager can help such youth create a plan for job hunting or housing. Many Wiyot youth require in-depth behavioral or mental healthcare. These services and temporary housing services may require traveling to cities hundreds of miles away. The Wiyot Tribe wants to serve as a social steward for younger generations (Goodluck, 2023).

## Impact on Health of Interaction with White Culture Then

After contact with White culture in the second half of the nineteenth century, the Wiyot population significantly decreased due to loss of homelands, frequent relocation, diseases, slavery, and genocide. In 1991, drinking water contamination and sanitation issues resulted in movement to another reservation where they reside today (Wiyot Tribe, n.d.).

## Impact on Health of Interaction with White Culture Now

The Wiyot Tribe is creating transitional housing units in the coastal city of Eureka which was returned to the Tribe in 2019. Due to high housing costs in California, Native residents can't afford to live there. The Tribe created the first community land trust there in 2020. The trust uses private and public funds to develop the area. Residents can own or rent housing, but cannot own the land which is generally leased for up to 99 years. When the trust buys the land, it is off the market and rental or mortgage rates can be kept low. The Wiyot Tribe showed good faith to Eureka residents, and they helped the Tribe obtain deeds of 40 acres in 2004 and over 200 acres in 2019. The Tribe received a grant from the EPA to help remediate the contaminated soil on Tuluwat Island. The Tribe works with Uxo Architects to create plans for 39 bedroom units, green space and common areas, a medicinal and food garden, and offices for behavioral health practitioners. They plan to repurpose old buildings, installing heating and cooling systems, and updating appliances. Two small accessory dwelling units are also planned for children and young adults (Goodluck, 2023).

## Wintun (Wintu)

There are several federally recognized Wintun tribes in California. The Redding Rancheria and Round Valley tribes have already been discussed. This section will address the five remaining Wintun tribes.

| Wintun | Enterprises |
| --- | --- |
| Cachil DeHe Band of Wintun Indians of the Colusa Indian Community of the Colusa Rancheria | Colusa Band's enterprises include the Colusa Casino, River Valley Lodge, and Outdoor Adventures (Colusa Indian Community Council, 2013). |
| Grindstone Indian Rancheria of Wintun-Wailaki Indians | The Grindstone Rancheria attempted to develop a casino, but there no record of one currently (Arrigoni, 2006). The Rancheria employs 20+ people (ChamberofCommerce.com, 2023). |
| Kletsel Dehe Wintun Nation | The Kletsel Dehe Wintun Nation has an EPA funded environmental management program called the Kletsel Environmental Regulatory Authority. The Nation also participates in housing initiatives with Northern Circle Indian Housing Authority Consortium (Kletsel Dehe Wintun Nation, 2020). |

| Wintun | Enterprises |
|---|---|
| Paskenta Band of Nomlaki Indians | Paskenta Band's enterprises include the Rolling Hills Casino & Resort, TEPA Companies, a golf course, and an equestrian center (Paskenta Band of Nomlacki Indians, 2023). |
| Yocha Dehe Wintun Nation | The Yocha Dehe Wintun Nation's enterprises include the Seka Hills Olive Mill & Tasting Room, Yocha Dehe Golf Club, and Cache Creek Casino Resort (Yocha Dehe Wintun Nation, 2023). |

## Health & Healing Then

The Grindstone Tribe held a harvest-time ceremony in October at the sacred round house with a ritual lasting three days. In the spring, a dance and prayer asked for a good harvest. In the fall, they gave thanks for everything in the year. The dance was performed by men and women prepared a week before by cleaning and cooking. They could dance on the sidelines and watched to keep everything clean. Women couldn't touch the men's ceremonial garments because the ceremony was sacred. Separation extended throughout the ceremony even at meals (Arrigoni, 2006).

## Health & Healing Now

The Community Services Department of the Colusa Indian Community Council provides multiple programs for their members. They conduct field trips for Elders, youth events, and provide family support services. The Tribal Health Program helps with wellness information, nutrition choices, exercise programs, healthy lifestyle choices, safety information, and diabetes/health check-ups. Their annual health fair includes multiple vendors for health services. The Education Department provides tutoring, assists high school graduates and adults with scholarship applications, and holds an annual Education Fair where participants meet representatives of colleges, universities, and vocational schools. Family Support Services has an on-site counselor for mental health needs and conducts a weekly teen group that is a safe space to discuss age-specific issues (Colusa Indian Community Council, 2013).

## Impact on Health of Interaction with White Culture Then

When missionaries and White explorers arrived, many Wintun people experienced violence and disease and others were enslaved to maintain the missions. As they were forced from their homelands, they experienced legalized genocide, and the tribe was decimated. It was a struggle to survive, and they could only cultivate meager crops, forcing dependence on the Federal government (Yocha Dehe Wintun Nation, 2023).

## Impact on Health of Interaction with White Culture Now

The Yocha Dehe Community Fund has partnerships with over 400 organizations locally, regionally, and nationally. They provide grants for education, health & wellness, environmental protection, Native rights and sovereignty, and Native arts & culture. They consider supporting requests from nonprofits, public entities, and organizations with a three-year track record (Yocha Dehe Wintun Nation, 2023). The Paskenta Band partners with community organizations to help children succeed and has collaborated with the Tehama County Library to introduce a collection of Native American Literature written by Non-Native and Native authors. The collection is designed to promote literacy (Paskenta Band of Nomlacki Indians, 2023).

## *Yuhaaviatam of San Manuel Nation*

The Yuhaaviatam were called the "People of the Pines" and were a clan of the Serrano people. 'Serrano' means "highlander" in Spanish. The San Manuel Nation was previously federally recognized as the San Manuel Band of Mission Indians and is now recognized as Yuhaaviatam of San Manuel Nation (SMBMI, 2023). Tribal enterprises include the Yaamava' Resort & Casino at San Manuel, the San Manuel Investment Authority which partners with Ohana Real Estate Investors to own the Waldorf Astoria Monarch Beach Resort & Club, the Bear Springs Hotel, and Three Fires Residence Inn. The Nation also is part of Four Fires economic partnership with other tribes in California and Wisconsin to diversify the economy. In an interesting approach to create a positive working relationship with the U.S. Federal government, the Yuhaaviatam of San Manuel Nation also owns a three-story, 12,000 square-foot building near

Capitol Hill in Washington, D.C. for government relations and real estate purposes (SMBMI, 2023).

## Health & Healing Then

Music was integral to Serrano tradition, using gourd rattles instead of drums. Traditional plants were gathered for health and wellness. The Serrano considered the land and everything it provided was sacred (SMBMI, 2023).

## Health & Healing Now

Yawa' means "acting on one's beliefs" and the Nation has benefitted from this generosity in the past. Now that they are more prosperous, the Yuhaaviatam seek to improve the region for everyone. They fund several education initiatives, including after-school, scholarship, career readiness, and college access programs. They partner with local agencies, community groups and native-led organizations to fund career pathway programs, direct healthcare services, disaster response and mitigation, direct services to address and prevent homelessness, senior citizens programs, economic mobility of veterans and military families, accessible transitional housing, support for victims of domestic violence, direct services for missing and murdered indigenous women and girls, and supporting non-profit organizations providing civil legal aid (SMBMI, 2023).

## Impact on Health of Interaction with White Culture Then

When California Missions were established in the 1700s, many Serrano were placed in the San Gabriel Mission, baptized, and forced to give up their traditions. As haciendas were created, they were used for labor. The few Serrano who weren't in the Missions, fled genocide from the influx of Whites. Finally, they were sent to the San Manual Reservation where the federal government made decisions for them, and they fought to retain their culture and traditions (SMBMI, 2023).

## Impact on Health of Interaction with White Culture Now

The San Manuel Environmental Department provides stewardship for the natural resources and conducts community outreach. San Manuel and the neighboring community have a unique ecosystem and the Department has a mission to protect wildlife and preserve the habitat. They protect native plants by preserving, replanting, and removing non-Native species. They also monitor water quality of the water sources in the area as well as flow rates. The Tribe collaborates with the Federal and State EPA, Army Corps of Engineering, the U.S. Geological Survey, and Fish & Wildlife Service to ensure compliance with the Clean Air Act, the Clean Water Act, the Migratory Bird Treaty Act, and the Endangered Species Act (SMBMI, 2023).

## Indian Health Service

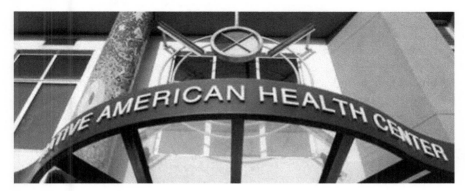

## Historic Perspective of Native Health

Native tribes had health and healing practices unique to their tribal societies to promote physical, social, emotional, spiritual, and intellectual health prior to interactions with White culture. They practiced ethnobotany, ate healthy diets, exercised regularly, used rituals and spiritual rites, and cared for the land they lived on communally.

The history of Native American/Alaska Native health disparities began with epidemics in the 1700s brought by European immigrants for which the Native people had no immunity. Tribal populations decreased by as much as 90% in the first century after contact with White trappers, traders, and settlers (Trahant, 2018). As stated in the previous addendum on Tribal Government, the United States Supreme Court in 1831 determined the trust doctrine in federal Indian law by recognizing tribes as "domestic dependent nations" (Bill of Rights Institute, 2023). Numerous treaties, laws, Executive Orders, and Supreme Court decisions since then have reinforced government responsibility for tribal health. In the 19th century, doctors were dispatched by the Army to military posts to protect the soldiers from infectious diseases. Since many tribal communities were located close to these outposts, Army doctors provided some care on an irregular basis. Since vaccination of the Native population could improve public health in these areas, Congress appropriated $12,000 in 1832 for smallpox vaccinations to these tribes (HIS, 1955-2023). That year a treaty with the Winnebago tribe promised two physicians as partial payment for ceded lands. That cost was budgeted at $200 annually while the Indian agent's salary there was $800 annually and that was considered low. Most treaties were not that specific, but the majority ratified by Congress included promises to send doctors and, in some cases, build and operate hospitals. Although the treaties made these promises, Congress neglected to appropriate the funding. In 1849, the Bureau of Indian Affairs was moved from the War Department to the Department of the Interior with responsibility for Native medical services, but this didn't solve the issue of competent, sufficient medical doctors (IHS, 1955-2023). Only 77 physicians served the entire Native American population in the United States and its territories by 1880. There also was significant disparity in allocated resources.  The Navy spent $48.10 per sailor, the Army spent $21.91 per soldier, and the government appropriated only $1.25 per Native patient (Trahant, 2018)

President William Howard Taft authorized the first direct appropriation for Indian health in 1911 and asked Congress to increase physicians' wages to attract better quality doctors to Indian service. At the time, the average salary for a physician there was less than half the average salary of a government employee (Trahant, 2018) The Snyder Act of 1921 authorized federal health services for tribes, but their health status remained poor for another three decades (HIS, 1955-2023). The Indian health care system suffered from inadequate funding, lack of supplies, low salaries, and undersupplied facilities. A doctor at the Navajo Medical Center named Michael J. Pijoan wrote in his resignation letter in 1951 that "the system is no longer medical. It is only bureaucratic. No more ceremonies are allowed in hospitals. Indians are now numbers, not people. We are machines. This is intolerable. We leave" (Trahant, 2018).

## Indian Health Service & the Indian Health Care Improvement Act

In 1955, Congress removed health programs from the Bureau of Indian Affairs to a  new agency called the Indian Health Service. The agency made a comprehensive survey of Native health in 1956-1957 and reported their results to Congress. This report concluded:

1.  "A substantial Federal Indian Health program will be required;
2.  "All community health resources should be developed in cooperation with Indian communities and done on a reservation-by-reservation basis;
3.  "Federal Indian Health programs should be planned in each community and services made available to Indians under State and local programs; and
4.  "Efforts should be made to recognize the obligations and responsibilities to Indian residents on a nondiscriminatory basis from the State and local communities" (IHS, 1955-2023).

The Indian Health Service (IHS) was still underfunded, and American Indians and Alaska Natives were living in poverty in areas with limited health services. Changes in their lifestyles after interaction with White culture resulted in poor nutritional intake, obesity, diabetes, cardiovascular disease, depression, alcoholism, drug-related deaths, and increased suicide rates. There was still an inadequate number of health professionals with low pay resulting in significant turnover. By 1974, the average age of death for Natives was more than 20 years less than for White Americans (Trahant, 2018). IHS began its work by establishing basic health services and seeking qualified medical professionals. In 1976, Congress approved the Indian Health Care Improvement Act to appropriate $1.6 billion new funding for Indian health. This included resources to improve staffing, modernize facilities, promote access to care for urban Indian populations, and open up Medicare and Medicaid revenue. The bill was signed into law by President Gerald Ford who stated "I am signing this bill because of my own conviction that our first Americans should not be last in opportunity " (Trahant, 2018).

The Act was not a panacea, but it enabled the IHS to make inroads into health issues impacting Native Americans and the tribes began involvement and participation leading to management of their own health systems (IHS, 1955-2023).

## Healthcare of Urban Populations

Many Native Americans did not live on reservations and resided in urban centers. This group had not been studied and health statistics were scarce. However, the known statistics painted a dismal picture.

1.  The urban Native infant mortality rate was 33% higher than the rest of the population;
2.  The accident death rate was 38% higher;
3.  The diabetes death rate was 54% higher;
4.  The alcohol related death rate was 178% higher;
5.  Depression affects 30% of all Native adults; and
6.  Cardiovascular disease, virtually unheard of 40 years ago, is now a leading cause of death (Trahant, 2018).

Urban Natives often live in poverty and have less access to health care due to bias against them and their distrust of government. The Indian Health Services only spends 1% of its budget on Indian health in urban areas (Trahant, 2018).

## Native American Health in the 1980s & 1990s

The Indian Health Care Improvement Act mandated the IHS to provide medical care and eliminate health disparities between the Native people and the rest of the population. Tribes and intertribal organizations formed health committees resulting in creation of the National Indian Health Board and the American Indian Health Care Association. These organizations began the focus on Native-directed healthcare programs. The IHS also collaborated with Native tribes to promote native healers as participants in community health. The 1990s saw increases in funding, construction of more modern facilities, and greater tribal involvement.

The IHS was elevated to Agency status in the US Public Health Service in1988 and formal consultation with tribes involved them in determining allocation for annual funds. The first political appointee held the IHS Director position and supported self-determination. Three distinct sectors emerged: IHS-managed, Tribal-managed, and Urban Indian Health programs (IHS, 1955-2023).

## Today's Indian Health Service System

Decentralized operations are integrated in 12 Area Offices and the basic service unit supports the local community with hospital units, clinics, and community care. 34 Urban programs are operated by local non-tribal and non-government organizations to help urban Natives access programs to provide clinical and outreach services (IHS, 1955-2023). The Indian Health Service is Indian Country's largest employer, and their employees exceed those of the Bureau of Indian Affairs. More than 60% of the health system is operated by intertribal organizations, nonprofits, and tribes themselves. Resources are still lacking. According to Don Berwick of Centers for Medicare & Medicaid Services Institute for Healthcare Improvement, "The Indian Health Service can and will be one of the leading prototypes of health care in America. The Indian Health Service is trying to deliver the same or better care with half the funding of other systems in the United States" (Trahant, 2018).

The Agency has had to be innovative and creative in chronic underfunding. This section would be incomplete without a Native example.

## Southcentral Foundation & the Alaska Native Medical Center

The Southcentral Foundation in Anchorage wanted to reinvent its program and started by surveying its patients. The answers were expected: primary care in the emergency room, long waits, and not patient-friendly. After reviewing the results, they replaced 'patients' with customer owners'. The board of directors are all Alaska Natives, and every patient is considered an owner. The Alaska Native Medical Center uses a team-based approach with smaller waiting rooms to reduce long waits. The customer-owners choose their own team that includes doctors, nurses, medical assistants, care coordinators, and even a behaviorist. A relationship is established with the team and the customer-owner can make changes if desired. This results in less return visits. The Southcentral Foundation's Nuka Model has resulted in 40% less urgent care and emergency room visits; a 20% decrease in primary care visits; a 50% decrease in specialty care visits; and over 35% decrease in admissions. The Model is not fully funded, and its funding includes 45% from Indian Health Service; 50% from billing of third-party insurers and Medicaid; and 5% from government or foundation grants. The Alaska Native Medical Center is the largest, most sophisticated location in the Indian health system. They have worked to optimize revenue and focus on controlling costs, delivering care smarter, and avoiding high care cost when possible. Early investment on prevention and focusing on the root causes of chronic diseases can reduce health disparities and the Nuka Model is a template for this change (Trahant, 2028).

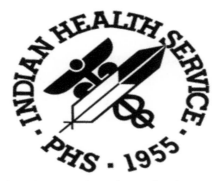

This Photo by Unknown Author is licensed under CC BY-NC-ND

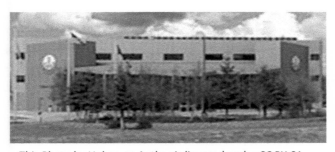

This Photo by Unknown Author is licensed under CC BY-SA

# Chapter 9
# Alaska Tribes

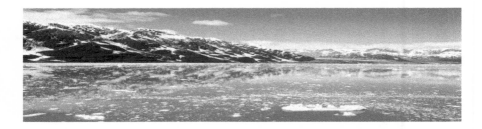

231 federally recognized tribes live in Alaska (Congressional Research Service, 2023). Since the number would significantly enlarge this book, the author has chosen to select representative tribes from each of the five identified regions: Far North/Arctic; Interior; Southwest; Southcentral; and Southeast (Handpicked Alaska, n.d.).

## *Far North/Arctic Region*

Four Native tribes in this region are the Nome Eskimo Community, the Inupiat Community of the Arctic Slopes, the Native Village of Venetie Tribal Government (Arctic Village and Village of Venetie) and the Native Village of Fort Yukon. The Inuit refer to themselves as "the human beings" and consider the word 'Eskimo' negative as it means "the eaters of raw flesh" (Inuit Circumpolar Council & Jessen Williamson, 2023).

| Tribe | Enterprises |
|---|---|
| Nome Eskimo Community | The Nome Eskimo Community has expanded social services to members and partners with community organizations to safeguard resources (Nome Eskimo Community, 2023). |
| Inupiat Community of the Arctic Slopes | The Community operates pull-tabs gambling in Barrow. Pull tabs have a predetermined and fixed quantity of winning chances. The Community also provides real estate services to owners |

| Tribe | Enterprises |
|-------|-------------|
|  | of restricted lands and is working on ice cellar thermosyphon (passive heat exchange) for communities of the Arctic Slope (Inupiat Community of the Arctic Slope, 2023). |
| Native Village of Venetie Tribal Government (Arctic Village and Village of Venetie | The residents of Arctic Village and Venetie live a subsistence existence, hunting for caribou and fishing (Alaskan Natives.com, n.d.). |
| Native Village of Fort Yukon | The residents of the Native Village of Fort Yukon also live a subsistence existence (Alaskan-Natives.com, n.d.). |

## Health & Healing Then

Living in a land with almost no vegetables, the Inuit hunted or fished for sustenance. They believed in multiple spiritual beings who could be helpful or harmful and their basic social unit was the nuclear family (Inuit Circumpolar Council & Jessen Williamson, 2023).

## Health & Healing Now

The Nome Eskimo Community provides welfare assistance for tribal members that includes financial support to meet shelter, food, and clothing needs. The Subsistence Reimbursement Program provides fuel, fishing and hunting supplies, and supplies to gather fruits. The Tribal Resources office is supported by a grant from the EPA and has several functions:

1. Water quality studies are performed in area streams;
2. Tribal members are taught about environmental issues;
3. Tribal members and other organizations participate in recycling activities; and
4. Tribal Resources staff represents the Nome Eskimo Community at environmental meetings to make the community environmentally safer (Nome Eskimo Community, 2023).

## Impact on Health of Interaction with White Culture Then

The Native tribes had some economic opportunities during the fur trade, whaling boom, and the Klondike Gold Rush in the 1800s, but these did not last. After White interaction, major epidemics of communicable diseases also decimated the Fort Yukon population from the 1860s to the 1920s (Alaskan-Natives.com, n.d.).

## Impact on Health of Interaction with White Culture Now

The Nome Eskimo Community's Tribal Transit Program provided public transportation in downtown Nome for residents and visitors prior to the Pandemic. The Transit Program was discontinued since then, but the Tribe has received a grant for operating assistance and indirect expenses from TTP Funding from the Federal Transit Administration to restart this service (FTA, 2021). The van is ADA-compliant and holds 16 passengers. Schedules have focused on typical work schedules and stops included residential areas, businesses, health facilities, schools, senior housing, and grocery stores (Nome Eskimo Community, 2023). Climate change has impacted the Inuit along with social and economic inequalities and colonialism has marginalized them compared to other populations (Inuit Circumpolar Council & Jessen Williamson, 2023).

## *Interior Region*

Three Native tribes in the Interior region are the Native Village of Tanana, Native Village of Tanacross, and Native Village of Kluti-Kaah (Copper Center). 'Tanana' means "straight water" and 'Athabaskan' means "trail people" (Wikipedia.org, n.d.).

| Tribe | Enterprises |
|---|---|
| Native Village of Tanana | The Tanana economy is a mixed subsistence-cash system. When wages are not available, they depend on moose hunting and fishing (Wikipedia.org, n.d.). |
| Native Village of Tanacross | The people of Tanacross live a substance existence depending on |

| Tribe | Enterprises |
|---|---|
|  | hunting and fishing (Tanana Chiefs Conference, 2023). |
| Native Village of Kluti-Kaah (Copper Center) | Kluti-Kaah residents live by hunting and fishing and the Tribe's Kluti-Kaah Memorial Hall is available for rental (Native Village of Kluti-Kaah, n.d.). |

## Health & Healing Then

They believed in animal spirits and the shaman/medicine man or woman was central to religious life. Practices and beliefs centered on certain animals and included charms, songs, amulets, omens, taboos, and supernatural beliefs.  Only dogs were pets. The Upper Tanana used lingonberries to treat coughs, colds, and sore throats. Potlatches or feasts of gift giving were held regularly to demonstrate luck or wealth. They lasted as long as a week and also were memorials for a deceased person one year after death (Wikipedia.org, n.d.).

## Health & Healing Now

The Chief Andrew Isaac Health Center provides services for the Tanana and Tanacross people. It is open daily Monday through Friday and includes the following outpatient services: primary care, women's health and obstetric care, orthopedics, pediatrics, diabetes, and behavioral health consultants. The Health Center also has pharmacy, radiology, dental, laboratory, eye clinic, and immunization services (Tanana Chiefs Conference, 2023). The Native Village of Kluti-Kaah has scholarships available for qualifying Tribal members with GPA of 2.0 to further their education. Full-time students can receive up to $2,000 for room and board, textbook, and tuition costs. Part-time/half-time qualifying Tribal members with GPA of 2.0 can receive up to $1,000 for room and board and tuition costs (Native Village of Kluti-Kaah, n.d.).

## Impact on Health of Interaction with White Culture Then

Traditional Athabaskan culture was disrupted by the arrival of missionaries, traders, miners, and explorers. Mission schools for Native children promoted new religious beliefs and resulted in loss of traditional practices and knowledge (Wikipedia.org, n.d.).

## Impact on Health of Interaction with White Culture Now

In November 2023, Tribal leaders testified to the Senate Committee on Indian Affairs about declining salmon and prohibited species catch of salmon adversely impacting their communities. Chief/Chairman Brian Ridley of Tanana Chiefs Conference asked Congress and federal agencies to maintain their trust responsibility to provide for the "survival and welfare of Indian Tribes and people." He requested that the Senate Committee on Indian Affairs do the following to protect salmon resources:

1. Quit subsidizing cod and pollock industries;
2. Stop minimizing the impact of waste (bycatch) and trawlers in fish harvesting;
3. Reauthorize and amend the Magnuson-Stevens Fishery Conservation & Management Act (MSA) to provide for Disaster Declaration and relief for subsistence fisheries' loss;
4. Add a minimum of two Tribal seats to the North Pacific Fisheries Management Council appointed by the Secretary of the Interior;
5. Move the Nation Marine Fisheries Service to the Department of the Interior to sustain ecosystems of fisheries from economic interests of industrial commercial fishing corporations; and
6. Recognize Alaska Native Tribal Hunting and Fishing Rights with legislation (Tanana Chiefs Conference, 2023).

## *Southwest Region*

Three Native tribes in the Southwest region are Native Village of Atka, Native Village of Nelson Lagoon, and Pribilof Islands Aleut Communities of St. Paul & St. George Islands. Aleut is a Russian name, and the people call themselves "Unangan" or "we the people" (Encyclopedia.com, 2019).

| Tribe | Enterprises |
|---|---|
| Native Village of Atka | The Atka economy is based on wages from the halibut industry and subsistence hunting and fishing (Alaskan-Natives.com, n.d.). |
| Native Village of Nelson Lagoon | Nelson Lagoon residents have boat docking facilities and are also involved in fishing. Two airlines also are available for charter trips (Eastern Aleutian Tribes, 2023). |
| Pribilof Islands Aleut Communities of St. Paul & St. George Islands | The Aleut Community of St. Paul Island's enterprises include the Aleut Community Store, St. Paul Restaurant & Lounge, St. Paul Real Estate, and ECO Enterprise (Aleut Community of St. Paul Island Tribal Government, 2017). |

## Health & Healing Then

Kinship was matrilineal and they worshipped spirits of animals and nature. Shamans foretold the future, created success in hunting and war, and cured the sick. The Aleut knowledge of medicine was extensive. They conducted autopsies to determine cause of death and used acupuncture and bloodletting to cure illnesses. They believed death was caused by natural and supernatural forces and interred corpses in various ways, including mummification, cave burial, special wooden or stone burial structures and in small holes in the ground by villages. Spirits of the dead continued to live (Encyclopedia.com, 2019).

## Health & Healing Now

Nelson Lagoon is a small village with health services from the Paul Marting Gunderson Memorial Clinic. The clinic is funded by the federal government and provides outpatient services along with immunizations, child care, pregnancy care, and mental and substance abuse treatment where applicable (Eastern Aleutian Tribes, 2023). Health Services on St. Paul Island include community & personal health, youth education &

training, personal & family services, and victim services (Aleut Community of St. Paul Island Tribal Government, 2017).

## Impact on Health of Interaction with White Culture Then

After first contact with Russians in 1747, Atka became an important trade site and in 1787 Atka hunters were enslaved by the Russians and relocated to harvest fur seals. Residents were evacuated in 1942 and the town was burned to prevent Japanese forces from using it (Alaskan-Natives.com, n.d.). Aleut people were relocated to a rundown gold mine and abandoned cannery with food shortages and lack of privacy. One in ten people died from pneumonia and tuberculosis. In 1945, the Alaska Territorial Legislature heard testimony about discrimination and segregation by White citizens. Signs in businesses read: "No Dogs, No Natives" and "We cater to White trade only". This resulted in the Anti-Discrimination Act of 1945 (Native Voices, n.d.). St. Paul families experienced cultural genocide in slavery, internment camps in World War II, boarding schools where children were punished for speaking their language, and condemnation of tribal spiritual practices. They suffered from disease epidemics and were forced to interact with non-Native corrections, justice, and child welfare systems (Aleut Community of St. Paul Island Tribal Government, 2017).

## Impact on Health of Interaction with White Culture Now

The Aleut Community of St. Paul Island Tribal Government partners with Advanced Aerial Education to provide drone certification and commercial licensing for Native Americans and Alaska Natives nationwide. The Community also has an Ecosystem Conservation Office (ECO) that partners with local, regional, state, and federal agencies to promote stewardship and conservation of land and marine environments. The Indigenous Sentinels Network includes ECO employees, volunteers, and contractors to monitor environmental conditions and wildlife in the Islands (Aleut Community of St. Paul Island Tribal Government, 2017).

## Southcentral Region

Three Native tribes in the Southcentral region are Alutiiq Tribe of Old Harbor, Native Village of Eyak (Cordova), and Wrangell Cooperative Association. Eyak means "Throat of the Lake, where the lake becomes the river" (Native Conservancy, 2021).

| Tribe | Enterprises |
|---|---|
| Alutiiq Tribe of Old Harbor | The Alutiiq Tribe uses a subsistence culture and has an airstrip and harbor for its fishing fleet (Alutiiq Tribe of Old Harbor, n.d.). |
| Native Village of Eyak (Cordova) | The Native Village of Eyak owns and operates the Prince William Sound Marina (Native Village of Eyak, n.d.). |
| Wrangell Cooperative Association | The Wrangell Cooperative Association uses a subsistence lifestyle and tourism to support the tribe economically (Wrangell Cooperative Association, 2023). |

### Health & Healing Then

There were two Eyak clans-the Eagle and the Raven. They had a matrilineal system and their shamans used painted figures of people, animals and drums to predict the future, heal, stop evil spirits, promote fertility, or help the dead travel into the spirit realm (Alaskan-Natives.com, n.d.).

### Health & Healing Now

The Native Village of Eyak's Elder Service Program encourages elders and youth to interact in summer activities to share culture and traditions across generations. Elders are provided with outreach, medication delivery, family support, services with chores, transportation, nutrition/dietary support, and subsistence. Elder activities include weekly Elder Sewing Circle, Sobriety Celebration Elder Hospitality Room, and monthly Elder Mug-ups to visit and enjoy healthy foods (Native Village of Eyak, n.d.).

## Impact on Health of Interaction with White Culture Then

When Americans arrived, their commercial canneries competed with the Eyak for salmon, which was the tribe's chief food. Introduction of communicable diseases also reduced the Eyak population (Alaskannatives.com, n.d.).

## Impact on Health of Interaction with White Culture Now

The Alutiq Tribe's Environmental Department Coordinator handles community outreach programs, reporting, and grant management. The Environmental Technician is responsible for landfill improvements, recycling, solid waste sorting, air and water quality, outreach support, and emergency environmental response. The Department has removed many hazardous materials from the village. It also received an Air Quality grant from the Alaska Native Tribal Health Consortium (ANTCH) and installed PurpleAir monitors to upload real time data about air quality issues. The Environmental Department conducts water sampling at recreational beaches to protect Native and non-Native people from bacteria such as enterococci and fecal coliform (Alutiq Tribe of Old Harbor, n.d.).

## *Southeast Region*

Three tribes of the Southeast region are Metlakatla Indian Community of Annette Island Reserve, Sitka Tribe of Alaska, and Skagway Village. Sitka means "people on the outside of shee" (Radcliffe, 2023).

| Tribe | Enterprises |
|---|---|
| Metlakatla Indian Community of Annette Island Reserve | The Metlakatla Indian Community's enterprises include tourism, forest products, fishing, and seafood processing (Metlakatla Indian Community, 2022). |
| Sitka Tribe of Alaska | The Sitka Tribe's enterprises include Sitka Tribal Enterprises (economic development), Sitka Tribal Tours, the Community House for local events, |

| Tribe | Enterprises |
|---|---|
|  | and the Cottage Industry Development Center for meetings or kitchen rental (Sitka Tribe of Alaska, 2011). |
| Skagway Village | Skagway Traditional Council contracts with the EPA and Bureau of Indian Affairs to provide services to citizens (Skagway Traditional Council, n.d.). |

## Health & Healing Then

Sitka had a connection to nature signifying harmony with the environment. The Sitka had respect for earth's resources and stewardship of the environment (Radcliffe, 2023). The Sitka Tribe used their traditional knowledge of plants for food and medicine by gathering, processing, using, and protecting traditional plants according to spiritual methods. They considered bark, roots, plants, moss, and mushrooms as special forest products (Sitka Tibe of Alaska, 2011).

## Health & Healing Now

The Skagway Village is starting a farm by growing starts in a garage and contracting for a new greenhouse. The farm has two goals: supply Tlingit potatoes for seed and harvest and to create greater food security for Skagway. Taiya Counseling Services LLC is also partnering with the Skagway Tribe to provide mental health services three days a week (Skagway Traditional Council, n.d.). The Sitka Tribe is concerned about the high dropout rate for Native students and lack of jobs for youth and older residents. The cost of living is 37.5% higher than the average in the United States and the unemployment rate is near 17%. The Education, Employment, and Training Student Support Specialist has relationships with school districts, head start, and other educational entities to assist with the GED program, higher education scholarships, and career preparation (Sitka Tribe of Alaska, 2011).

## Impact on Health of Interaction with White Culture Then

The Sitka population was decimated in the mid-1800s and early 1900s by tuberculosis and influenza epidemics (Sitka Tribe of Alaska, 2011).

## Impact on Health of Interaction with White Culture Now

The Skagway Village Environmental Department participates in the following projects:

1. Drone-based Light Detection & Ranging to collect data along Skagway's eastern ridge that will detect hazards there and at the active slide area (funded by the KLUTI Project of the Sitka Sound Science Center, the University of Washington, and other scientific organizations);
2. Weekly bacteria sampling at five Skagway recreational beaches to provide the community with information about water safety (funded by the Alaska Department of Environmental Conservation Alaska Beach Monitoring Program);
3. Air testing (24-hour tests every other day) to determine pollutants in the air; and
4. Teaching youth at summer camp about invasive species (Skagway Traditional Council, n.d.).

The Metlakatla Indian Community's Tourism Department serves as cultural ambassadors to positively represent the Community's culture to outside guests (Metlakatla Indian Community, 2022).

# Subsistence Management; An Alaska Tradition

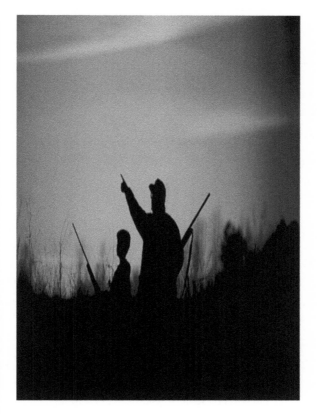

## Subsistence in Alaska

Subsistence means "harvest, use, and sharing of wild, renewable plant and animal resources for food, shelter, fuel, clothing, tools, or transportation as part of long-standing practices that are an important foundation of Alaska Native cultures (Bureau of Indian Affairs, n.d.). While many people consider hunting and fishing as sport, Alaska Natives consider these resources as social, cultural, spiritual, and economic necessities from the land. Living a subsistence lifestyle means living with and from the land. Each average rural Alaska resident harvests about 18,000 tons of wild foods annually or an average 295 pounds. Fish is about 56% of these harvests (Bureau of Land Management, n.d.).

## History of Federal Subsistence Management

Alaska Natives harvested wildlife and fish for thousands of years before the arrival of White culture. Here is the timeline after 1867:

| Dates | Actions |
|---|---|
| 1867-1959 | After the United States made the Alaska Purchase, the federal government managed the fish and wildlife resources there. |
| 1960 | The authority to manage fish and wildlife resources in Alaska was transferred to the new State of Alaska government. |
| 1971 | The Alaska Native Claims Settlement Act (ANCSA) was passed by Congress with the following provisions: <br> • Title to greater than 40 million acres of land for Alaska Natives; <br> • Nearly $ one billion in compensation to Alaska Natives; and <br> • Termination of aboriginal fishing and hunting rights with the expectation that the State of Alaska and the Secretary of the Interior would protect Native Alaskans' subsistence needs (U.S. Department of the Interior, n.d.). |
| 1978 | Alaska creates a subsistence law making subsistence use a priority that does not define subsistence users. |
| 1980 | Congress passes the Alaska National Interest Lands conservation Act (ANILCA) to protect rural Alaskans' subsistence needs. This Act prioritizes fish and wildlife harvests by rural Alaskans over commercial and sport/recreational users on federal lands (Bureau of Indian Affairs, n.d.). |
| 1982 | A rural subsistence priority is created in the Alaska Board of Fisheries and Game regulations. |
| 1989 | The rural residency preference is ruled in violation of the Alaska Constitution by the Alaska Supreme Court. |
| 1990 | The federal government manages subsistence trapping, fishing, and hunting on non-navigable waters and federal public lands. |
| 1992 | Final subsistence management regulations are adopted. |
| 1993 | Federal Regional Advisory Councils begin. |
| 1995 | A ruling of the Ninth Circuit Court of Appeals permits the Federal Subsistence Board to manage subsistence fisheries in all navigable waters where the U.S. has reserve water rights. This ruling cannot take effect until October 1, 1999. |

| Dates | Actions |
|---|---|
| 1999 | Fisheries on all federal public waters and lands are under federal subsistence management. |
| 2009 | A comprehensive review of the Federal Subsistence Management Program is begun by the Secretary of the Interior. |
| 2010-2011 | The Secretary of the Interior and Secretary of Agriculture direct the Federal Subsistence Board to add two public members who represent rural subsistence users. |
| 2012 | Two public members are appointed to the Federal Subsistence Board and the Tribal consultation policy is adopted on ANILCA. |
| 2015 | Federal Subsistence Board can define communities or areas of Alaska that are nonrural so the Board can have more flexibility in decisions about regional differences. This process enhances input from Subsistence Advisory Councils, Alaska Native Corporations, federally-recognized Alaska Tribes, and the public (National Park Service, 2017). |

(U.S. Department of the Interior, n.d.).

Today, a public member chairs the Federal Subsistence Board and Alaska is the only state where about 60% of the state's public land and water (about 230 million acres) is managed by the federal government. The goal is to preserve and prioritize the Native Alaskan way of life (Bureau of Land Management, 2021).

## The Subsistence Tradition

To Alaska Natives, subsistence is spiritual and cultural where the sky, land, rivers, and waters provide resources for the people. They share these resources with others, including family and friends, developing relationships that are lasting. This unique connection to the land and these resources is traditional and links the past to the present. Subsistence activities occur all year and vary by the season (National Park Service, 2016). Hunting, trapping ,and fishing are only part of the subsistence tradition. Indigenous plant knowledge also is used in harvesting traditional plants for food and medicine. There is a spiritual meaning in this harvesting that fosters a reciprocal relationship between the individual and the plants themselves. Each must take care of the other. Beyond simple nutrition, plants benefit physical, emotional, mental, and spiritual health and Alaska Natives respect them along with other wild, renewable resources (Alaska Pacific University, 2023).

Alaska Natives also make optimal use of their resources through direct and indirect personal or family uses. Besides nutrition, these resources provide shelter, clothing, fuel, transportation, tools, bartering opportunities, and trade items. Even non-edible parts of animals and fish are used to make and sell as handicrafts. Alaska is unique because wild subsistence foods are economical and healthier than processed foods. Replacing subsistence supplies with other means of sustenance would be very expensive. Non-Native Alaskans also use subsistence in rural areas to sustain their way of life (National Park Service, 2016).

## Alaska Native Perceptions

Traditions and ceremonies vary among Alaska Natives depending on each tribe's subsistence practices, but it is essential to their communities beyond the physical aspects. Here are some perspectives by Alaska Natives themselves that illustrate the importance of subsistence living.

- Hallehana Alagum Ayagaa Stepetin is Unangax and teaches at the University of Alaska Anchorage: "We don't think about subsistence as merely a quantifiable event. Subsistence is a whole structure, it's a way of life. It's an embodied knowledge, an embodied way of life. And when we dance about these activities, we're extending that process of subsistence. It's always surprising to me that people don't know what subsistence is, which is really just living a balanced and sustainable lifestyle with your local ecosystem, and stewarding that ecosystem for returns to come for generations in the future. All of our pedagogy revolves around transfers of subsistence, which included sharing, storytelling, dance, song, and eating together. It permeates every single part of an Alaskan Native existence" (Sullivan, 2021).
- Rosita Worl is Tlingit and currently is President of Sealaska Institute. She is renowned in subsistence research and advocacy: "A major issue is that the general public, overall, does not understand the full significance of subsistence hunting as one, our basic food security, and then also the cultural dimensions of it. These spiritual things, they're important to our cultural survival" (Sullivan, 2021).

These perspectives show that subsistence living is vital to the Native Alaska culture.

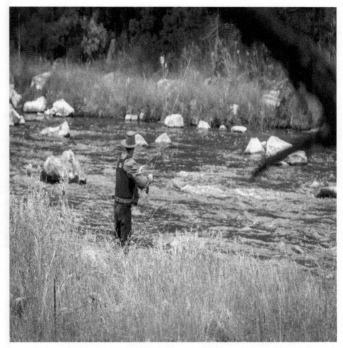

# Chapter 10
# Hawaiian Tribes

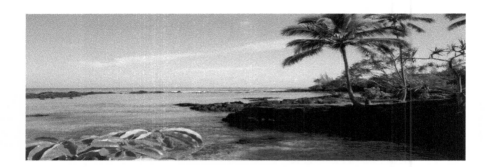

## *Aboriginal People*

There are no federally recognized Native Hawaiians because they are not considered indigenous. Instead, they are considered aboriginal or members of the first human migration to arrive in the Hawaiian Islands. According to the history of Hawaii, these first Natives were Polynesian who came from central Polynesia. Indigenous Natives lived in their lands prior to arrival of pre-colonial societies (Hawaiian Kingdom Blog, 2016). According to the National Park Service, the Polynesians sailed across 2,400 miles of ocean in double-hulled canoes between 1000 and 1200 A.D. The unique Hawaiian culture developed over 400 years of isolation prior to the arrival of Captain James Cook in 1778.

In the nineteenth century, the Hawaiian Kingdon was recognized as an independent and sovereign State whose citizens were called Hawaiian subjects. These citizens included pure Hawaiians and naturalized non-Natives, such as Japanese, Chinese, Portuguese, Whites, and 60 other nationalities. In her will, Princess Bernice Pauahi Bishop referenced aboriginal Hawaiians when she provided for establishing the Kamehameha Schools: "I direct my trustees to invest the remainder of my estate in such manner as they may think best…in maintenance of said schools…and to devote a portion of each year's income to the support and education of orphans, and others in indigent circumstances, giving the preference to Hawaiians of pure or part aboriginal blood" (Hawaiian Kingdom Blog, 2016).

## Health & Healing Then

The Native Hawaiians lived in a caste system. The ali'i or chiefs were the rulers over the land. The kahuna were experts on herbal medicine, healing, and religious rituals. They were respected and sometimes feared. The maka'ainana or commoners were farmers, fishermen, and builders who paid taxes to the chiefs. The lowest caste was kauwa who were slaves or outcasts. Kanawai or laws maintained the social order. Sacred places, things, people, and times were forbidden or kapu. Women did not eat with men and were not to eat coconuts, bananas, pork, or some other foods. Fishing, planting, and harvesting were strictly regulated by kapu to ensure resource conservation. Guardian spirits and gods were worshipped, and history was described through songs, chanting, and dancing the hula (National Park Service, 2011).

## Health & Healing Now

Many Native Hawaiians consider their culture to be their identity. One aspect of their culture is the land where they live which connects them to their ancestors. Today, much of the traditional lands are gone and 42% of Hawaii's homeless population is Native Hawaiian, They have higher rates of poverty and lower incomes. Their health statistics reflect disparities between them and other members of the United States' population:

1. Native Hawaiians are twice as likely to develop Type 2 diabetes;
2. They are eight times more likely to die from diabetes than non-Hawaiians;
3. They are five times more likely to die from heart disease; and
4. They have the second highest mortality rate for all cancers in the United States (Kauana Osorio, 2021).

According to the Office of Hawaiian Affairs in 2017, "Today, Native Hawaiians are perhaps the single racial group with the highest health risk in the State of Hawaii. This risk stems from high economic and cultural stress, lifestyle and risk behaviors, and late or lack of access to health care" (Kauana Osorio, 2021).

## Impact on Health of Interaction with White Culture Then

After Captain Cook's arrival in 1778, the Native Hawaiians experienced epidemics for which they had no immunity. Diseases like measles, smallpox, and whooping cough decimated the population and only 10% remained by 1890. As many of the Natives died, other cultures migrated reducing the dominance of the Native culture. As White culture increased, missionaries began to influence Native Hawaiians by discouraging use of their language and cultural practices. Children were forbidden to speak Hawaiian in schools and were taught patriotic exercises to Americanize them. They were severely punished if caught speaking Hawaiian. The hula, an important religious and cultural tradition, was banned from 1830-1886 (Kauana Osorio, 2021).

## Impact on Health of Interaction with White Culture Now

Higher living costs in Hawaii have resulted in lack of affordable housing for Native Hawaiians who live in overcrowded locations with extended family members. They frequently undertake additional jobs and move to areas further from employment. Although the Kuelana Act appropriated about 200,000 acres on less populated islands for Natives who are at least 50% Hawaiian, only 11% of Native Hawaiians live on Hawaiian Homestead land (Kauana Osorio, 2021)`.

## Powwows and Tribal Regalia

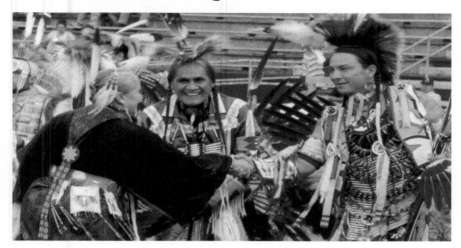

## Historic Perspective

Powwow is an Algonquian term meaning "medicine man". Native communities always held ceremonial gatherings, but powwows originated when Plains tribes were forced to relocate in the late 1800s. Intertribal contact resulted in solidarity among the tribes. Two new intertribal traditions emerged: the Grass Dance and the Drum Religion. The Grass Dance reflected ancient warrior dances and the Drum Religion fostered friendship and peace by a sacred drum ritual. Both shared gift exchanges and generosity and were adopted and adapted to reflect each tribe's culture. These celebrations preceded today's powwows (Smithsonian Institution, 2023).

In the early twentieth century, the word powwow began to appear in advertising shows of "war dances" for non-Native audiences. Stereotypes of Native people emerged, and powwows became commercialized. In the beginning, vendors only sold beads, shoes, and other supplies to the dancers. American Indian veterans returning from World War I and II brought back warrior traditions to powwows which celebrated and commemorated American Indian veterans. These veterans became involved in organizing these events. In the 1950s, thousands of Plains tribal members were relocated to cities across the United States where they created new communities to connect with each other. This included powwows. Students in government boarding schools also learned about powwows from their Great Plains peers and classmates (Smithsonian Institution, 2023).

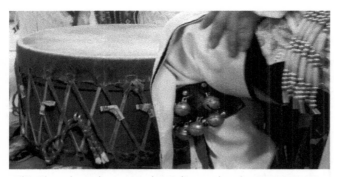

## Modern Powwows

Today's powwows are held every weekend in multiple venues for local, regional, national, and international audiences. Drumming is vital to each powwow, but specific traditions vary from tribe to tribe. The echoes of the drum call to the spirits and bring singers, dancers, and the audience into shared rhythm. Drumming traditions vary and songs are passed down orally for each tribe from generation to generation. Women who are Northern style singers may sit beside the men and beat the drum. Eight or more musicians sit at a drum, drumming in unison and singing non-lyrical powwow songs. Northern and Southern traditions have distinct singing styles.

There are also diverse powwow dances. Only warriors danced at original powwows. Today, dances involve women, elders, youth, and children. Powwow dances reflect both tradition and individual community identities. Here are common dances.

1. The Men's and Women's Traditional Dance follows a two-beat pattern and the Men's version now allows more self-expression in its movements;
2. The Men's Fancy Dance is a modern dance where dancers wear feathered, circular bustles on their backs and jump, shake, and twist to make the bustles become a blur of texture and color; and
3. The Women's Fancy Shawl Dance is a physically challenging dance that is the most popular newer dance for women and girls (Smithsonian Institution, 2023).

## Regalia

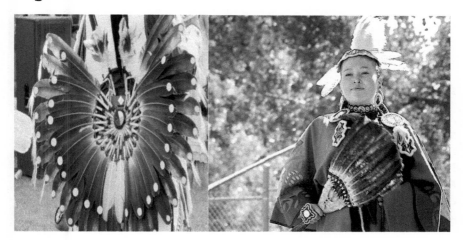

Regalia represents personal tastes and community traditions. This clothing is not a costume. It is special, reflecting the dancer's family background, interests, and life. Regalia evolves over time and incorporates modern elements as well as traditional garments. Dancers always wear headgear to signify formality. This varies from a headdress, war bonnet, band, porcupine head roach, or ribbon. Dancers also carry objects, such as staffs, fur-wrapped hoops, or feathered fans. Dancers only wear the regalia of their own tribe and do not dance or sing songs of other tribes. Taking the sacred elements of other tribes is disrespectful.

Dancers also must be sure their adornments are securely fastened before stepping into the dance circle. If an accessory comes off during the dance, protocol and particular ceremonies ensure that the spiritual balance of the dance is not disturbed, If an eagle feather falls, it cannot be touched until it is properly retrieved, cleaned, and returned. During the dance, others dance around the eagle feather and protect it until it can be properly cared for. Regalia is a mode of self-expression combining modern and historical dress (Smithsonian Institution, 2023).

## Spirituality and Community

Powwow rituals and reflection enhance the spirituality for participants. Circle imagery, sacred objects, and the drum as a central focus have spiritual meaning and powwows can evoke spiritual awakening. Many community members also attend and participate in powwows for an opportunity to socialize and enjoy being with others. These gatherings celebrate tribal identity and welcome other Native community members.

When there are needs, a member of the host tribe may lay down a blanket, request an honor song, and ask for donations to be placed on the blanket. The donation blanket expresses traditional values by gift exchange and generosity. Every powwow reflects its community and is valuable and authentic for its people (Smithsonian Institution, 2023).

## Financial Aspects

Attracting drum groups and popular dancers often requires honorariums and prize money from dance competitions. Since financial issues are a reality for today's Native communities, attracting attendance of non-Natives is a revenue source. This enables performers and craftsmen to be reimbursed for their time and travel expenses and powwows continue to address cultural, spiritual, and financial needs (Smithsonian Institution, 2023).

# Afterword

In *Native American Health—Then and Now*, Dr. Johnson's personal experiences form the foundation for guiding us through a deep understanding of the historical and contemporary successes and challenges of Native Americans. Throughout this narrative and the accompanying examples, Dr. Johnson has provided a comprehensive view of the journey of Native American tribes in relation to their health and healing practices, as well as the impact of interaction with the White culture that enhanced (occasionally), changed (frequently), or negatively impacted (often) the physical, social, emotional, and mental health of Native Americans. With data from north to south and east to west across America, the experiences of Indigenous people in regard to health practices are explained in detail.

After reading the compelling narrative, we are now challenged to explore the next chapter of the Indigenous people story – what is the "next" that follows "then" and "now"? Startling awareness of injustices that have been committed and lack of respect and value that have occurred over time provide us with knowledge to move into the future with a commitment to change. From local neighborhood connections to federal government actions, what are the opportunities for improvement? This book serves as a call to action for each of us to reflect on our own perspectives, contemplate the challenges faced by Indigenous people who have been disenfranchised throughout American history, and resolve to be part of a brighter future that builds bridges and unites us all in a spirit of caring, health, and healing.

Pam Dickerson, PhD, RN, NPDA-BC®, FAAN
Nursing Professional Development Specialist and Consultant
Westerville, Ohio

# Appendix

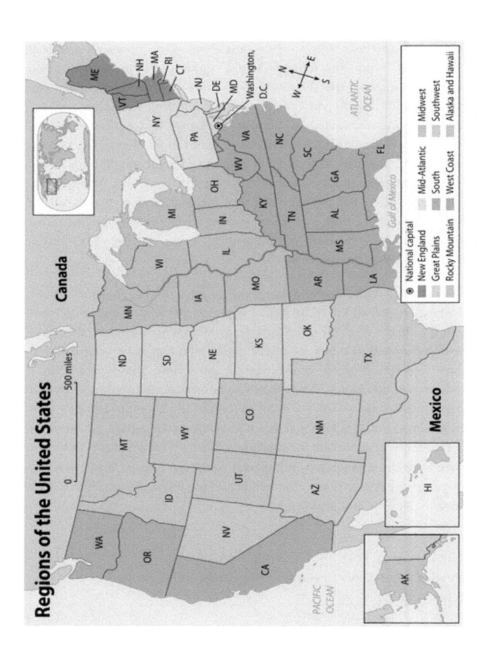

# References

500Nations.com. (1999-2023). *Desert Rose Casino*. Retrieved September 20, 2023, from 500nations.com: https://500nations.com/casinos/caDesert Rose.asp

AAA Native Arts. (1999-2023). *Big Lagoon Rancheria*. Retrieved September 24, 2023, from AAA Native Arts: https://www.aaanativearts.com/big-lagoon-rancheria-index

AAANativeArts.com. (1999-2023). *Accohannock Indian Tribe*. Retrieved April 22, 2023, from AAANativeArts.com: https://www.aaanativearts.com/accohannock-indian-tribe

AAANativeArts.com. (1999-2023). *Arapaho Tribe of the Wind River Reservation*. Retrieved July 29, 2023, from AAANativeArts.com: https://www.aaanativearts.com/arapahoe-tribe-wind-river-index

Abenaki Arts & Education Center. (2018). *Welcome to the Abenaki Arts & Education Center*. Retrieved April 17, 2023, from abenaki-edu.org: https://abenaki-edu.org/

abenaki.edu.org. (2023, April 13). *Abenaki Alliance Statement in Support of Vermont's Truth and Reconciliation Commission*. Retrieved April 17, 2023, from Abenaki Arts & Education Center: https://abenaki-edu.org/abenaki-alliance-statement-in-support-of-vermonts-truth-and-reconciliation-commission/

Absentee Shawnee Tribe of Indians of Oklahoma. (2021). *Hi Ho ne ho wa se we ki ni*. Retrieved June 13, 2023, from https://www.astribe.com/: https://www.astribe.com/

Access Genealogy. (2023). *Ioway Tribe*. Retrieved May 31, 2023, from Access Genealogy: https://accessgenealogy.com/native/ioway-tribe.htm

Access Genealogy. (2023). *Pennsylvania Indian Tribes*. Retrieved April 23, 2023, from Access Genealogy: https://accessgenealogy.com/pennsylvania/pennsylvania-indian-tribes.htm

AccessGenealogy. (n.d.). *Saluda Tribe*. Retrieved April 26, 2023, from AccessGenealogy: https://accessgenealogy.com/pennsylvania/saluda-tribe.htm

accessgenealogy.com. (2023). *Huron Tribe*. Retrieved May 30, 2023, from
    Access Genealogy: https://accessgenealogy.com/illinois/huron-tribe.htm

Administration for Native Americans. (2010). *Accohannock Indian Tribe, Inc.*
    Retrieved June 24, 2023, from Maryland: https://www.acf.hhs.gov/sites/
    default/files/documents/ana/maryland.pdf

Agua Caliente Band of Cahuilla Indians. (2023). *Agua Caliente Band of Cahuilla
    Indians*. Retrieved September 25, 2023, from www.aguacaliente.org:
    https://www.aguacaliente.org/

Ak-Chin Indian Community. (2021). *Ak-Chin Indian Community*. Retrieved
    September 3, 2023, from ak-chin.nsn.us: http://ak-chin.nsn.us/

Akridge, S. (2020, May 27). *For Decades the U.S. Punished Indigenous Healers.
    Now the Indian Health Service Wants to Hire Tem*. Retrieved August 1, 2023,
    from In These Times: https://inthesetimes.com/article/indigenous-
    medicine-traditional-healers-indian-health-service-fort-belknap

Alaska Pacific University. (2023). *Alaska Native Plants and Traditional Uses*.
    Retrieved November 21, 2023, from www.alaskapacific.edu:
    https://www.alaskapacific.edu/stories/alaska-native-plants-and-
    traditional-uses/

Alaska Travel Industry Association. (2023). *Alaska Native Culture*. Retrieved
    November 14, 2023, from www.travelalaska.com:
    https://www.travelalaska.com/Things-To-Do/Alaska-Native-Culture

Alaskan-Natives.com. (n.d.). *Eyak Culture Area*. Retrieved November 16, 2023,
    from www.alaskan-natives.com: https://www.alaskan-
    natives.com/2152/eyak-culture-area/

Alaskan-Natives.com. (n.d.). *Native Village of Atka*. Retrieved November 16,
    2023, from www.alaskan-natives.com: https://www.alaskan-
    natives.com/663/native-village-atka/

Alaskan-Natives.com. (n.d.). *Native Village of Fort Yukon*. Retrieved November
    15, 2023, from www.alaskan-natives.com: https://www.alaskan-
    natives.com/700/native-village-fort-yukon/

Alaskan-Natives.com. (n.d.). *Native Village of Venetie Tribal Government*.
    Retrieved November 15, 2023, from /www.alaskan-natives.com:
    https://www.alaskan-natives.com/834/native-village-venetie-tribal/

Alatidd, J. (2022, May 12). *Native American boarding schools in Kansas supported US land grab and forced cultural assimilation.* Retrieved July 20, 2023, from Topeka Capital-Journal: https://www.cjonline.com/story/news/state/2022/05/12/report-native-american-boarding-schools-kansas-child-labor/9733760002/

Alchin, L. (2017). *Mandan Tribe.* Retrieved May 9, 2023, from warpaths2peacepipes.com: https://www.warpaths2peacepipes.com/indian-tribes/mandan-tribe.htm

Alchin, L. (2017). *Narragansett Tribe.* Retrieved April 19, 2023, from warpaths2peacepipes.com: https://www.warpaths2peacepipes.com/indian-tribes/narragansett-tribe.htm

Aleut Community of St. Paul Island Tribal Government. (2017). *The Aleut Community of St. Paul Island Tribal Government.* Retrieved November 16, 2023, from www.aleut.com: https://www.aleut.com/

Alexander, K. (2019, Febraury). *Susquehannock Tribe of the Northeast.* Retrieved April 28, 2023, from Legends of America: https://www.legendsofamerica.com/susquehannock-tribe/#:~:text=The%20Susquehannock%20people%2C%20also%20called%20the%20Conestoga%20by,has%20also%20been%20found%20in%20northern%20West%20Virginia.

Alexander, K. (2023, May). *Maidu Indians of Northern California.* Retrieved October 14, 2023, from www.legendsofamerica.com: https://www.legendsofamerica.com/maidu-indians/

Alexander, K. (2023, January). *The Sac and Fox Tribe.* Retrieved May 27, 2023, from Legends of America: https://www.legendsofamerica.com/sac-and-fox/

Alexander, K. (2023). *The Shasta Indians.* Retrieved October 23, 2023, from /www.legendsofamerica.com/: https://www.legendsofamerica.com/shasta-indians/

Alonso, L., Decora, L., & Bauer, U. (2019, August 8). *Obesity and Diabetes in the Winnebago Tribe of Nebraska: From community Engagement to Action, 2014-2019.* Retrieved July 28, 2023, from cdc.gov: https://www.cdc.gov/pcd/issues/2019/19_0181.htm

Alutiq Tribe of Old Harbor. (n.d.). *Alutiq Tribe of Old Harbor.* Retrieved November 16, 2023, from alutiiqtribe.org: https://sites.google.com/alutiiqtribe.org/main/home

ANCSA Regional Association. (n.d.). *ANCSA Regional Association.* Retrieved November 14, 2023, from ancsaregional.com: https://ancsaregional.com/

Anderson, M. (2022, October 17). *Conservationists begin to remove thousands of invasive trees at the Bear River Massacre site.* Retrieved July 28, 2023, from KSL-TV: https://www.ksl.com/article/50497312/conservationists-begin-to-remove-thousands-of-invasive-trees-at-the-bear-river-massacre-site

Anzalone, C. s. (2020, January 28). Retrieved July 9, 2023, from UB News Center: https://www.buffalo.edu/news/releases/2020/01/026.html

Apache Tribe of Oklahoma. (2020, March). *Apache Tribe of Oklahoma Injury Prevention Program.* Retrieved August 20, 2023, from ihs.gov: https://www.ihs.gov/sites/injuryprevention/themes/responsive2017/display_objects/documents/tipcap-funded/Apache_Tribe_of_Oklahoma_Program_Profile_2020.pdf

Apache Tribe of Oklahoma. (2023). *Welcome to the Apache Tribe of Oklahoma.* Retrieved August 4, 2023, from apacetribe.org: https://apachetribe.org/

Apache Tribe of Oklahome. (2023). *Welcome to the Apache Tribe of Oklahoma.* Retrieved August 4, 2023, from apachetribe.org: https://apachetribe.org/

apachetribe.org. (2020, March). *Injury Prevention Program.* Retrieved August 5, 2023, from apachetribe.org: https://www.ihs.gov/sites/injuryprevention/themes/responsive2017/display_objects/documents/tipcap-funded/Apache_Tribe_of_Oklahoma_Program_Profile_2020.pdf

Arnold, M., Bennett, S., Christensen, M., Harmon, Z., Hatch, C., & Reid, M. (2010). Shoshone Culture. In S. Bennett, *Transcultural Nursing.* Orem, UT: Utah Valley University. Retrieved June 18, 2023, from http://freebooks.uvu.edu/NURS3400/index.php/ch09-shoshone-culture.html

Arrigoni, B. (2006, September 30). *Grindstone Centennial: Tribal eldert shares history, traditions.* Retrieved November 2, 2023, from www.chicoer.com: https://www.chicoer.com/2006/09/30/grindstone-centennial-tribal-elder-shares-history-traditions/

Asylum Projects. (2021, December 21). *Pawnee Boarding School.* Retrieved September 14, 2023, from Asylum Projects: https://www.asylumprojects.org/index.php/Pawnee_Boarding_School

Augustine Band of Cahuilla Indians. (2018). *Cahuilla.* Retrieved September 25, 2023, from augustinetribe-nsn.gov/cahuilla-people: https://augustinetribe-nsn.gov/cahuilla-people/

Bacich, D. (2023). *The Luiseño of Southern California.* Retrieved October 13, 2023, from www.californiafrontier.net: https://www.californiafrontier.net/the-luiseno-of-southern-california/#The_Luiseno_Name

Baddour, D. (2022). *Coming Home.* Retrieved August 5, 2023, from The Nature Conservancy: https://www.nature.org/en-us/magazine/magazine-articles/texas-buffalo-project/

bahkhoje.com. (2023). *Bah Kho-Je.* Retrieved May 31, 2023, from Iowa Tribe of Oklahoma: https://www.bahkhoje.com/

Baker, M. (1981). *The Ethnobotany of the Yurok, Tolowa, and Karok Indians of northwest California.* Thesis, Arizona State University. doi:10.13140/RG.2.2.12690.66240

Barona Ban of Mission Indians. (2020). *Barona Band of Mission Indians.* Retrieved September 25, 2023, from www.barona-nsn.gov: https://www.barona-nsn.gov/

Bear River Band of the Rohnerville Rancheria. (2021). *Bear River Band of the Rohnerville Rancheria.* Retrieved September 22, 2023, from /www.bearriverrancheria.org: https://www.bearriverrancheria.org/

Benjamin, M. (2023). *Judge Upholds Decision Allowing Madera, CA Casino/Hotel Project to Proceed.* Retrieved 2023, from www.hotel-online.com: https://www.hotel-online.com/press_releases/release/judge-upholds-decision-allowing-madera-casino-project/

Benjamin, M. (2023, March 15). *Judge Upholds Decision Allowing Madera, CA Casino/Hotel Project to Proceed.* Retrieved October 20, 2023, from Today's News: https://www.hotel-online.com/press_releases/release/judge-upholds-decision-allowing-madera-casino-project/

Bennett, S., Barney, T., Hill, R., Hilton, L., StepaYananova, Taylor, T., & Young, D. (2010). Ute Culture. In S. N. Bennett, *Transcultural Nursing.* Utah Valley University. Retrieved August 18, 2023, from http://freebooks.uvu.edu/NURS3400/index.php/ch08-ute-culture.html

Benton Paiute Reservation. (2023). *Utu Utu Gwaitu Paiute Tribe*. Retrieved September 20, 2023, from www.bentonpaiutereservation.org: https://www.bentonpaiutereservation.org/

Berry Creek Rancheria of Maidu Indians. (n.d.). *Berry Creek Rancheria of Maidu Indians of California*. Retrieved October 15, 2023, from www.berrycreek maiduindians.org: https://www.berrycreekmaiduindians.org/

Big Sandy Rancheria. (2023). *Big Sandy Rancheria*. Retrieved October 19, 2023, from www.bigsandyrancheria.com: https://www.bigsandyrancheria.com/

Big Valley Band of Pomo Indians. (n.d.). *Big Valley Band of Pomo Indians*. Retrieved Ovtober 22, 2023, from www.bvrancheria.com: https://www.bvrancheria.com/

bigorrin.org. (n.d.). *Shawnee Mythology*. Retrieved June 13, 2023, from http://www.bigorrin.org/archive123.htm: http://www.bigorrin.org/archive123.htm

Bill of Rights Institute. (2023). *A Deep Stain on the American Character: John Marshall and Justice for Native Americans*. Retrieved August 22, 2023, from Bill of Rights Institute: https://billofrightsinstitute.org/activities/a-deep-stain-on-the-american-character-john-marshall-and-justice-for-native-americans-handout-a-narrative

Bird Grinnell, G. (1905). Some Cheyenne Plant Medicines. *American Anthropologists, 7*, 37-43. Retrieved May 16, 2023, from https://archive.org/details/jstor-659332

Bishop Paiute Tribe. (2022). *Welcome to our Tribe*. Retrieved June 11, 2023, from Bishop Paiute Tribe: https://www.bishoppaiutetribe.com/

Black Horse, Bree; Kilpatrick Townsend & Stockton LLP. (2023, June 26). *Oklahoma Tribel Regalia Bill Represents Restorative Justice for Oklahoma Native Students*. Retrieved July 10, 2023, from Kilpatrick Townsend: https://www.jdsupra.com/legalnews/oklahoma-tribal-regalia-bill-represents-1154568/

*Blackfeet Nation*. (2023). Retrieved May 13, 2023, from blackfeetnation.com: https://blackfeetnation.com/

Blue Lake Rancheria. (2023). *Blue Lake Rancheria*. Retrieved September 24, 2023, from www.bluelakerancheria-nsn.gov: https://www.bluelakerancheria-nsn.gov/

Bolton, A. (2022, May 24). *The Blackfeet Nation's struggles underscore the fentanyl crisis on Native American reservations.* Retrieved July 13, 2023, from Montana Public Radio: https://www.npr.org/sections/health-shots/2022/06/01/1101799174/tribal-leaders-sound-the-alarm-after-fentanyl-overdoses-spike-at-blackfeet-natio

Brasser, T. (1991). The Sarsi: Athapaskans on the Northern Plains. *Arctic Anthropology, 28*(1), 67-73. Retrieved August 7, 2023, from https://www.jstor.org/stable/40316293

britannica.com. (n.d.). *Diegueno.* Retrieved September 25, 2023, from www.britannica.com: https://www.britannica.com/topic/Diegueno

Bruchac, M. (2005). *Founding of Schaghticoke and Odanak.* Retrieved April 20, 2023, from Penn Libraries: https://repository.upenn.edu/cgi/view content.cgi?article=1146&context=anthro_papers

Buena Vista Rancheria Me-Wuk Indians. (2023). *Buena Vista Rancheria Me-Wuk Indians.* Retrieved October 17, 2023, from bvtribe.com: https://bvtribe.com/

Bureau of Indian Affairs. (n.d.). *Alaska Subsistence Program.* Retrieved November 21, 2023, from www.bia.gov: https://www.bia.gov/ service/alaska-subsistence-program

Bureau of Indian Affairs. (n.d.). *Indian Affairs.* Retrieved August 22, 2023, from Department of the Interior: https://www.bia.gov/

Bureau of Indian Education. (n.d.). *Bureau of Indian Education.* Retrieved September 16, 2023, from bie.edu: https://www.bie.edu/

Bureau of Land Management. (2021, August 17). *More than survival, the subsistence tradition sustains meaning for rural Alaska Natives abd non-native residents alike.* Retrieved November 21, 2023, from www.blm.gov: https://www.blm.gov/blog/2021-08-17/more-survival-subsistence-tradition-sustains-meaning-rural-alaska-natives-and-non

Burgess, K., & Spilde, K. (2004). *Indian Gaming and Community Building: A History of the Intergovernmental Relations of the Mohegan Tribe of Connecticut.* Case Study, Harvard University, The Harvard Project on American Indian Economic Development. Retrieved April 19, 2023, from https://hwpi. harvard.edu/files/hpaied/files/nigacasestudymohegan.pdf?m=1639579131

Burns Paiute Tribe. (2023). *Welcome to the Burns Paiute Tribe!* Retrieved June 11, 2023, from https://burnspaiute-nsn.gov/: https://burnspaiute-nsn.gov/

Cabazon Tribal Utility Authority. (2023). *Cabazon Tribal Utility.* Retrieved September 25, 2023, from cabazon-tu.com: https://cabazon-tu.com/

Cabeen, I. (2021, May 17). *Paiute Indian Cure for Warts.* Retrieved June 11, 2023, from UCS Digital Folklore Archives: http://folklore.usc.edu/paiute-indian-cure-for-warts/

Caddo Nation. (2023). *Caddo Nation.* Retrieved May 15, 2023, from mycaddonation.com: https://mycaddonation.com/

Cahuilla Band of Indians. (2023). *Cahuilla Band of Indians.* Retrieved September 25, 2023, from cahuilla-nsn.gov: https://cahuilla-nsn.gov/

CAL ICH. (2023, September 22). *California Tribes Receive $20 milliom in Funding for Homelessness and Housing Projects.* Retrieved September 24, 2023, from www.bcsh.ca.gov: https://www.bcsh.ca.gov/media/press_releases/calich_20230922.pdf

California Department of Parks and Recreation. (2023, April 26). *California State Parks and Cher-Ae-Heights Indian Community of the Trinidad Rancheria sign Memorandum of Understanding.* Retrieved October 3, 2023, from www.parks.ca.gov: https://www.parks.ca.gov/NewsRelease/1168

California Valley Miwok Tribe. (2003-2019). *California Valley Miwok Tribe.* Retrieved October 17, 2023, from californiavalleymiwok.us: https://californiavalleymiwok.us/

Campo Kumeyaay Nation. (2013). *Campo Kumeyaay Nation.* Retrieved September 26, 2023, from www.campo-nsn.gov: http://www.campo-nsn.gov/

Cannon, C. C. (2018, March). Ancient Wisdom, Modern Times: Decolonizing Eduycation Paradigms in a Southwestern Tribal Community. *Journal of Sustainability Education, 18.* Retrieved September 2, 2023, from http://www.susted.com/wordpress/content/ancient-wisdom-modern-times-decolonizing-education-paradigms-in-a-southwestern-tribal-community_2018_04/

Carlisle Indian Project. (2020). *Giving Voice to the Legacy.* Retrieved April 22, 2023, from Carlisle Indian School Project: https://carlisleindianschoolproject.com/

Carlisle, J. (1952). *Creek Indians*. Retrieved April 30, 2023, from Texas State Historical Association: https://www.tshaonline.org/handbook/entries/creek-indians

CasinosAvenue. (2023, May 27). *La Jolla Trading Post and Casino, Pauma Valley*. Retrieved October 13, 2023, from www.casinosavenue.com: https://www.casinosavenue.com/en/casino/la-jolla-trading-post-casino-pauma-valley/9624

Cassar, C. (2023, August 20). *Doiscovering the Rich History of the Quechan Tribe*. Retrieved September 10, 2023, from Anthropology Review: https://anthropologyreview.org/anthropology-archaeology-news/quechan-tribe/

Cassar, C. (2023, August 20). *Exploring the History and Culture of the Hupa Tribe*. Retrieved October 7, 2023, from anthropologyreview.org: https://anthropologyreview.org/anthropology-archaeology-news/hupa-tribe-history-culture/

catawba.com. (n.d.). *The Catawba Nation*. Retrieved April 28, 2023, from Catawba Indian Nation: https://www.catawba.com/

Cato Institute. (2013). *The Declaration of Independence and the Constitution of the United States of America*. Retrieved August 22, 2023, from Cato Institute: .https://www.cato.org/books/cato-pocket-constitution

cayuganation-nsn.gov. (n.d.). *Cayuga Nation*. Retrieved April 23, 2023, from Cayuga Nation of New York: https://cayuganation-nsn.gov/index.html

CDC.gov. (2010). *The Cherokee Nation Obesity and Tobacco Use Prevention*. Retrieved July 12, 2023, from CDC.gov: https://www.cdc.gov/nccdphp/dch/programs/communitiesputtingpreventiontowork/communities/profiles/pdf/CPPW_CommunityProfile_B1_CherokeeNation_FINAL_508.pdf

Cedarville Rancheria. (n.d.). *Cedarville Rancheria*. Retrieved September 20, 2023, from cedarvillerancheria.com: https://cedarvillerancheria.com/

Central NY News. (2022). *Meet the "Creek Rats" as they try to turn a stinky Syracuse stream into an attraction*. Retrieved July 7, 2023, from Central NY News: https://www.syracuse.com/news/2022/09/meet-the-creek-rats-as-they-try-to-turn-a-stinky-syracuse-stream-into-an-attraction.html

Chamberlin, R. (1911). *The Ethno-Botany of the Gosiute Indians of Utah.* Philadelphia: Academy of Natural Sciences. Retrieved August 14, 2023, from fs.usa.gov: https://www.jstor.org/stable/pdf/4063364.pdf

Chamberofcommerce.com. (2023). *Grindstone Indian Rancheria.* Retrieved November 5, 2023, from www.chamberofcommerce.com: https://www.chamberofcommerce.com/united-states/california/elk-creek/tribal-headquarters/32573109-grindstone-indian-rancheria

Chemehuevi Indian Tribe. (2023). *Chemehuevi Indian Tribe.* Retrieved September 27, 2023, from chemehuevi.org: https://chemehuevi.org/

cherokee.org. (2023). *Cherokee Nation.* Retrieved April 30, 2023, from Cherokee Nation: https://www.cherokee.org/

Cheyenne and Arapaho Tribes. (2022). *Tsistsistas | Hinono'ei.* Retrieved May 16, 2023, from cheyenneand arapaho-nsn.gov: https://www.cheyenne andarapaho-nsn.gov/

Cheyenne River Sioux Tribe. (n.d.). *Cheyenne River Sioux Tribe.* Retrieved June 4, 2023, from cheyenneriversioux.com: https://www.cheyenne riversioux.com/

chickasaw.net. (2023). *Chikasha saya.* Retrieved April 29, 2023, from The Chickasaw Nation: https://chickasaw.net/

Chicken Ranch Rancheria Me-Wuk Indians of California. (n.d.). *The mountains and streams are our home. Welcome to our land.* Retrieved October 17, 2023, from chickenranchrancheria.org: https://chickenranchrancheria.org/home

Chippewa Cree Tribe. (2011-2019). *Chippewa Cree Tribe Human Services Division.* Retrieved August 5, 2023, from ccthumanservices.org: http://www.ccthumanservices.org/

choctawnation.com. (2023). *Choctaw Nation of Oklahoma.* Retrieved April 30, 2023, from Choctaw Nation of Oklahoma: https://www.choctaw nation.com/

Citizen Potawatomi Nation. (2023). *People of the Place of Fire.* Retrieved June 12, 2023, from https://www.potawatomi.org/: https://www.potawatomi.org/

Coarsegold Historic Museum. (2023). *The Chukchansi People.* Retrieved October 21, 2023, from coarsegoldhistoricalsociety.com: https://coarsegoldhistoricalsociety.com/the-chukchansi-people/

Coeur d'Alene Tribe. (n.d.). *Coeur d'Alene Tribe.* Retrieved August 11, 2023, from cdatribe-nsn.gov: https://www.cdatribe-nsn.gov/

Colusa Indian Community Council. (2013). *Colusa Indian Community Councvi.* Retrieved November 2, 2023, from www.colusa-nsn.gov: https://www.colusa-nsn.gov/

Comanche Nation. (2023). *Comanche Nation Lords of the Plains.* Retrieved July 31, 2023, from comanchenation.com: https://comanchenation.com/

Confederated Salish & Kootenai Tribes. (2022). *Confederated Salish & Kootenai Tribes of the Flathead Reservation.* Retrieved August 15, 2023, from csktribes.org: https://www.csktribes.org/

Confederated Tribes of Siletz Indians. (2023). *Confederated Tribes of Siletz Indians.* Retrieved October 3, 2023, from www.ctsi.nsn.us: https://www.ctsi.nsn.us/

Congressional Research Service. (2023, February 8). *The 574 Federally Recognized Indian Tribes in the United States.* Retrieved August 22, 2023, from Congressional Research Service: https://crsreports.congress.gov/product/pdf/R/R47414

Countries and their Cultures. (2023). *Tolowa.* Retrieved September 24, 2023, from www.everyculture.com: https://www.everyculture.com/North-America/Tolowa.html

Coyote Valley Band of Pomo Indians. (2021). *Coyote Valley Band of Pomo Indians.* Retrieved October 22, 2023, from www.coyotevalleytribe.org: https://www.coyotevalleytribe.org/

Crow Canyon Archeological Center. (2023). *The Origin of the Name "Navajo".* Retrieved September 5, 2023, from crowcanyon.org: https://lcontent.crowcanyon.org/EducationProducts/peoples_mesa_verde/post_pueblo_navajo_name.php

crow-nsn.gov. (2023). *Executive Branck of the Apsáalooke Nation.* Retrieved May 27, 2023, from Crow Tribe: http://www.crow-nsn.gov/

Cultural Resources. (2015, January). *Saguaro Fruit: A Traditional Harvest.* Retrieved September 4, 2023, from Cultural Resources: https://www.nps.gov/sagu/learn/historyculture/upload/Saguaro-Fruit-A-Traditional-Harvest-Brief.pdf

Dakota Wicohan. (2020). *History on the Dakota of Minnesota.* Retrieved May 27, 2023, from Dakota Wicohan: https://dakotawicohan.org/dakota-of-minnesota-history/

D'Angelo, P. (2022, May 11). *One year into a new health clinic, the Upper Mattaponi Tribe is expanding and buying back lands.* Retrieved July 8, 2023, from Radio IQ: https://www.wvtf.org/news/2022-05-11/one-year-into-a-new-health-clinic-the-upper-mattaponi-tribe-is-expanding-and-buying-back-lands

Deerfield History Museum. (2020). *Glossary.* Retrieved April 20, 2023, from Deerfield History Museum: http://1704.deerfield.history.museum/list/glossary/all.do

Delaware Public Media. (2015, June 26). *History Matters: Nanticoke tribe seeks to sustain its identity.* Retrieved April 25, 2023, from Delaware Public Media: https://www.delawarepublic.org/culture-lifestyle-sports/2015-06-26/history-matters-nanticoke-tribe-seeks-to-sustain-its-identity

delawarenation-nsn.gov. (n.d.). *Delaware Nation.* Retrieved July 5, 2023, from delawarenation-nsn.gov: https://www.delawarenation-nsn.gov/

delawaretribe.org. (2023). *Official Web Site of the Delaware Tribe of Indians.* Retrieved April 23, 2023, from delawaretribe.org: https://delawaretribe.org/

Diamond Mountain Casino & Hotel. (2023). *Diamond Mountain Casino.* Retrieved October 15, 2023, from dmcah.com: http://dmcah.com/

Diaz-Gonzalez, M. (2020, January 30). *The complicated history of the Kinzua Dam and how it changed life for the Seneca people.* Retrieved June 23, 2023, from Environmental Health News: https://www.ehn.org/seneca-nation-kinzua-dam-2644943791.html

Dockter, M. (2021 [updated May 24, 2023], October 26). Omaha Tribe to provide housing aid, buys Walthill grocery store. *Sioux City Journal.* Retrieved June 8, 2023, from https://siouxcityjournal.com/news/local/omaha-tribe-to-provide-housing-assistance-for-tribal-residents-buys-walthill-grocery-store/article_bc54edb1-6e5c-5515-9a81-b15baa7baade.html#:~:text=--%20The%20Omaha%20Tribe%20of%20Nebraska%20said%20Tuesday,grocery%

Dolton-Thornton, N. (2019). *The Elem Tribe's Last Stand.* Retrieved October 22, 2023, from earthisland.org/journal: https://earthisland.org/journal/index.php/magazine/entry/the-elem-tribes-last-stand

Dressler, A. (2022, May 10). *"No More Stolen Sisters": A March to Remember Those Lost to Violence.* Retrieved July 26, 2023, from The Rapidian: https://therapidian.org/no-more-stolen-sisters-a-march-to-remember-those-lost-to-violence

Dry Creek Rancheria. (n.d.). *Dry Creek Rancheria of Pomo Indians.* Retrieved October 22, 2023, from drycreekrancheria.com: https://drycreekrancheria.com/

*Duckwater Shoshone Tribe.* (n.d.). Retrieved June 18, 2023, from https://www.duckwatertribe.org/: https://www.duckwatertribe.org/

Duren, J. (2023, January 9). *Pascua Yaqui Tribe Announces New Casino After Feds Expand Land Trust.* Retrieved September 11, 2023, from Play USA: https://www.playusa.com/pascua-yaqui-tribe-announces-new-arizona-casino/#:~:text=There%20are%20four%20casinos%20in%20the%20Tucson%20area%3A,Xavier%29%204%20Desert%20Diamond%20Casino%20Tucson%20%28San%20Xavier%29

East County News Service. (2021, October). *Former Manzanita tribal police chief admits to stealing over $300,000 from local tribe by selling fake badges.* Retrieved September 26, 2023, from eastcountymagazine.org: https://www.eastcountymagazine.org/former-manzanita-tribal-police-chief-admits-stealing-over-300000-local-tribe-selling-fake-badges

Eastern Aleutian Tribes. (2023). *Nelson Lagoon.* Retrieved November 16, 2023, from www.eatribes.org: https://www.eatribes.org/communities/nelson-lagoon/

Eastern Shawnee Tribe of Oklahoma. (2022). *Eastern Shawnee Tribe of Oklahoma.* Retrieved June 13, 2023, from https://estoo-nsn.gov/enterprises: https://estoo-nsn.gov/enterprises/

Eastern Shoshone. (2023). *Eastern Shoshone Tribe.* Retrieved June 18, 2023, from https://easternshoshone.org/: https://easternshoshone.org/

easternpequottribalnation.org. (2021). *Eastern Pequot Tribal Nation.* Retrieved April 18, 2023, from easternpequottribalnation.org: https://www.easternpequottribalnation.org/

Eggert, A. (2021). *New mining claims at Zortman prompt push for investigation.* Retrieved August 1, 2023, from Montana Free Press: https://montana freepress.org/2021/10/06/mine-claims-in-zortman-promp-call-for-investigation/

Elem Indian Colony. (2023). *Elem Indian Colony.* Retrieved October 22, 2023, from www.elemindiancolony.org: http://www.elemindiancolony.org/

Elk Valley Rancheria. (2023). *Elk Valley Rancheria.* Retrieved October 5, 2023, from elk-valley.com: https://elk-valley.com/

Elsworth, T. (2022, March 15). *Most Common Pacific Northwest Native Plants and their traditional/cultural uses.* Retrieved October 30, 2023, from www.recreationnorthwest.org: https://www.recreationnorthwest.org/recreation-northwest/most-common-pacific-northwest-native-plants-and-their-traditional-cultural-uses/

Ely Shoshone Tribe. (n.d.). *Ely Shoshone Tribe.* Retrieved June 18, 2023, from https://www.elyshoshonetribe.com/: https://www.elyshoshonetribe.com/

encyclopedia.com. (2018, May 21). *Abenaki-U\*X\*L Encyclopedia of Native American Tribes.* Retrieved April 17, 2023, from encyclopepia.com: https://www.encyclopedia.com/history/united-states-and-canada/north-american-indigenous-peoples/abnaki

encyclopedia.com. (2019). *Achumawi.* Retrieved September 20, 2023, from encyclopedia.com: https://www.encyclopedia.com/humanities/encyclopedias-almanacs-transcripts-and-maps/achumawi

Encyclopedia.com. (2019). *Aleut.* Retrieved November 16, 2023, from www.encyclopedia.com: https://www.encyclopedia.com/history/united-states-and-canada/north-american-indigenous-peoples/aleut

encyclopedia.com. (2019). *Chumash.* Retrieved October 7, 2023, from encyclopedia.com: https://www.encyclopedia.com/humanities/encyclopedias-almanacs-transcripts-and-maps/chumash

encyclopedia.com. (2019). *Karok.* Retrieved October 23, 2023, from encyclopedia.com: https://www.encyclopedia.com/humanities/encyclopedias-almanacs-transcripts-and-maps/karok

Encyclopedia.com. (2019). *Miwok.* Retrieved October 16, 2023, from www.encyclopedia.com/: https://www.encyclopedia.com/humanities/encyclopedias-almanacs-transcripts-and-maps/miwok-0 encyclopedia.com. (2019). *Modoc.* Retrieved October 18, 2023, from encyclopedia.com: https://www.encyclopedia.com/humanities/encyclopedias-almanacs-transcripts-and-maps/modoc

Encyclopedia.com. (2019). *Pit River Indians.* Retrieved October 21, 2023, from /www.encyclopedia.com: https://www.encyclopedia.com/humanities/encyclopedias-almanacs-transcripts-and-maps/pit-river-indians

Encyclopedia.com. (2019). *Quechan.* Retrieved September 10, 2023, from Encyclopedia.com: https://www.encyclopedia.com/humanities/encyclopedias-almanacs-transcripts-and-maps/quechan

encyclopedia.com. (2019). *Siletz.* Retrieved October 3, 2023, from encyclopedia.com: https://www.encyclopedia.com/humanities/encyclopedias-almanacs-transcripts-and-maps/siletz

encyclopedia.com. (2019). *Yahi and Yana.* Retrieved October 24, 2023, from www.encyclopedia.com: https://www.encyclopedia.com/humanities/encyclopedias-almanacs-transcripts-and-maps/yahi-and-yana

encyclopedia.com. (2019). *Yurok.* Retrieved September 24, 2023, from /www.encyclopedia.com/: https://www.encyclopedia.com/history/united-states-and-canada/north-american-indigenous-peoples/yurok

Encyclopedia.ocm. (2019). *Tohono O'odham.* Retrieved September 4, 2023, from encyclopedia.com: https://www.encyclopedia.com/humanities/encyclopedias-almanacs-transcripts-and-maps/tohono-oodham

Enterprise Rancheria. (2023). *Enterprise Rancheria.* Retrieved October 15, 2023, from enterpriserancheria.org: https://enterpriserancheria.org/

EPA.gov. (2021, August 31). *EPA and Justice Department reach settlement with Northern Cheyenne Utilities Commission to address Clean Water Act Violations in Montana.* Retrieved July 14, 2023, from EPA.gov: https://www.epa.gov/newsreleases/epa-and-justice-department-reach-settlement-northern-cheyenne-utilities-commission

epa.gov. (2023, June 23). *Superfund Sites in Reuse in Oklahoma.* Retrieved September 8, 2023, from epa.gov: https://www.epa.gov/superfund-redevelopment/superfund-sites-reuse-oklahoma

Evans, H. (2023, August 31). *Whu are the Miwok Indians?* Retrieved October 5, 2023, from www.unitedstatesnow.org: https://www.unitedstatesnow.org/who-are-the-miwok-indians.htm

everyculture.com. (2023). *Hidatsa-Religion and Expressive Culture.* Retrieved
    May 9, 2023, from everyculture.com: https://www.everyculture.com/
    North-America/Hidatsa-Religion-and-Expressive-Culture.html

everyculture.com. (2023). *Kickapoo-Religion and Expressive Culture.* Retrieved
    June 1, 2023, from everyculture.com: https://www.everyculture.com/
    North-America/Kickapoo-Religion-and-Expressive-Culture.html

Everything Explained Today. (2009-2023). *La Posta Band of Diegueno Mission
    Indians Explained.* Retrieved September 26, 2023, from
    /everything.explained.today: https://everything.explained.today/
    La_Posta_Band_of_Diegue%c3%b1o_Mission_Indians/

Everything Explained Today. (2009-2023). *Tolowa Explained.* Retrieved
    September 24, 2023, from everything.explained.today:
    https://everything.explained.today/Tolowa/

Fallon Paiute-Shoshone Tribe. (n.d.). *The Fallon Paiute-Shoshone Tribe.*
    Retrieved June 11, 2023, from https://www.fpst.org/: https://www.fpst.org/

Fanta, B. (2022, May 10). *The first years of Genoa Industrial School.* Retrieved July
    24, 2023, from history.nebraska.gov: https://history.nebraska.gov/the-first-
    years-of-genoa-indian-industrial-school/

Federated Indians of Graton Rancheria. (2023). *Federated Indians of Graton
    Rancheria.* Retrieved October 5, 2023, from gratonrancheria.com:
    https://gratonrancheria.com/

Feller, W. (n.d.). *Chemehuevi Indians.* Retrieved September 27, 2023, from
    /mojavedesert.net: http://mojavedesert.net/chemehuevi-indians/

Feller, W. (n.d.). *Timbisha Shoshone.* Retrieved June 18, 2023, from
    https://mojavedesert.net/timbisha-shoshone/: https://mojavedesert.net/
    timbisha-shoshone/

Ferris, K. (2012). *Plants and Medicines of the Chippewa.* Retrieved May 27, 2023,
    from Turtle Mountain Chippewa Heritage Center: http://www.chippe
    waheritage.com/heritage-blog2/plants-and-medicines-of-the-chippewa

Flathead Watershed Source Book. (2010-2023). *Ql'spe (Pend d'Oreille or
    Kalispel) and Selis (Salish or Flathead).* Retrieved August 16, 2023, from
    flatheadwatershed.org: http://www.flatheadwatershed.org/
    cultural_history/pend_salish.shtml

Forest County Potawatomi. (2023). *Forest County Potawatomi.* Retrieved June 12, 2023, from https://www.fcpotawatomi.com/: https://www.fcpotawatomi.com/

Fort Belknap Indian Community. (2023). *Welcome to Fort Belknap Indian Community.* Retrieved July 31, 2023, from ftbelknap.org: https://ftbelknap.org/

Fort Independence Indian reservation. (2020). *Fort Independence Indian Reservation.* Retrieved June 11, 2023, from Fort Independence: https://fortindependence.com/

Fort McDowell Yavapai Nation. (2013-2020). *Fort McDowell Yavapai Nation.* Retrieved September 12, 2023, from www.fmyn.org: https://www.fmyn.org/

Fort Mojave Indian Tribe. (2023). *Pipa Aha Macav.* Retrieved October 18, 2023, from www.fortmojaveindiantribe.com: https://www.fortmojaveindiantribe.com/

Fort Peck Tribes. (n.d.). *Fort Peck Tribes.* Retrieved June 4, 2023, from fortpecktribes.org: https://fortpecktribes.org/

Fort Sill Apache Tribe. (2020). *Fort Sill Apache Tribe.* Retrieved August 30, 2023, from fortsillapache-nsn.gov: https://fortsillapache-nsn.gov/

Foster, N. (2023, August 10). *What is an Indian Reservation?* Retrieved September 14, 2023, from unitedstatesnow.org: https://www.https://www.unitedstatesnow.org/what-is-an-indian-reservation.htm

FourStar, R. (. (1992-2003). *History of the Assiniboine People from the Oral Tradition.* Retrieved July 30, 2023, from msun.edu: https://mtprof.msun.edu/Win2003/r4star.html

Frey, R. (n.d.). *Coeur d'Alene (Schitsu'umsh).* Retrieved August 12, 2023, from University of Washington.edu: https://content.lib.washington.edu/aipnw/frey.html

Ft McDermitt Piute-Shoshone TRB. (2023). *Ft McDermitt Piute-Shoshone TRB.* Retrieved July 25, 2023, from fmcdwc.org: https://www.fmcdwc.org

FTA. (2021). *FTA Application.* Retrieved November 15, 2023, from www.dol.gov:

https://www.dol.gov/sites/dolgov/files/olms/regs/compliance/DSP/2021/08
aug/AK-2021-030-00_Nome_Eskimo_Community.pdf

Gebauer, A. (2020, April 15). *The slow clean up of Midnite Mine*. Retrieved
October 26, 2023, from outthereoutdoors.com:
https://outthereoutdoors.com/the-slow-clean-up-of-midnite-mine/

Genco, J. (2021, March 30). *Volunteers deliver precious commodity to Tuscorara
Nation residents*. Retrieved April 28, 2023, from Niagara Gazette:
https://www.niagara-gazette.com/news/local_news/volunteers-deliver-
precious-commodity-to-tuscarora-nation-residents/article_15dfc374-f9c0-
5d66-a146-fcd9fec3cb84.html

Gershon, L. (2021, January 15jstor.org). *Native Nations and the BIA: It'd
Complicated*. Retrieved September 15, 2023, from jstor.org:
https://daily.jstor.org/native-nations-and-the-bia-its-complicated/

Gifford, E. (1936). *Yavapai*. Retrieved September 13, 2023, from naeb.brit.org:
http://naeb.brit.org/uses/tribes/284/

Gila River Indian Community. (n.d.). *Discover the Gila River Indian Community*.
Retrieved September 3, 2023, from www.gilariver.org:
https://www.gilariver.org/

Gillis, E. (2021). *Radicalized Health Disparities for North Carolina's Unrecognized
Tribes*. Retrieved April 26, 2023, from Healers and Patients in North
Carolina: https://healersandpatients.web.unc.edu/2021/05/racialized-
health-disparities-for-north-carolinas-unrecognized-tribes/

Gillis, E. (2021, May 3). *Radicalized Health Disparities for North Carolina's
Unrecognized Tribes*. Retrieved July 8, 2023, from Healers and Patients in
North Carolina: https://healersandpatients.web.unc.edu/2021/05/
racialized-health-disparities-for-north-carolinas-unrecognized-tribes/

Gilmore, M. (1919). *Ponca*. Retrieved September 8, 2023, from Native
American Ethnobotany DB: http://naeb.brit.org/uses/tribes/205/

Goodluck, K. (2023, May 10). *The Wiyot Tribe Is Getting Its Land Back and*.
Retrieved October 31, 2023, from znetwork.org:
https://znetwork.org/znetarticle/the-wiyot-tribe-is-getting-its-land-back-
and-making-california-more-affordable/

Goshute Indian Tribe. (2023). *Goshute Indian Tribe*. Retrieved August 14, 2023,
from ctgr.us/home: https://ctgr.us/home/

Government Accountability Office. (2022, June 28). *Bureau if Indian Education has Addressed Some Management Weaknesses, but Additional Work is Needed on Others*. Retrieved September 16, 2023, from GAO.gov: https://www.gao.gov/assets/730/721392.pdf

GovTribe.com. (2022). *Project Grant OK2022005*. Retrieved July 31, 2023, from govtribe.com: https://govtribe.com/award/federal-grant-award/project-grant-ok2022005

Graetz, R. (2023). *The Blackfeet Nation has long, epic history*. Retrieved May 14, 2023, from This is Montana: https://www.umt.edu/this-is-montana/columns/stories/blackfeet.php

Grand Traverse Band of Ottawa and Chippewa Indians. (n.d.). *Grand Traverse Band of Ottawa and Chippewa Indians*. Retrieved June 6, 2023, from https://www.gtbindians.org/: https://www.gtbindians.org/

Great Falls Tribune. (2022, August 6). *Zortman-Landusky mine owner fined more than $500K for mining violations*. Retrieved Aigust 1, 2023, from Great Falls Tribune: https://www.greatfallstribune.com/story/news/2022/08/06/zortman-landusky-mine-owner-fined-more-than-500k-for-mining-violations/65394320007/

Greenville Rancheria. (2023). *Greenville Rancheria*. Retrieved October 15, 2023, from www.grth.org: https://www.grth.org/

grist.org. (2023, July 22). *In Arizona Water Ruling, the Hopi Tribe sees limits on its future*. Retrieved September 1, 2023, from grist.org: https://grist.org/drought/in-arizona-water-ruling-the-hopi-tribe-sees-limits-on-its-future/

Growing Magazine. (2018, October 8). *Urban Farming Operation Thrives*. Retrieved September 14, 2023, from Growing Magazine: https://www.growingmagazine.com/urban-farming-operation-thrives/

Gun Lake Tribe. (2017). *Gun Lake Tribe*. Retrieved June 12, 2023, from https://gunlaketribe-nsn.gov/: https://gunlaketribe-nsn.gov/

Habematolel Pomo of Upper Lake. (2023). *Habematolel Pomo of Upper Lake*. Retrieved October 22, 2023, from www.hpultribe-nsn.gov: https://www.hpultribe-nsn.gov/

haliwa-saponi.org. (2022). *Official Site of the Haliwa Saponi Tribe*. Retrieved April 26, 2023, from haliwa-saponi.org: https://www.haliwa-saponi.org/

Hamilton, T. (2018). Piscataway-Conoy: Rejuvenating ancestral ties to southern parks. *Maryland Natural Resopurce Magazine*. Retrieved April 26, 2023, from https://news.maryland.gov/dnr/2018/10/01/piscataway-conoy/

Hamilton, T. (2018, Fall). *Piscataway-Conoy: Rejuvenating ancestral ties to southern parks*. Retrieved July 7, 2023, from Maryland Natural Resource Magazine: https://news.maryland.gov/dnr/2018/10/01/piscataway-conoy/

Handpicked Alaska. (n.d.). *Handpicked Alaska*. Retrieved November 14, 2023, from handpickedalaska.com: https://handpickedalaska.com/

Hanes, R., & Pifer, M. (2023). *Blackfoot*. Retrieved May 14, 2023, from Countries and their Cultures: https://www.everyculture.com/multi/A-Br/Blackfoot.html

Hannahville Indian Community. (n.d.). *Hannahville Potawatomi*. Retrieved June 12, 2023, from https://hannahville.net/: https://hannahville.net/

Hard Rock Hotel and Casino Sacramento at Fire Mountain. (2023). *Hard Rock Hotel and Casino Sacramento at Fire Mountain*. Retrieved October 15, 2023, from www.hardrockhotelsacramento.com: https://www.hardrockhotelsacramento.com/

Hardy, N. (2021). Eugenics at UVM: Why Abenaki leaders feel the apology wasn't enough. *The Vermont Cynic*, May. Retrieved April 17, 2023, from https://vtcynic.com/news/eugenics-at-uvm-why-abenaki-leaders-feel-the-apology-wasnt-enough/

Harrington, M. (1913, September). A Visit to the Otoe Indians. *The Museum Journal, IV*(3). Retrieved June 6, 2023, from The Museum Journal: https://www.penn.museum/sites/journal/285/

Harrington, W. (1914). *Sacred Bundles of the Sac and Fox Indians* (Vol. IV No. 2). Philadelphia: The University Museum Anthropological Publications.

haudenosauneeconfederacy.com. (2023). *Haudenosaunee Confederacy*. Retrieved April 28, 2023, from haudenosauneeconfederacy.com: https://www.haudenosauneeconfederacy.com/

Havasupai Tribe. (2017-2020). *The Havasupai Tribe*. Retrieved September 3, 2023, from theofficialhavasupaitribe.com: https://theofficial havasupaitribe.com/

Hawaiian Kingdom Blog. (2016, Febraury 26). *Natives of the Hawaiian Islands are not Indigenous Peopele, They're Aboriginal*. Retrieved November 22, 2023, from Hawaiian Kingdom Blog: https://hawaiiankingdom.org/blog/natives-of-the-hawaiian-islands-are-not-indigenous-theyre-aboriginal/

Hays, G. (2022, April 28). *Researcher unearth the painful history of a Native boarding school in Missouri.* Retrieved May 29, 2023, from PBS news Hour: https://www.pbs.org/newshour/education/uncovering-the-traumatic-history-of-one-native-american-boarding-school-in-the-midwest

Herrera, A. (2022, March 1). *'This is our backyard': Quapaw Nation asserts more control over environment withgin its reservation.* Retrieved September 8, 2023, from KOSU: https://www.kosu.org/energy-environment/2022-03-01/this-is-our-backyard-quapaw-nation-asserts-more-control-over-environment-within-its-reservation

Herrington, A. (2020, February 28). *In Historic First, California Weed Grow Receives License to Operate on Tribal Lands.* Retrieved October 5, 2023, from merryjane.com: https://merryjane.com/culture/in-historic-first-california-weed-grow-receives-license-to-operate-on-tribal-lands

Herrington, A. (2023, August 3). *Red Lake Nation Opens Minnesota's First Adult-Use Dispensary.* Retrieved August 6, 2023, from HighTimes: https://hightimes.com/dispensaries/red-lake-nation-opens-minnesotas-first-adult-use-dispensary/

Heutmaker, M. (2017, September 29). The Spiritual or Religious Beliefs of the Powhaten. *Classroom.* Retrieved April 26, 2024, from https://classroom.synonym.com/the-spiritual-or-religious-beliefs-of-the-powhatan-12087579.html

Hewitt, J. N. (1939). Notes on the Creek Indians. (J. R. Swanson, Ed.) *Anthropological Papers, 10*(123). Retrieved April 30, 2023

Hicks, P., Haaland, B., Feehan, M., Crandall, A., Pettey, J., Nuttall, E., . . . DeAngelis, M. (2020). Systemic Disease and Ocular Comorbidity Analysis of Geographically Isolated Federally Recognized American Indian Tribes of the Intermountain West. *Journal of Clinical Medicine*, 1-24. Retrieved August 14, 2023, from https://www.mdpi.com/2077-0383/9/11/3590

Hirst, K. K. (2020, August 29). *Cheyenne People: History, Culture, and Current Status.* Retrieved May 16, 2023, from ThoughtCo.: https://www.thoughtco.com/cheyenne-people-4796619

History.com Editors. (2023, April 20). *Trail of Tears*. Retrieved April 30, 2023, from History: https://www.history.com/topics/native-american-history/trail-of-tears

Hobson, J. (2019, August 13). *Guardians of the Grand Canyon: The Havasupai Tribe's Long Connection to the Canyon's Red Rocks*. Retrieved September 3, 2023, from wbur.org: https://www.wbur.org/hereandnow/2019/08/13/grand-canyon-havasupai-tribe

Ho-Chunk Nation Department of Health. (2023, June). *Health Profile Report*. Retrieved July 20, 2023, from health.ho-chunk.com: https://health.ho-chunk.com/index.htm

ho-chunknation.com. (2023). *Ho-Chunk Nation*. Retrieved May 29, 2023, from ho-chunknation.com: https://ho-chunknation.com/

Hoffmann, M. (2023, May 18). Omaha Tribe of Nebraska opens new casino in hopes of attracting visitors, new business. Retrieved June 8 2023, from https://www.ktiv.com/2023/05/18/omaha-tribe-nebraska-opens-new-casino-hopes-attracting-visitors-new-business/

Holmes, E. (1884). *Medicinal Plants Used by the Cree Indians, Hudson's Bay Territory*. Retrieved August 5, 2024, from Henriette's Herbal Homepage from American Journal of Pharmacy: https://www.henriettes-herb.com/eclectic/journals/ajp/ajp1884/12-cree.html

Holmes, J. (2011, July 21). *A Brief History of the Ponca People*. Retrieved September 8, 2023, from www.powwows.com: https://www.powwows.com/a-brief-history-of-the-ponca-people/

Hoopa Valley Tribe. (2003-2020). *Hoopa Valley Tribe*. Retrieved October 7, 2023, from www.hoopa-nsn.gov: https://www.hoopa-nsn.gov/

Hopi Tribe Economic Development Corporation. (n.d.). *Making Economic Development Impacts on Behalf of the Hopi People*. Retrieved August 31, 2023, from htedc.com: https://htedc.com/

Hopland Band of Pomo Indians. (2023). *Our Culture*. Retrieved October 22, 2023, from www.hoplandtribe.com: https://www.hoplandtribe.com/

hualapai-nsn.gov. (n.d.). *The Hualapai Tribe*. Retrieved September 2, 2023, from hualapai-nsn.gov: https://hualapai-nsn.gov/

HUD. (2022). *Cold Springs Rancheria of Mono Indians*. Retrieved October 19, 2023, from ihbgformula.com:

https://ihbgformula.com/FRFinalAllocationFY2022/Cold%20Springs%20Ra
ncheria%20of%20Mono%20Indians.pdf

IHS. (1955-2023). *Indian Health Service*. Retrieved November 12, 2023, from
www.ihs.gov: https://www.ihs.gov/

ihs.gov. (2020, June). *Ak-Chin Indian Community Injury Prevention Program*.
Retrieved September 4, 2023, from ihs.gov: https://www.ihs.gov/sites/
injuryprevention/themes/responsive2017/display_objects/documents/tipca
p-funded/Ak-Chin_Program_Profile_2020.pdf

ihs.gov. (n.d.). *Colorado Service Unit*. Retrieved September 3, 2023, from
ihs.gov: https://www.ihs.gov/phoenix/healthcarefacilities/coloradoriver/

Iipay Nation of Santa Ysabel. (n.d.). *Iipay Nation of Santa Ysabel*. Retrieved
September 26, 2023, from iipaynationofsantaysabel-nsn.gov:
https://www.iipaynationofsantaysabel-nsn.gov/

Illinois State Museum Society. (2000). *The Illinois*. Retrieved May 30, 2023,
from MuseumLink Illinois: https://www.museum.state.il.us/muslink/
nat_amer/post/htmls/hi_decline.html

indianaffairs.nd.gov. (2002). *The History and Culture of the Manbdan, Hidatsa,
Sahnish (Arikara)*. Retrieved May 2, 2023, from North Dakota Department
of Public Instruction: https://www.indianaffairs.nd.gov/sites/www/
files/documents/pdfs/History_and_Culture_Mandan_Hidatsa_and_Arikar
a.pdf

Inter Tribal Council of Arizona. (2011-2023). *Salt River Pima-Maricopa Indian
Community*. Retrieved September 3, 2023, from itcaonline.com:
https://itcaonline.com/member-tribes/salt-river-pima-maricopa-indian-
community/

International Indian Treaty Council. (2021, November 17). *The International
Indian Treaty Council Joins the Pit river Tribe in Celebrating Historic Land and
Cultural rights Victories*. Retrieved October 22, 2023, from www.iitc.org:
https://www.iitc.org/the-international-indian-treaty-council-joins-the-pit-
river-tribe-in-celebrating-historic-land-and-cultural-rights-victories/

Inter-Tribal Council of Arizona. (2011-2023). *San Carlos Apache Tribe-Tonto
Apache Tribe*. Retrieved August 30, 2023, from itcaonline.com:
https://itcaonline.com/member-tribes/

Inuit Circumpolar Council, & Jessen Williamson, J. (2023, October 16). *Inuit People*. Retrieved November 15, 2023, from www.britannica.com: https://www.britannica.com/topic/Inuit-people

Inupiat Community of the Arctic Slope. (2023). *ICAS*. Retrieved November 15, 2023, from icas-nsn.gov: https://icas-nsn.gov/

Iowa Tribe of Kansas and Nebraska. (2023). *Welcome to the Iowa Tribe of Kansas and Nebraska*. Retrieved May 31, 2023, from iowatrib ofkansasandnebraska .com: https://iowatribeofkansasandnebraska.com/

Ioway Cultural Institute. (n.d.). *Medicine Plants used by the Ioway and Otoe*. Retrieved May 31, 2023, from Ioway Cultural Institute: http://ioway.nativeweb.org/culture/medicineplants.htm

Island Mountain Development Group. (2023). *IMDG*. Retrieved July 31, 2023, from islandmtn.com: https://www.islandmtn.com

Jackson Rancheria Casino Resort. (2023). *Jackson Rancheria Casino Resort*. Retrieved October 17, 2023, from jacksoncasino.com: https://jacksoncasino.com/

Jakober, A. (2023). *Cochiti's Return to Native Foods Brigns Better Health & Economy*. Retrieved September 6, 2023, from firstnations.org: https://www.firstnations.org/stories/cochitis-return-to-native-foods-brings-better-health-economy/

James, I. (2020, December 15). *"We need water to survive": Hopi Tribe pushes for solutions in long struggle for water*. Retrieved September 1, 2023, from Arizona Republic: https://www.waternewsnetwork.com/we-need-water-to-survive-hopi-tribe-pushes-for-solutions-in-long-struggle-for-water/

Jamul Indian Village. (2021). *Jamul Indian Village*. Retrieved September 26, 2023, from jamulindianvillage.com: https://jamulindianvillage.com/

Jannen, B. J. (2012, April). *Manzanita Tribe and others at risk from 'dirty electricity' from wind turbines, expert warns*. Retrieved September 26, 2023, from www.eastcountymagazine.org: https://www.eastcountymagazine .org/manzanita-tribe-and-others-risk-dirty-electricity-wind-turbines-expert-warns

Johnson, A. (n.d.). *Th Hualapai Tribe*. Retrieved September 3, 2023, from Prezi.com: https://prezi.com/wh_ufyfrwkvv/hualapai-tribe/

Jones, N. (2023, September 6). *Isleta Casino sees health and business benefits after going non-smoking2-23.* Retrieved September 7, 2023, from kunm.org: https://www.kunm.org/local-news/2023-09-06/isleta-casino-sees-health-and-business-benefits-after-going-non-smoking

Jones, W. (1939). *Ethnography of the Fox Indians.* (M. Welpley Fisher, Ed.) Retrieved May 29, 2023, from Smithsonian Institution Bureau of American Ethnology Bulletin 125: bulletin1251939smit.pdf

Jordan, J. (2008). *Plains Apache Ethnobotany.* University of Oklahoma Press. Retrieved August 6, 2023

Justice Murphy for the U.S. Supreme Court. (1942). *Seminole Nation v. United States.* Retrieved August 22, 2023, from Marquette.edu: https://law.marquette.edu/sites/default/files/Seminole%20Nation%20v.%20United%20States%20%281942%29%20%28edited%29.pdf

Justo. (2023, May 4). *Cultural Traditions of Kalispel Tribe: Insights into Native American Practices.* Retrieved October 8, 2023, from nativetribe.info: https://nativetribe.info/cultural-traditions-of-kalispel-tribe-insights-into-native-american-practices/

Justo. (2023, March24). *Explore the Culture of the Miwok Tribe: History, Traditions, and Beliefs.* Retrieved October 5, 2023, from nativetribe.info: https://nativetribe.info/explore-the-culture-of-the-miwok-tribe-history-traditions-and-beliefs/

Kalispel Tribe of Indians. (2023). *We are Kalispel.* Retrieved October 8, 2023, from kalispeltribe.com: https://kalispeltribe.com/

Kapoor, M. (2021, June 29). Mining for lithium, at cost to Indigenous religions. *High Country News.* Retrieved September 2, 2023, from https://www.hcn.org/issues/53.7/indigenous-affairs-mining-for-lithium-at-a-cost-to-indigenous-religions

Karuk Tribe. (2015). *Karuk Tribe.* Retrieved October 23, 2023, from /www.karuk.us: https://www.karuk.us/

Kashia Band of Pomo Indians. (n.d.). *About the Kashia Band of Pomo Indians.* Retrieved October 22, 2023, from www.stewartspoint.org: https://www.stewartspoint.org/wp2/

Kauana Osorio, E. (2021). *Struggle for Hawaiian Cultural Survival.* Retrieved November 24, 2023, from Ballardbrief@byu.edu:

https://ballardbrief.byu.edu/issue-briefs/struggle-for-hawaiian-cultural-survival#:~:text=Native%20Hawaiians%20lost%20their%20homes%2C%20health%2C%20resources%2C%20and,residents%20of%20Hawaii%2C%20and%20still%20lack%20affordable%20housing.

Kaur, H. (2021, November 5). *An indigenous tribe in Texas is getting its sacred burial ground back.* Retrieved August 3, 2023, from CNN: https://edition.cnn.com/2021/11/05/us/lipan-apache-cemetery-presidio-texas-cec/index.html

Kesler, S., Aronczyk, A., Romer, K., & Rubin, W. (2023, March 24). *Blood, oil, and the Osage Nation: The battle over headrights.* Retrieved June 8, 2023, from NPR: https://www.npr.org/2023/03/23/1165619070/osage-headrights-killers-of-the-flower-moon-fletcher-lawsuit

Ketchum, D. (2017, September 29). *Religious Beliefs of the Pueblos.* Retrieved September 7, 2023, from classroon-synonym.com: https://classroom.synonym.com/mikmaq-religious-beliefs-12085356.html

KFF Health News. (2021, October 22). *Montana Tribes want to stop jailing people for suicide attempts but lack a safer alternative.* Retrieved July 30, 2023, from US News & World Report: https://www.usnews.com/news/health-news/articles/2021-10-22/montana-tribes-want-to-stop-jailing-people-for-suicide-attempts-but-lack-a-safer-alternative

Kickapoo Tribe of Oklahoma. (n.d.). *A HO PI TI KE NO.* Retrieved May 31, 2023, from Kickapoo Tribe of Oklahoma: https://www.kickapootribeofoklahoma.com/

kickapootexas.org. (2021). *Kickapoo Traditional Tribe of Texas.* Retrieved May 31, 2023, from kickapootexas.org: https://kickapootexas.org/

Kiowa Tribe. (2023). *Beautiful People.* Retrieved August 1, 2023, from kiowatribe.org: https://www.kiowatribe.org/

Klauk, E. (2023). *Human Health Impacts at Fort Belknap from Gold Mining.* Retrieved August 1, 2023, from carlton.edu: https://serc.carleton.edu/research_education/nativelands/ftbelknap/humanhealth.html

Kletsel Dehe Wintun Nation. (2020). *Kletsel Dehe Wintun Nation.* Retrieved November 2, 2023, from www.kletseldehe.org: https://www.kletseldehe.org/

Kootenai Tribe of Idaho. (2022). *Kootenai Tribe of Idaho.* Retrieved August 15, 2023, from kootenai.org: https://www.kootenai.org/

Kraker, D. (2004, March 15). *Tribe defeted a dam and won back its water.* Retrieved September 14, 2023, from High Country News: https://www.hcn.org/issues/270/14627

Krasnow, B. (2016, September 29). *'Heart and soul' returns to Cochiti Pueblo in land swap with state.* Retrieved September 6, 2023, from The New Mexican: https://www.santafenewmexican.com/news/local_news/heart-and-soul-returns-to-cochiti-pueblo-in-land-swap-with-state/article_7fc9886b-3465-5e59-8b20-86932f3261e6.html

ktik-nsn.gov. (n.d.). *Kansas Kickapoo Tribe.* Retrieved May 31, 2023, from ktik-nsn.gov: https://www.ktik-nsn.gov/

Kumeyaay. (2023). *Kumeyaay.* Retrieved Septermber 26, 2023, from www.kumeyaay.com/capitan-grande-band-of-indians: https://www.kumeyaay.com/capitan-grande-band-of-indians.html

La Flesche, F. (n.d.). *The Omaha Buffalo Medicine Men.* Retrieved June 8, 2023, from omahatribe.unl.edu: http://omahatribe.unl.edu/etexts/oma.0017/

La Posta Band of Mission Indians. (n.d.). *La Posta Band of Mission Indians.* Retrieved September 26, 2023, from www.lptribe.net: https://www.lptribe.net/

LaMore, J. (2021, May 18). *Survival of the Southern Piute.* Retrieved July 25, 2023, from National Park Service: https://www.nps.gov/articles/survival-of-the-southern-paiute.htm

LaRock, M. (n.d.). Saw-Whet Owl and the Origin of Menominee Medicine. Retrieved June 4, 2023, from The Menominee Clans Story: https://www3.uwsp.edu/menominee-clans/dedications/MenomineeMedicine.html

Las Vegas Paiute Tribe. (n.d.). *Las Vegas Paiute Tribe.* Retrieved June 11, 2023, from https://www.lvpaiutetribe.com/: https://www.lvpaiutetribe.com/

Lauer, K. (2022, May 18). *Richmond: Ppoint Molate to be sold for $400 to Native American tribe after 270-acre development plan fizzles.* Retrieved October 22, 2023, from East Bay Times: https://www.eastbaytimes.com/2022/05/18/richmond-point-molate-to-be-sold-for-400-to-native-american-tribe-after-270-acre-development-plan-fizzles/

Ledford, C. R. (2012, December). A Preliminary Pawnee Ethnobotany Checklist. *Oklahoma Native Plant Record, 12*, pp. 33-42. doi:https://doi.org/10.22488/okstate.17.100090

Legends of America. (2023). *Lenape-Delaware Tribe.* Retrieved April 23, 2023, from Legends of America: https://www.legendsofamerica.com/lenape-delaware-tribe/

Legends of America. (2023). *The Hopi-Peaceful Ones of the Southwest.* Retrieved September 1, 2023, from Legends of America: https://www.legendsofamerica.com/na-hopi/

lenapeindiantribeof delaware.com. (2010). *Lenape Indian Tribe of Delaware.* Retrieved April 23, 2023, from lenapeindiantriabeofdelaware.com: http://www.lenapeindiantribeofdelaware.com/

Lipan Apache Tribe. (2023). *Official Website of the Lipan Apache Tribe.* Retrieved August 3, 2023, from lipanapache.org: http://www.lipanapache.org/

Lipan Apache Tribe. (n.d.). *Lipan Apache Tribe of Texas.* Retrieved August 2, 2023, from lipanapache.org: http://www.lipanapache.org/

Little Missouri Headwaters Cultural Heritage Project. (2018). *Gros Ventre.* Retrieved July 31, 2023, from Little Missouri Headwaters Cultural Heritage Project: https://lmheadwatersproject.com/gros-ventre/

Little River Band of Ottawa Indians. (2-23). *Little River Band of Ottawa Indians.* Retrieved June 6, 2023, from https://lrboi-nsn.gov/: https://lrboi-nsn.gov/

Little Traverse Bay Bands of Odawa Indians. (n.d.). *Little Traverse Bay Bands of Odawa Indians.* Retrieved June 6, 2023, from https://ltbbodawa-nsn.gov/: https://ltbbodawa-nsn.gov/

Longtoe Sheehan, V. (2022, June 26). *Nebizun: Water is life curatorial statement.* Retrieved April 17, 2023, from Abenaki Arts & Education Center: https://abenaki-edu.org/nebizun-water-is-life-curator-statement/

Los Coyotes Band of Cahuilla & Cupeno Indians. (2021). *Los Coyotes Reservation.* Retrieved 25 2023September, from www.loscoyotestribe.org: https://www.loscoyotestribe.org/

Lovelock Paiute Tribe. (n.d.). *Lovelock Paiute Tribe.* Retrieved June 11, 2023, from Lovelock Paiute Tribe: https://www.paiutetribelovelock.org/

Lower Brule Sioux Tribe. (2019). *Kul Wikasa Oyate*. Retrieved June 4, 2023, from lowerbrulesiouxtribe.com: https://www.lowerbrulesiouxtribe.com/

Lower Sioux Indian Community. (2023). *Lower Sioux Indian Community*. Retrieved June 21, 2023, from https://lowersioux.com/: https://lowersioux.com/

lowersioux.com. (2023). *Lower Sioux Indian Community*. Retrieved May 27, 2023, from lowersioux.com: https://lowersioux.com/

Lytton Rancheria of California. (2022). *Lytton Rancheria*. Retrieved October 22, 2023, from www.lyttonrancheria.com: https://www.lyttonrancheria.com/

Magagnini, S. (2015, April 28). *Tiny California casino tribe adopts white men in failed attempt to profit*. Retrieved September 20, 2023, from Merced Sun-Star: https://www.mercedsunstar.com/news/weird/article19784055.html

Magee, M. (2021). *An Exploration of Ethnobotanically Significant Plants to the Native American Tribes of Montana*. Retrieved August 6, 2023, from ScholarWorks at University of Montana: https://scholarworks.umt.edu/ cgi/viewcontent.cgi?article=1366&context=utpp

Malinowski, K. (n.d.). *Report on the Health, Diet, and Old Ways of the Blackfeet*. Retrieved July 13, 2023, from American Indian Health & Diet Project: https://aihd.ku.edu/foods/Blackfeet.html

Manchester Point-Arena of Pomo Inbdians. (2023). *Manchester Point-Arena of Pomo Inbdians*. Retrieved October 22, 2023, from www.mpapomotribe.org: https://www.mpapomotribe.org/

Mandewo, A. (2020). *a Brie History on the Trail of Tears*. Retrieved April 30, 2023, from The Inigenous Foundation: https://www.theindigenous foundation.org/articles/a-brief-history-on-the-trail-of-tears

Mark, J. (2021, April 27). *Cahokia*. Retrieved May 16, 2023, from World History Encyclopedia: https://www.worldhistory.org/cahokia/

Marsteller, D., & Marsteller, T. (2021, July 10). *History of the Chetco People*. Retrieved October 5, 2023, from HMdb.org: https://www.hmdb.org/m.asp?m=176836

Martin, J. (2016). *The Tuscarora*. Retrieved April 28, 2023, from North Carolina History Project: https://northcarolinahistory.org/encyclopedia/the-tuscarora/

Maryland Archives. (2022, March 14). *Maryland at a Glance: Native Americans.* Retrieved April 22, 2023, from Mrayland Manual On-Line: https://msa. maryland.gov/msa/mdmanual/01glance/native/html/01native.html

mashpeewampanoagtribe-nsn.gov. (n.d.). *Mashpee Wampanoag Tribe.* Retrieved April 21, 2023, from mashpeewampanoagtribe-nsn.gov.: https://mashpeewampanoagtribe-nsn.gov/

Mattaponi Tribe. (2022). *Mattaponi Tribe.* Retrieved July 8, 2023, from Mattaponi Tribe.Org: https://www.mattaponitribe.org/

McCartlin, G., & Rementer, J. (1986). Lenape Indian Medicine. *Bulletin of the Archaeological Society of New Jersey, 40.* Retrieved April 23, 2023, from Bulletin of the Archeological Society of New Jersey: https://delawaretribe.org/wp-content/uploads/LENAPE-MEDS.pdf

McTighe, F. (2018, April 3). *Medicine wheel key in traditional Blackfoot wellness.* Retrieved May 14, 2023, from Macleod Gazette: https://www.fortmacleodgazette.com/2018/medicine-wheel-key-in-traditional-blackfoot-wellness/

Mechoopda Indian Tribe. (2023). *Mechoopda Indian Tribe of Chico Rancheria.* Retrieved October 15, 2023, from www.mechoopda-nsn.gov: https://www.mechoopda-nsn.gov/

menominee-nsn.gov. (2023). *The Menominee Indian Tribe of Wisconsin.* Retrieved June 4, 2023, from menominee-nsn.gov: https://menominee-nsn.gov/

Merriam-Webster. (2023). *Mattole.* Retrieved September 22, 2023, from merriam-webster.com: https://www.merriam-webster.com/dictionary/Mattole

Merriam-Webster Dictionary. (2023). *Maricopa.* Retrieved September 3, 2023, from Merriam-Webster.com: https://www.merriam-webster.com/dictionary/Maricopa

Mesa Grande. (2023). *Haawka.* Retrieved September 26, 2023, from mesagrandeband-nsn.gov: https://www.mesagrandeband-nsn.gov/

Mescalero Apache Tribe. (2023). *Mescalero Apache Tribe.* Retrieved August 30, 2023, from mescaleroapachetribe.com: https://mescaleroapachetribe.com/

meskwaki.org. (2023). *Meskwaki Nation.* Retrieved May 27, 2023, from Sac and Fox Tribe of Mississippi: https://www.meskwaki.org/

Metlakatla Indian Community. (2022). *Welcome to Metlakatla, Alaska.* Retrieved November 16, 2023, from www.metlakatla.com: https://www.metlakatla.com/

Meyer, D. (2011). *Plains Crees.* Retrieved August 5, 2023, from Encyclopedia of the Great Plains: http://plainshumanities.unl.edu/ encyclopedia/doc/egp.na.086

mhanation.com. (2018). *MHA Nation.* Retrieved May 2, 2023, from MHA Nation: https://www.mhanation.com/

miamiindians.org. (n.d.). *The Miami Nation of Indiana.* Retrieved June 5, 2023, from miamiindians.org: http://www.miamiindians.org/

Miamination.com. (2023). *The Miami Tribe of Oklahoma.* Retrieved June 5, 2023, from miamination.com: https://www.miamination.com/

micmac-nsn.gov. (2023). *Mi'kmaq Nation.* Retrieved April 17, 2023, from micmac-nsn.gov: http://micmac-nsn.gov/

Middletown Rancheria of Pomo Indians of California. (2021). *Middletown Rancheria.* Retrieved October 22, 2023, from middletownrancheria-nsn.gov: https://middletownrancheria-nsn.gov/

Miewald, C. (1995, February). The Nutritional Impacts of European Contact on the Omaha: A Continuing Legacy. *Great Plains Research, 5*(1), 71-113. Retrieved June 8, 2023, from https://www.jstor.org/stable/23777767

Milkawkee Public Museum. (2022). *Ho-Chunk Culture.* Retrieved May 29, 2023, from Milwaukee Public Museum: https://www.mpm.edu/content/ wirp/ICW-52

Miller, V. (1982). The Decline of Nova Scotia Micmac Population, A.D. 1600-1850. *Culture, 2*(3). Retrieved April 17, 2023, from Culture: https://www.erudit.org/en/journals/culture/1900-v1-n1-culture06111/1078116ar.pdf

Milwaukee Public Museum. (2022). *Federal Acknowledgement or Recognition.* Retrieved August 29, 2023, from Milwaukee Public Museum: https://www.mpm.edu/educators/wirp/nations/tribe/federal-acknowledgement

Milwaukee Public Museum. (2022). *Menominee History.* Retrieved June 5, 2023, from Milwaukee Public Museum: https://www.mpm.edu/content/

wirp/ICW-153#:~:text=The%20Menominee%20lived%20around%20
Green,mouth%20of%20the%20Menominee%20River.

Milwaukee Public Museum. (2022). *Ojibwe History*. Retrieved May 27, 2023,
from Milwaukee Public Museum: https://www.mpm.edu/content/
wirp/ICW-151

Minnesota Chippewa Tribe. (n.d.). *Welcome to the Minnesota Chippewa Tribe*.
Retrieved May 18, 2023, from Minnesota Chippewa Tribe:
https://www.mnchippewatribe.org/

Mistequa Casino Hotel. (2023). *Mistequa Casino Hotel*. Retrieved October 26,
2023, from mistequa.com: https://mistequa.com/

Mobley, A. (2020, Novemnber 12). *Oklahoma's Environmentally Toxic Ghost
Town*. Retrieved September 10, 2023, from advocate.jbu.edu:
https://advocate.jbu.edu/2020/11/12/oklahomas-environmentally-toxic-
ghost-town/#:~:text=Children%20in%20Picher%20got%20sick%20
very%20often%20and,high%20infant%20mortality%20rates%20to%20the%
20chat%20piles.

Modoc Nation. (2023). *Modoc Nation*. Retrieved October 18, 2023, from
modocnation.com: https://modocnation.com/

Mojave Desert.net. (n.d.). *Timbisha Shoshone*. Retrieved July 28, 2023, from
MojaveDesert.net: https://mojavedesert.net/timbisha-shoshone/

Montana Cowboy Hall of Fame. (2021). *The Sacred Medicine Tree of the Salish*.
Retrieved August 16, 2023, from Montana Cowboy Hall of Fame:
https://montanacowboyfame.org/inductees/2009/11/the-sacred-medicine-
tree-of-the-salish

Montana Little Shell Chippewa Tribe. (n.d.). *Who we are*. Retrieved July 14,
2023, from https://www.montanalittleshelltribe.org/:
https://www.montanalittleshelltribe.org/

montanakids.com. (2020). *Crow Indian Reservation*. Retrieved May 27, 2023,
from http://montanakids.com: https://montanakids.com/history_and_
prehistory/indian_reservations/crow.htm

Mooretown Rancheria of Maidu Indians. (2022-2023). *Mooretown Rancheria*.
Retrieved October 15, 2023, from www.mooretownrancheria-nsn.gov:
https://www.mooretownrancheria-nsn.gov/

Morongo Band of Mission Indians. (2022). *Morongo*. Retrieved September 25, 2023, from morongonation.org: https://morongonation.org/

mptn-nsn.gov. (2023). *The Mashantucket (Western) Pequot Tribal Nation*. Retrieved April 18, 2023, from Mashantucket Pequot Tribal Nation: https://www.mptn-nsn.gov/default.aspx

mt.gov. (n.d.). *Chippewa Cree Tribe*. Retrieved Auguist 5, 2023, from tribalnations.mt.gov: https://tribalnations.mt.gov/Directory/ ChippewaCreeTribe

Murphy, C. (2017, August 14). *Navajo Herbal Remedies*. Retrieved September 5, 2023, from healthfully.com: https://healthfully.com/440145-navajo-herbal-remedies.html

muscogeenation.com. (2023). *The Muscogee Nation*. Retrieved April 30, 2023, from The Muscogee Nation: https://www.muscogeenation.com/

Nambé Pueblo. (2014). *Nambé Pueblo*. Retrieved September 7, 2023, from www.nambepueblo.org: https://www.nambepueblo.org/

nanticokeindians.org. (2011). *Nanticoke Indian Home Page*. Retrieved April 24, 2023, from nanticokeindians.org: http://www.nanticokeindians.org/

nanticokelenapemuseum.org. (2017). *Plant Medicine*. Retrieved April 25, 2023, from Nanticoke and Lenape Confederation: Learning Center and Museum: https://nanticokelenapemuseum.org/learning-center/742/plant-medicine/

Narragansett Indian Tribe. (2022). *Narragansett Indian Tribe*. Retrieved April 19, 2023, from narragansettindiannation.org: https://narragansettindiannation.org/

National Conference of State Legislatures. (2016, October 10). *State Recognition of American Indian Tribes*. Retrieved August 29, 2023, from National Conference of State Lergislatures: https://www.ncsl.org/quad-caucus/state-recognition-of-american-indian-tribes

National Congress of American Indians. (2021). *Food Sovereignty San Carlos Apache Tribe*. Retrieved August 30, 2023, from National Congress of American Indians: https://www.ncai.org/ptg/SCAT.Case.Study.pdf#:~: text=Through%20military%20and%20civilian%20authorities%2C%20the% 20federal%20government,society%20by%20micromanaging%20every%20a spect%20of%20Apache%20life.

National Park Service. (2015). *Mojave Tribe: Culture*. Retrieved October 18, 2023, from www.nps.gov: https://www.nps.gov/moja/learn/ historyculture/mojave-culture.htm

National Park Service. (2016, July 28). *Gates of the Arctic*. Retrieved November 21, 2023, from www.nps.gov: https://www.nps.gov/gaar/learn/ historyculture/subsistence.htm

National Park Service. (2017, May 9). *History of Subsistence Management in Alaska*. Retrieved November 21, 2023, from www.nps.gov: https://www.nps.gov/subjects/alaskasubsistence/education.htm

National Park Service. (2021, February 18). *People of the Islands*. Retrieved November 22, 2023, from www.nps.gov: https://www.nps.gov/havo/learn/ historyculture/native-hawaiians.htm

National Park Service. (2023, August 14). *Mojave Tribe*. Retrieved October 18, 2023, from home.nps.gov: https://home.nps.gov/moja/learn/ historyculture/mojave-tribe.htm

*Native Alliance Against Violence*. (2023). Retrieved August 7, 2023, from oknaav.org: https://oknaav.org/

Native Conservancy. (2021). *Eyak History*. Retrieved November 16, 2023, from www.nativeconservancy.org: https://www.nativeconservancy.org/eyak-history.html

*Native Hope*. (2022). Retrieved August 9, 2023, from nativehope.org: https://www.nativehope.org

Native Ministries International. (2022). *Skull Valley Band of Goshute Indians of Utah*. Retrieved August 14, 2023, from Native Ministeries International: https://data.nativemi.org/tribal-directory/Details/skull-valley-band-of-goshute-indians-of-utah-198481

Native Village of Eyak. (n.d.). *Native Village of Eyak*. Retrieved November 16, 2023, from www.eyak-nsn.gov: https://www.eyak-nsn.gov/

Native Village of Kluti-Kaah. (n.d.). *Welcome to the Native Village of Kluti-Kaah*. Retrieved November 16, 2023, from www.klutikaah.com: http://www.klutikaah.com/

Native Voices. (n.d.). *1942. Unangan evacuated, interned during WWII*. Retrieved November 16, 2023, from Native Voices: https://www.nlm.nih.gov/native voices/timeline/469.html#:~:text=It%20was%20something%20they%20had

%20to,in%20Southeast%20Alaska%2C%20where%20many%20died.&text=
It%20was%20something%20they,Alaska%2C%20where%20many%20died.
&text=something%20they%20had%20to,in%2

Native-Americans.com. (2012, July 10). *Table Mountain Rancheria of California.*
Retrieved October 20, 2023, from native-americans.com: https://native-
americans.com/table-mountain-rancheria-index

native-languages.org. (1998-2000). *Original Tribal Names of Native North
American People.* Retrieved June 3, 2023, from Native Languages of the
Americas Website: http://www.native-languages.org/original.htm

native-net.org. (2005-2020). *Lakota Indians.* Retrieved June 4, 2023, from native-
net.org: https://www.native-net.org/tribes/lakota-indians.html

nau.edu. (2023, March 8). *Community partner highlight: the Crow Tribe.*
Retrieved July 15, 2023, from nau.edu: https://nau.edu/cher/partner-crow-
tribe/

New Mexico Tourism Department. (2023). *Santa Clara.* Retrieved September 8,
2023, from www.newmexico.org: https://www.newmexico.org/native-
culture/native-communities/santa-clara-pueblo/

New Mexico Tourism Department. (2023). *Tesuque Pueblo.* Retrieved
September 8, 2023, from www.newmexico.org: https://www.newmexico
.org/native-culture/native-communities/tesuque-pueblo/

New Mexico Tourism Department. (2023). *Zia Pueblo.* Retrieved September 8,
2023, from www.newmexico.org: https://www.newmexico.org/native-
culture/native-communities/zia-pueblo/

New World Encyclopedia. (2023, May 22). *Yaqui.* Retrieved September 12,
2023, from New World Encyclopediau: https://www.newworld
encyclopedia.org/entry/Yaqui

NewsCenter1 Staff. (2022, January 24). *Tribes to assume control of all tribal
healthcare in Pennington County.* Retrieved July 20, 2023, from
NewsCenter1: https://www.newscenter1.tv/news/tribes-to-assume-
control-of-all-tribal-healthcare-in-pennington-county/article_a883934b-
dcb7-5385-bf29-43bd10c6c8e5.html

NIDC. (n.d.). *Food Assessment.* Retrieved June 24, 2023, from https://nippi.org/:
https://nippi.org/

niehs.nih.gov. (2021). *Environmental Exposures of the Northenr Arapaho Tribe: An Exploratory Study.* Retrieved July 30, 2023, from niehs.nih.gov: https://tools.niehs.nih.gov/portfolio/index.cfm?do=portfolio.grantDetail&grant_number=R21ES032137

NIGC.gov. (2022). *National Indian Gaming Commission.* Retrieved June 20, 2023, from https://www.nigc.gov/: https://www.nigc.gov/

nihb.org. (n.d.). *Local Impact-South Carolina.* Retrieved July 10, 2023, from National Indian Health Board: https://www.nihb.org/sdpi/local_impact_catawba.php

nimhd.nih.gov. (2019, November 12). *Sharing the Message of Health, Fighting Chronic Disease in the Crow Nation: A Q&A.* Retrieved July 15, 2023, from nimhd.nih.gov: https://www.nimhd.nih.gov/news-events/features/community-health/crow-nation.html

nipmucnation.org. (2021). *Tribal Government of the Nipmuc Nation.* Retrieved April 20, 2023, from Nipmuc Nation Tribal Council, Inc.: https://www.nipmucnation.org/

nippi.org. (2023). *Nipmuc Indian Development Corporation.* Retrieved April 20, 2023, from nippi.org: https://nippi.org/

NIWRC.org. (2023). *National Indigenous Women's Resource Center.* Retrieved August 9, 2023, from niwrc.org: https://www.niwrc.org/

NOAA Fisheries. (2020, November 25). *Endangered Sturgeon get help from Pamunkey Indian Tribe in Virginia.* Retrieved July 8, 2023, from NOAA Fisheries: https://www.fisheries.noaa.gov/feature-story/endangered-sturgeon-get-help-pamunkey-indian-tribe-virginia

Nome Eskimo Community. (2023). *Nome Eskimo Community.* Retrieved November 15, 2023, from www.necalaska.org: https://www.necalaska.org/

North Fork Rancheria of Mono Indians. (2020). *North Fork Rancheria of Mono Indians of California.* Retrieved October 20, 2023, from www.northforkrancheria-nsn.gov: https://www.northforkrancheria-nsn.gov/

Northern Arapaho Tribe. (n.d.). *Northern Arapaho Tribe.* Retrieved June 22, 2023, from https://www.northernarapaho.com/: https://www.northernarapaho.com/

Northern Arapaho Tribe. (n.d.). *Northern Arapaho Tribe*. Retrieved July 29, 2023, from northernarapaho.com: https://northernarapaho.com/

Northern Cheyenne Tribe. (2013). *Breaking Free from Fort Dependency*. Retrieved May 16, 2023, from cheyennenation.com: http://www.cheyennenation.com/

Northwestern Band of the Shoshone Nation. (n.d.). *Northwestern Band of the Shoshone Nation*. Retrieved June 18, 2023, from http://www.nwbshoshone.com/: http://www.nwbshoshone.com/

Nottawaseppi Huron Band of the Potawatomi. (2022). *Nottawaseppi Huron Band of the Potawatomi*. Retrieved June 12, 2023, from https://nhbp-nsn.gov/: https://nhbp-nsn.gov/

NPS.gov. (n.d.). *Early Choctaw History*. Retrieved April 30, 2023, from National Park Service: https://www.nps.gov/natr/learn/historyculture/choctaw.htm#:~:text=The%20Choctaw%20people's%20ancestral%20homeland,important%20to%20the%20Choctaw%20people.

obsn.org. (2021). *Occaneechi Band of the Saponi Nation*. Retrieved April 26, 2023, from obsn.org: https://obsn.org/

Odell, J. (2017-2023). *History-Andrew Taylor Still, MD, DO*. Retrieved June 13, 2023, from Bioregulatory Medicine Institute: https://www.biologicalmedicineinstitute.com/andrew-taylor-still

Oglala Sioux Tribe. (2022). *Oglala Sioux Tribe*. Retrieved June 4, 2023, from oglalalakotanation.net: https://oglalalakotanation.net/

Ohio History Central. (n.d.). *Wea Indians*. Retrieved June 19, 2023, from Ohio History Central: https://ohiohistorycentral.org/w/index.php?title=Wea_Indians

Ohkay Owingeh. (2018). *Ohkay Owingeh*. Retrieved September 7, 2023, from ohkay.org: http://ohkay.org/

Ojibwe. (2015, April 16). *Indiana 101: Kootenai Origins and Spirituality*. Retrieved August 15, 2023, from Daily Kos: https://www.dailykos.com/stories/2015/4/16/1378060/-Indians-101-Kootenai-Origins-and-Spirituality

ok.gov. (2010, November 1). *Oklahoma Statutes on Smoking in Public Places and Indoor Workplaces*. Retrieved July 12, 2023, from ok.gov: https://www.ok.gov/breatheeasyok/documents/Oklahoma%20Laws%20on%20Secondhand%20Smoke%20effective%20Nov%201%202010.pdf

Oklahoma Historical Society. (n.d.). *Folk Medicine*. Retrieved May 16, 2023, from The Encyclopedia of Oklahoma History and Culture: https://www.okhistory.org/publications/enc/entry.php?entry=FO009

Oklahoma Historical Society. (n.d.). *Kiowa*. Retrieved August 2, 2023, from Oklahoma Historical Society: https://www.okhistory.org/publications/enc/entry.php?entry=KI017

Oklahoma Historical Society. (n.d.). *Peoria*. Retrieved May 30, 2023, from The Encyclopedia of Oklahoma History and Culture: https://www.okhistory.org/publications/enc/entry?entry=PE013#:~:text=The%20Peoria%20tribe%20belong%20to,practiced%20a%20nature%2Dcentered%20religion.

Oklahoma Indian Tribe Education Guide. (2014, July). *Ottawa Tribe of Oklahoma*. Retrieved June 11, 2023, from Oklahoma Indian Tribe Education Guide: https://sde.ok.gov/sites/ok.gov.sde/files/documents/files/Tribes_of_OK_Education%20Guide_Ottawa_Tribe.pdf

Oklahoma Wildlife Department. (n.d.). *Neosho Mucket*. Retrieved July 25, 2023, from Oklahoma Wildlife Department: ttps://www.wildlifedepartment.com/wildlife/field-guide/invertebrates/neosho-mucket

okstate.edu. (1845). *Treaty with the Creeks and Seminole, 1845*. Retrieved April 30, 2023, from Tribal Treaties Database: https://treaties.okstate.edu/treaties/treaty-with-the-creeks-and-seminole-1845-0550

Olade, M., & Smith, A. (2023, July 6). *The Colorado River Flooded Chemehuevi Land. Decades Later, the Tribe Still Sturggles to Take Its Share of Water*. Retrieved September 27, 2023, from mavensnotebook.com/: https://mavensnotebook.com/2023/07/06/pro-publica-the-colorado-river-flooded-chemehuevi-land-decades-later-the-tribe-still-struggles-to-take-its-share-of-water/

Oleson, E. (2014, November 21). *Nipmuc artifacts tell tale of their role in early Massachusetts*. Retrieved April 20, 2023, from Telegram & Gazette: https://www.telegram.com/story/news/local/south-west/2014/11/21/nipmuc-artifacts-tell-tale-their/35910645007/

Omaha Public Schools. (2014). *Pre-statehood Interaction of Native Americans and Europeans*. Retrieved June 8, 2023, from Omaha Public Schools: https://www.ops.org/Page/1874

Omaha Tribe of Nebraska. (2023). *Omaha Tribe of Nebraska*. Retrieved June 8, 2023, from https://www.omahatribe.com/: https://www.omahatribe.com/

Omaha Tribe of Nebraska. (2023). *Omaha Tribe of Nebraska*. Retrieved June 6, 2023, from https://www.omahatribe.com/: https://www.omahatribe.com/

Oneida Nation of Wisconsin. (2023). *Oneida*. Retrieved June 21, 2023, from https://oneida-nsn.gov/: https://oneida-nsn.gov/

oneidaindiannation.com. (2020). *Oneida*. Retrieved april 25, 2023, from oneidaindiannation.com: https://www.oneidaindiannation.com/

oneida-nsn.gov. (2023). *Clan Systems*. Retrieved April 28, 2023, from Oneida Nation: https://oneida-nsn.gov/our-ways/our-story/clan-systems/

Onondaganation.org. (2023). *Onondaga Nation: People of the Hills*. Retrieved April 25, 2023, from Onondaga Nation: https://www.onondaganation.org/

Osage Nation. (n.d.). *The Osage Nation*. Retrieved June 8, 2023, from osgaenation-nsn.gov: https://www.osagenation-nsn.gov/

Otoe Missouria Tribe. (n.d.). *Otoe Missouria Tribe*. Retrieved June 5, 2023, from omtribe.org: https://www.omtribe.org/

Ottawa Tribe of Oklahoma. (2021). *The Adawe of Oklahoma*. Retrieved June 10, 2023, from Ottawa Tribe of Oklahoma: https://www.ottawatribe.gov/

OVC. (2022, September 21). *FY 2022 Tribal Victim Services Set-Aside Project: Tonkawa Tribe*. Retrieved August 7, 2023, from ovc.ojp.gov: https://ovc.ojp.gov/funding/awards/15povc-22-gg-01271-tvag

Paiute Indian Tribe of Utah. (2021). *Paiute Indian Tribe of Utah*. Retrieved June 11, 2023, from https://pitu.gov/: https://pitu.gov/

Pala Band of Mission Indians. (2023). *Pala Band of Mission Indians*. Retrieved October 13, 2023, from wwwpalatribe.com: http://www.palatribe.com/

Pamunkey Indian Tribe. (2021). *We are the Pamunkey Indian Tribe*. Retrieved July 8, 2023, from Pamunkey Indian Tribe: https://pamunkey.org/

Pascua Yaqui Tribe. (2023). *Pascua Yaqui Tribe*. Retrieved September 11, 2023, from www.pascuayaqui-nsn.gov: https://www.pascuayaqui-nsn.gov/

Paskenta Band of Nomlacki Indians. (2023). *Paskenta Band of Nomlacki Indians*. Retrieved November 2, 2023, from paskenta-nsn.gov: https://paskenta-nsn.gov/

Pauma Band of Luiseno Indians. (n.d.). *Pauma Band of Luiseno Indians*. Retrieved October 13, 2023, from wwwpaumatribe.com: https://www.paumatribe.com/

Pawnee Nation. (2023). *Pawnee Nation*. Retrieved September 14, 2023, from pawneenation.org: https://pawneenation.org/

Pawnee Nation College. (n.d.). *Pawnee Nation College*. Retrieved September 14, 2023, from pawneenationcollege.org: https://pawneenationcollege.org/

Pawnee Tribal Development Corporation. (n.d.). *Pawnee Tribal Development Corporation*. Retrieved September 14, 2023, from www.pawneetdc.com: https://www.pawneetdc.com

Pechanga Band of Indians. (2023). *Pechange Band of Indians*. Retrieved October 13, 2023, from /www.pechanga-nsn.gov: https://www.pechanga-nsn.gov/

Peoria Tribe of Indians of Oklahoma. (n.d.). *Peoria Tribe of Indians of Oklahoma*. Retrieved May 30, 2023, from peoriatribe.com: https://peoriatribe.com/

Perez, J. (2022, November 24). *Arizona's Indigenous communities are reviving millenia-old food that was nearly lost*. Retrieved September 4, 2023, from azcentral.com: https://www.azcentral.com/story/news/local/arizona/2022/11/24/arizonas-indigenous-communities-are-reclaiming-ways-farm-grow-food/10401816002/

Perttula, T. (1952 (updated 10/8/2020)). *Caddo Indians*. Retrieved May 16, 2023, from TSHA Texas State Historical Association: https://www.tshaonline.org/handbook/entries/caddo-indians

Picard, K. (2019, May 16). *A Traditional Abenaki Elder Helps Those in Need*. Retrieved April 17, 2023, from sevendaysvt.com: https://www.sevendaysvt.com/vermont/a-traditional-abenaki-elder-helps-those-in-need/Content?oid=2510557

Picayune Rancheria of the Chukchansi Indians. (2023). *Picayune Rancheria of the Chukchansi Indians*. Retrieved October 21, 2023, from /chukchansi-nsn.gov: https://chukchansi-nsn.gov/

Picuris Pueblo. (n.d.). *Picuris Pueblo*. Retrieved September 7, 2023, from www.picurispueblo.org: http://www.picurispueblo.org/

Pinoleville Pomo Nation. (2020, October 22). *Pinoleville Pomo Nation*. Retrieved 2023, from pinoleville-nsn.gov: https://pinoleville-nsn.gov/

*Pipa Aha Macav*. (2023). Retrieved from www.fortmojaveindiantribe.com: https://www.fortmojaveindiantribe.com/

piscatawayindians.com. (2022). *Cedarville Band of the Piscataway Indians, Inc.* Retrieved April 25, 2023, from piscatawayindians.com: https://www.piscatawayindians.com/

Piscawatawayconoytribe.com. (n.d.). *Piscataway Conoy Tribe.* Retrieved April 25, 2023, from Piscatawayconoytribe.com: http://www.piscatawayconoytribe.com/

Pit River Tribe. (n.d.). *Official Home of the Pit River Tribe.* Retrieved October 21, 2023, from pitrivertribe.gov: https://pitrivertribe.gov/

Poff, B. (n.d.). *The Paiute & Shoshone of Fort McDermitt, Nevada.* Retrieved June 11, 2023, from Sierra Service Project: https://oregonexplorer.info/ data_files/OE_location/lakes/documents/fortmcdermitt.history.pdf

Pokagon Band of Potawatomi. (2023). *Welcome to Pokagon Band of Potawatomi.* Retrieved June 12, 2023, from https://www.pokagonband-nsn.gov/: https://www.pokagonband-nsn.gov/

Pokagon, Simon 1898 collection. (1998-2020). *Native languages of the Americas: Ottawa Legends, Myths & Stories.* Retrieved June 11, 2023, from http://www.native-languages.org/ottawa-legends.htm: http://www.native-languages.org/ottawa-legends.htm

Ponca Tribe of Indians of Oklahoma. (2022). *Ponca Tribe of Indians of Oklahoma.* Retrieved September 8, 2023, from www.ponca-nsn.gov: https://www.ponca-nsn.gov/

Ponca Tribe of Nebraska. (2023). *Ponca Tribe of Nebraska.* Retrieved September 8, 2023, from www.poncatribe-ne.org: https://www.poncatribe-ne.org/

Potter Valley Tribe. (2023). *Potter Valley Tribe.* Retrieved October 22, 2023, from pottervalleytribe.com: https://pottervalleytribe.com/

Prairie Band Potawatomi Nation. (2023). *Prairie Band Potawatomi Nation.* Retrieved June 12, 2023, from https://www.pbpindiantribe.com/: https://www.pbpindiantribe.com/

prairieisland.org. (2023). *Bdewkantunwan. Born of the Waters.* Retrieved May 27, 2023, from Prairie Island Indian Community: https://prairieisland.org/

Pueblo de Cochiti. (n.d.). *Pueblo de Cochiti Administration.* Retrieved September 6, 2023, from www.cochiti.org/: http://www.cochiti.org/

Pueblo of Acoma. (n.d.). *Welcome to the Pueblo of Acoma, Haaku.* Retrieved Septmeber 5, 2023, from puebloofacoma.org: https://www.puebloofacoma.org/

Pueblo of Isleta. (n.d.). *Welcome to the Pueblo of Isleta.* Retrieved September 6, 2023, from isletapueblo.com: https://www.isletapueblo.com/

Pueblo of Isleta. (n.d.). *Welcome to the Pueblo of Isleta.* Retrieved September 7, 2023, from www.isletapueblo.com: https://www.isletapueblo.com/

Pueblo of Jemez. (2023). *Pueblo of Jemez.* Retrieved September 7, 2023, from www.jemezpueblo.org: https://www.jemezpueblo.org/

Pueblo of Laguna. (n.d.). *Pueblo of Laguna.* Retrieved September 7, 2023, from www.lagunapueblo-nsn.gov: https://www.lagunapueblo-nsn.gov/

Pueblo of Pojoaque. (n.d.). *Pueblo of Pojoaque.* Retrieved September 7, 2023, from Pojoaque: Pojoaque

Pueblo of Sandia. (n.d.). *Pueblo of Sandia.* Retrieved September 7, 2023, from sandiapueblo.nsn.us: https://sandiapueblo.nsn.us/

Pueblo of Zia. (n.d.). *Home of the Zia Sun symbol.* Retrieved September 8, 2023, from www.ziapueblo.org: https://www.ziapueblo.org/

Pueblo of Zuni. (2016). *Keshi!* Retrieved September 8, 2023, from www.ashiwi.org: http://www.ashiwi.org/

Quapaw Nation. (n.d.). *Welcome to Ogahpah.* Retrieved September 8, 2023, from quapawtribe.com: http://quapawtribe.com/

Quartz Valley Indian Resewrvation. (n.d.). *Quartz Valley Indian Reservation.* Retrieved October 23, 2023, from www.qvir.com: http://www.qvir.com/

Radcliffe, D. (2023, November 10). *Sitka Namne Meaning.* Retrieved November 16, 2023, from techsslash.com: https://techsslash.com/sitka-name-meaning/

Ramona Band of Cahuilla. (2021). *Ramona Band of Cahuilla.* Retrieved September 25, 2023, from ramona-nsn.gov/: https://ramona-nsn.gov/

Rancheria of Pomo Indians. (2008). *Cloverdale Rancheria of Pomo Indians.* Retrieved October 22, 2023, from www.cloverdalerancheria.com: http://www.cloverdalerancheria.com/

RCAC. (2020). *Cold Springs Rancheria of Mono Indians.* Retrieved October 19, 2023, from www.rcac.org: https://www.rcac.org/

Red Corn, L. (2022, November 1). *Osage Nation moving forward with multi-million dollar Sports Complex.* Retrieved July 24, 2023, from Osage News: https://osagenews.org/osage-nation-moving-forward-with-multi-million-dollar-sports-complex/

Red Lake Nation. (2023). *Red Lake Nation.* Retrieved August 6, 2023, from redlakenation.org: https://www.redlakenation.org/

Red Lake Nation College. (2022). *Red Lake Nation College.* Retrieved August 6, 2023, from rlnc.edu: https://www.rlnc.edu/

Redding Rancheria. (2023). *Redding Rancheria.* Retrieved October 24, 2023, from www.reddingrancheria-nsn.gov: https://www.reddingrancheria-nsn.gov/

Redfern, J. (2023, September 5). *After a Century, Oil and Gas Problems Persist on Navajo Lands.* Retrieved September 5, 2023, from capitalandmain.com: https://capitalandmain.com/after-a-century-oil-and-gas-problems-persist-on-navajo-lands

Redwood Valley Rancheria. (2023). *Redwood Valley Little River Band of Pomo Indians.* Retrieved October 22, 2023, from www.rvrpomo.net: https://www.rvrpomo.net/

Reid, S., Wishingrad, V., & McCabe, S. (2009). *Native American Uses of California Plants: Ethnobotany.* Retrieved October 20, 2023, from arboretum.ucsc.edu: https://arboretum.ucsc.edu/pdfs/ethnobotany-webversion.pdf

Reno-Sparks Indian Colony. (2019). *Reno-Sparks Indian Colony.* Retrieved October 30, 2023, from www.rsic.org: https://www.rsic.org/

Resighini Rancheria. (n.d.). *'O' Lomah!* Retrieved October 24, 2023, from resighinirancheria.com: http://resighinirancheria.com/

revwartalk.com. (2014, March 8). *Iroquois-Mingo Tribe.* Retrieved April 24, 2023, from RevWarTalk: https://www.revwartalk.com/iroquois-mingo-tribe/

Reyhner, J. (2013 [updated 2019]). *1819-2013 A History of American Indian Education.* Retrieved September 16, 2023, from Education Week: https://www.edweek.org/leadership/1819-2013-a-history-of-american-indian-education/2013/12

Rincon Band of Luiseno Indians. (2023). *Rincon Band of Luiseno Indians.* Retrieved October 13, 2023, from rincon-nsn.gov: https://rincon-nsn.gov/

Ritter, B. (2011). *Poncas.* Retrieved September 8, 2023, from Encylcopedia of the Great Plains: http://plainshumanities.unl.edu/encyclopedia/doc/egp.na.088

Roberta, E. (2013, July 23). *Pima and Maricopa Indians of Arizona.* Retrieved September 3, 2023, from nstiveheritageproject.com: https://nativeheritageproject.com/2013/07/23/pima-and-maricopa-indians-of-arizona/

Robinson Rancheria. (2020). *Robinson Rancheria.* Retrieved October 22, 2023, from rrcbc-nsn.gov: https://rrcbc-nsn.gov/

Roscoe, J. (1985). *An Ethno history of the Mattole.* California: The Digital Archaelogical Record. doi:doi:10.6067/XCV8T72FX0

Rosebud Sioux Tribe. (2023). *Rosebud Sioux Tribe.* Retrieved June 4, 2023, from rosebudsiouxtribe-nsn.gov: https://www.rosebudsiouxtribe-nsn.gov/

Round Valley Indian Tribes. (n.d.). *Tribal Territory Since Time Began.* Retrieved October 22, 2023, from www.rvit.org: https://www.rvit.org/

Roy, L. (n.d.). *Ojibwa.* Retrieved August 6, 2-23, from Countries & Their Cultures: https://www.everyculture.com/multi/Le-Pa/Ojibwa.html#:~:text=The%20Ojibwa%20met%20non-Native%20Americans%20in%20the%201600s%2C,by%20French%20explorers%20and%20fur%20traders%2C%20who%20were

sacand foxks.com. (2023). *Sac and Fox Nation iof Missouri in Kansas and Nebraska.* Retrieved May 27, 2023, from sacandfoxks.com: http://www.sacandfoxks.com/

sacandfoxnation-nsn.gov. (2023). *Sac & Fox Nation.* Retrieved May 27, 2023, from sacandfoxnation-nsn.gov: https://www.sacandfoxnation-nsn.gov/

Sacred Circle Healthcare. (2021). *Redefining Compassionate Healthcare.* Retrieved August 14, 2023, from SacredCircle.com: https://sacredcircle.com/about-us/

sagchip.org. (1998-2023). *Saginaw Chippewa Indian Tribe.* Retrieved May 26, 2023, from Saginaw Chippewa Indian Tribe of Michigan: http://www.sagchip.org/

Sage-Answers. (2023). *What traditions did the Shasta tribe have?* Retrieved October 23, 2023, from sage-answers.com: https://sage-answers.com/what-traditions-did-the-shasta-tribe-have/#:~:text=Shastan%20villages%2C%20 dwellings%2C%20and%20communal%20sweat%20houses%20were,Shasta n%20religion%20centred%20on%20guardian%20spirits%20and%20shama nism.

Samish Indian Nation. (2017). *Samish Indian Nation.* Retrieved October 25, 2023, from www.samishtribe.nsn.us: https://www.samishtribe.nsn.us/

San Felipe Pueblo. (2023). *Pueblo of San Felipe.* Retrieved September 7, 2023, from sfpueblo.com: https://sfpueblo.com/

San Ildefonso Pueblo. (2023). *Pueblo de San Ildefonso.* Retrieved September 8, 2023, from sanipueblo.org: https://sanipueblo.org/

San Juan Southern Paiute Tribe. (2019). *San Juan Southern Paiute Tribe.* Retrieved June 11, 2023, from https://www.sanjuanpaiute-nsn.gov/: https://www.sanjuanpaiute-nsn.gov/

San Pasqual Band of Mission Indians. (2018). *San Pasqual Band of Mission Indians.* Retrieved September 26, 2023, from sanpasqualbandof missionindians.org: https://www.sanpasqualbandofmissionindians.org/

Sanchez, L. (2018, July 9). *The role revealed of sacred pollen for the Mescalero Apache.* Retrieved August 30, 2023, from Ruidoso News: https://www.ruidosonews.com/story/news/local/community/2018/07/09/ro le-sacred-pollen-mescalero-apache/767949002/

Santa Ana Pueblo. (2023). *Santa Ana Pueblo.* Retrieved September 8, 2023, from snantana-nsn.gov: https://santaana-nsn.gov/

Santa Rosa Band of Cahuilla Indians. (2023). *Santa Rosa Band of Cahuilla Indians.* Retrieved September 25, 2023, from santarosa-nsn.gov: https://santarosa-nsn.gov/

Santa Ynez Band of Chumash Indians. (n.d.). *Santa Ynez Band of Chumash Indians.* Retrieved October 25, 2023, from chumash.gov: https://chumash.gov/

Santa Ynez Reservation. (n.d.). *Our Community.* Retrieved October 7, 2023, from chumash.gov: https://chumash.gov/the-santa-ynez-reservation

Santiago, E. (2019, April 8). *Narragansett medicine woman remembered as wisdom keeper.* Retrieved April 19, 2023, from The Westerly Sun:

https://www.thewesterlysun.com/news/narragansett-medicine-woman-
remembered-as-wisdom-keeper/article_240dcfc6-ec7a-532b-a513-
73fb9afcf55b.html

Santo Domingo Pueblo. (n.d.). *Santo Dom ingo Pueblo.* Retrieved September 8,
2023, from santodomingopueblo.com: https://santodomingopueblo.com/

sappony.org. (n.d.). *Sappony.* Retrieved April 26, 2023, from sappony.org:
https://www.sappony.org/

Sault Ste. Marie Tribe of Chippewa Indians. (2023). *Sault Tribe of Chippewa
Indiana.* Retrieved May 18, 2023, from saulttribe.com:
https://www.saulttribe.com/

Scott, B. (2023, August 28). *What is the Pima Tribe?* Retrieved September 4,
2023, from unitedstatesnow.org: https://www.unitedstatesnow.org/what-
is-the-pima-tribe.htm

Scott, D. (2023, June 27). *HHS Roundup: Overdose4 Prevention; Healt Exams.*
Retrieved July 12, 2023, from The Seminole Tribune: https://seminole
tribune.org/hhs-roundup-overdose-prevention-health-exams/

Scotts Valley Band of Pomo Indians. (n.d.). *Scotts Valley Band of Pomo Indians.*
Retrieved October 22, 2023, from www.scottsvalley-nsn.gov:
https://www.scottsvalley-nsn.gov/

Seaver, C. (2023). *The History and Culture of the Mohawk Dribe.* Retrieved April
24, 2023, from History DEfined: https://www.historydefined.net/the-
history-and-culture-of-the-mohawk-tribe/

semtribe.com/stof. (n.d.). *Seminole Tribe of Florida.* Retrieved April 30, 2023,
from semtribe.com/stof: https://www.semtribe.com/stof

Seneca-Cayuga Nation. (n.d.). *Seneca-Cayuga Nation.* Retrieved June 22, 2023,
from https://sctribe.com/: https://sctribe.com/

senecanation.weebly.com. (n.d.). *Seneca Traditions and Beliefs.* Retrieved April
26, 2023, from Seneca Nation: https://senecanation.weebly.com/the-
senecas-traditions-and-beliefs.html

Setzer, W. (2018, November 12). The Phytochemistry of Cherokee Aromatic
Medicinal Plants. *Medicines, 5*(4). doi:10.3390/medicines5040121

shakopeedakota.org. (2023). *Shakopee Mdewakanton Sioux Community.* Retrieved May 27, 2023, from Shakopee Mdewakanton Sioux Community: https://www.shakopeedakota.org/

Shanley, J. (1999). Traditional Assiniboine Family Values: Let us bring back something beautiful. *Tribal College Journal of American Indian Higher Education, 11*(1). Retrieved July 30, 2023, from Tribal College: https://tribalcollegejournal.org/traditional-assiniboine-family-values-bring-beautiful/

Shaw Duty, S. (2021, August 21). *Osage Nation requests community input for Outdoor Health Complex.* Retrieved July 24, 2023, from Osage News: https://osagenews.org/osage-nation-requests-community-input-for-outdoor-health-complex/#:~:text=Putting%20Osages%20at%20risk%20on%20the%20reservation%20include,WahZhaZhe%20Health%20Center%20as%20their%20primary%20care%20provider.

Shawnee Tribe. (n.d.). *Shawnee Tribe.* Retrieved June 13, 2023, from https://www.shawnee-nsn.gov/: https://www.shawnee-nsn.gov/

Sherwood Valley Band of Pomo Indians. (n.d.). *Sherwood Valley Band of Pomo Indians.* Retrieved October 22, 2023, from www.sherwood valleybandofpomo.com: https://www.sherwoodvalleybandofpomo.com/

Shingle Springs Band of Miwok Indians. (n.d.). *Welcome to Shingle Springs Band of Miwok Indians.* Retrieved October 18, 2023, from www.shinglespringsrancheria.com: https://www.shinglesprings rancheria.com/

Sho-Pai Tribes. (2023). *Shoshone-Paiute Tribes of Duck Valley Indian Reservation.* Retrieved June 11, 2023, from https://www.shopaitribes.org/spt/: https://www.shopaitribes.org/spt/

Shoshone-Bannock Tribes. (2023). *Shoshone-Bannock Tribes.* Retrieved Auguist 11, 2023, from sbtribes.com: http://www.sbtribes.com/

Simaratana, R. W. (2011). *Medicine Wheel Matrix.* Retrieved April 21, 2023, from http://medicinewheelmatrix.com/

Sitka Triobe of Alaska. (2011). *Sitka Triobe of Alaska.* Retrieved November 16, 2023, from www.sitkatribe.org: https://www.sitkatribe.org/

Skagway Traditional Council. (n.d.). *Skagway Traditional Council.* Retrieved November 16, 2023, from www.skagwaytraditional.org: http://www.skagwaytraditional.org/

skngov.com. (2020). *Skaroreh Katenuaka.* Retrieved April 28, 2023, from Tuscarora Nation of Indians: https://www.skngov.com/

SMBMI. (2023). *San Manuel Band of Mission Indians.* Retrieved November 6, 2023, from sanmanuel-nsn.gov: https://sanmanuel-nsn.gov/

Smith, H. H. (1932, May 2). Ethnobotany of the Ojibwe Indians. *Bulletin of the Public Museum of the City of Milwaukee, 4*(3), pp. 327-525. Retrieved August 6, 2023, from nwic.edu: http://blogs.nwic.edu/briansblog/files/2013/02/ Ethnobotany-of-the-Ojibwe-Indians.pdf

Smithsonian Institution. (2023). *American Indian Powwows.* Retrieved November 25, 2023, from Smithsonian Institution: https://folklife.si.edu/ online-exhibitions/american-indian-powwows/smithsonian

sni.org. (2023). *Welcome-We are the Seneca Nation.* Retrieved April 26, 2023, from sni.org: https://sni.org/

sno-nsn.org. (2023). *The Great Seminole Nation of Oklahoma.* Retrieved April 30, 2023, from sno-nsn.org: https://www.sno-nsn.org/

Soboba Band of Luiseno Indians. (n.d.). *Soboba Band of Luiseno Indians.* Retrieved October 13, 2023, from soboba-nsn.gov: https://soboba-nsn.gov/

Solis, J. (2023, July 20). *9th Circuit says Thacker Pass lithium mine can proceed.* Retrieved July 25, 2023, from This Reno.com-Nevada Current: https://thisisreno.com/2023/07/9th-circuit-says-thacker-pass-lithium-mine- can-proceed/

Somerset County. (2023). *Acchohannock Water Trail-Marion.* Retrieved June 24, 2023, from Trail Mix: http://www.somersettrailmix.com/kayaking- trails/accohannock-water-trail-marion/

Southern Ute Indian Tribe. (2023). *Southern Ute Indian Tribe.* Retrieved August 18, 2023, from www.southernute-nsn.gov/: https://www.southernute- nsn.gov/

Speck, F. (1944). Catawba Herbals and Curative Practices. *Journal of American Folklore, 57*(223), 37-50. Retrieved April 29, 2023

Speck, F. (1950). *Midwinter Rites of the Cayuga Long House.* University of Pennsylvania Press. Retrieved April 23, 2023, from https://www.penn press.org/9781512813791/midwinter-rites-of-the-cayuga-long-house/

Spokane Tribe . (n.d.). *Spokane Tribe of Indians.* Retrieved October 26, 2023, from www.spokanetribe.com: https://www.spokanetribe.com/

SpottedBird, J. (2000, February 27). *Ethnobotanical Information Chihuahuan Desert Gardens, Centennial Museum, University of Texas El Paso.* Retrieved September 26, 2023, from www.utep.edu/: https://www.utep.edu/leb/pdf/ethnobot.pdf

SpottedBird, J. (2000, February 27). *Ethnobotanical Information, Chichuahuan Desert Gardens, Centennial Museum, University of Texas at El Paso.* Retrieved September 4, 2023, from https://www.utep.edu/leb/pdf/ethnobot.pdf

SPRC.org. (2020, October). *Omaha Tribe of Ne3braska.* Retrieved July 24, 2023, from SPRC.org: https://sprc.org/grantee/omaha-tribe-of-nebraska/

Springer, P. (2023, May 27). *Lake Sakakawea hinders medicine access at Fort Berthold. How drones could offer a fix.* Retrieved July 12, 2023, from InForum: https://www.inforum.com/news/north-dakota/lake-sakakawea-hinders-medicine-access-at-fort-berthold-how-drones-could-offer-a-fix

srmt-nsn.gov. (n.d.). *Saint Regis Mohawk Tribe.* Retrieved April 23, 2023, from Saint Regis Mohawk Tribe (en-us): https://www.srmt-nsn.gov/

Stamper, V. (2023, September 17). *11 Surprising Facts About Chemehuevi.* Retrieved September 27, 2023, from facts.net: https://facts.net/general/11-surprising-facts-about-chemehuevi/#:~:text=They%20have%20a%20 strong%20spiritual%20belief%20system.%20The,and%20a%20close-knit%20relationship%20with%20the%20spiritual%20realm.

Standing Rock Sioux Tribe. (n.d.). *Standing Rock Sioux Tribe.* Retrieved June 4, 2023, from standingrock.org: https://www.standingrock.org/

Stargazer, S. (2023, September 11). *'Protecting our sacred lands".* Retrieved September 11, 2023, from Yuma Sun: https://yumasun.pressreader.com/article/281522230678939

stcroixojibwe-nsn.gov. (n.d.). *St. Croix Chippewa Indians of Wisconson.* Retrieved May 18, 2023, from stcroixojibwe-nsn.gov: https://stcroixojibwe-nsn.gov/

Stebbins, S. (2012, April). *Historic Jamestowne: Chronology of Powhatan Indian Activity.* Retrieved April 26, 2023, from National Park Service: https://www.nps.gov/jame/learn/historyculture/chronology-of-powhatan-indian-activity.htm

Sterling, R. (2011, February). Genetic Research among the Havasuypai: A Coutionary Tale. *AMA Journal of Ethics, 13*(2), 113-117. Retrieved September 3, 2023, from https://journalofethics.ama-assn.org/article/genetic-research-among-havasupai-cautionary-tale/2011-02

Stillaguamish Tribe of Indians. (2020). *Stillaguamish Tribe of Indians.* Retrieved October 26, 2023, from www.stillaguamish.com: https://www.stillaguamish.com/

stolaf.edu. (2020). *Dakota and Ojibwe Uses of Native Plants.* Retrieved May 27, 2023, from St. Olaf Natural Lands: https://wp.stolaf.edu/naturallands/files/2020/09/indigenousplants-brochure-1.pdf

Stone Child College. (2022). *Stone Child College.* Retrieved August 5, 2023, from stonechild.edu: https://www.stonechild.edu/

Storytellers, C. (Writer). (2023). *Winter Fire Episode 1 Traditional Medicine* [Motion Picture]. Chickasaw TV. Retrieved April 29, 2023, from https://www.chickasaw.tv/videos/oeta-winter-fire-episode-1-traditional-medicine

Sullivan, M. (2021, October 14). *Can indigenous subsistence rights still be protected in Alaska?* Retrieved November 22, 2023, from Indian Country Today: https://alaskapublic.org/2021/10/14/subsistence-is-absolutely-critical-to-our-survival-can-indigenous-subsistence-rights-still-be-protected-in-alaska/#:~:text=%E2%80%9CSubsistence%20is%20absolutely%20critical%20to%20our%20survival.%20Without,community%20g

Summit Lake Paiute Tribe. (n.d.). *Summit Lake Paiute Tribe.* Retrieved June 11, 2023, from https://www.summitlaketribe.org/: https://www.summitlaketribe.org/

Suryabarayanan, S. (2019, December). *Ho-Chunk Nation Community Health Assessment 2017-2019.* Retrieved July 19, 2023, from University of Wisconsin Population Health Institute: https://health.ho-chunk.com/docs/CHA2020.pdf#:~:text=The%20survey%20also%20highligh

ted%20health%20disparities%2C%20particularly%20in,population%20nor
ms%20in%20Wisconsin%20and%20the%20United%20States.

Susanville Indian Rancheria. (2023). *Susanville Indian Rancheria.* Retrieved
October 15, 2023, from www.sir-nsn.gov: https://www.sir-nsn.gov/

Swan, D., & Simons, L. (2014, August 23). *An Ethnobotany of Firewood in Osage
Big Moon Peyotism: Practical knowledge, ritual participation, and aesthetic
preference.* Retrieved June 9, 2023, from Ethnobotany Journal:
www.ethnobotanyjournal.org/vol12/i1547-3465-12-325.pdf

Sycuan Casino Resort. (n.d.). *Sycuan Casino Resort.* Retrieved September 26,
2023, from www.sycuan.com: https://www.sycuan.com/

Tachi Yokut Tribe. (n.d.). *Tachi Yokut Tribe.* Retrieved October 25, 2023, from
www.tachi-yokut-nsn.gov: https://www.tachi-yokut-nsn.gov/rancheria

Tanana Chiefs Conference. (2023). *Tanana Chiefs Conference.* Retrieved
November 16, 2023, from www.tananachiefs.org:
https://www.tananachiefs.org/

Taos Pueblo. (2023). *Taos Peublo.* Retrieved September 8, 2023, from
taospueblo.com: https://taospueblo.com/

Tayac, G. (2019, November 7). *Indigenous Voices: Discover the hidden beauty of
Nanjemoy Creek.* Retrieved July 7, 2023, from Conservancy:
https://potomac.org/blog/2019/11/nanjemoy-creek

Te-Moak Tribe of Western Shoshone. (2004-2022). *Te-Moak Tribe of Western
Shoshone.* Retrieved June 18, 2023, from https://www.temoaktribe.com/:
https://www.temoaktribe.com/

Ten Tribes Partnership. (2023). *Jicarilla Apache Nation.* Retrieved August 30,
2023, from tentribespartnership.org:
https://tentribespartnership.org/tribes/jicarilla-apache-nation/

Texas Band of Yaqui Indians. (2021). *Welcome to Texas Banbd of Yaqui Indians.*
Retrieved September 12, 2023, from www.tbyi.gov: https://www.tbyi.gov/

Texas Monthly. (1997, February). The Forgotten People. *Texas Monthly.*
Retrieved June 1, 2023, from https://www.texasmonthly.com/being-
texan/the-forgotten-people/

The American History.org. (2022). *The Comanche Religion.* Retrieved July 31, 2023, from theamericanhistory.org: https://theamericanhistory.org/the-comanche-religion.html

The Clothesline Project. (2023). *Clothesline Project.* Retrieved October 30, 2023, from www.theclotheslineproject.org: https://www.theclotheslineproject.org/

The Free Dictionary. (n.d.). *Pueblo.* Retrieved September 5, 2023, from thefreedictionary.com: https://www.thefreedictionary.com/Pueblo

*The Goshutes: Ddid You Know?* (2008). Retrieved August 14, 2023, from utahindians.org: https://utahindians.org/archives/goshute/didYouKnow.html

The Historic round Rock Collection. (1991). *The Tonkawa Indians.* Retrieved August 7, 2023, from Round Rock Texas: https://www.roundrock texas.gov/city-departments/planning-and-development-services/historic-preservation-2/historic-round-rock-collection/tonkawa-indians/

The Hopi Tribe. (2023). *Welcome to the Hopi Tribe.* Retrieved August 31, 2023, from www.hopi-nsn.gov: https://www.hopi-nsn.gov/

The Klamath Tribes. (2023). *Waq lis ?aat.* Retrieved October 18, 2023, from klamathtribe.org: https://klamathtribes.org/

The Koi Nation of Northern California. (2023). *Welcome.* Retrieved Octoberr 22, 2023, from www.koinationsonoma.com: https://www.koinationsonoma.com/

The Mohegan Tribe. (2023). *Honoring the past, building for the future.* Retrieved April 19, 2023, from Mohegan Tribe: https://www.mohegan.nsn.us/

The Navajo Nation. (2023). *The Official Site of the Navajo Nation.* Retrieved September 5, 2023, from https://www.navajo-nsn.gov/: https://www.navajo-nsn.gov/

The Plant Lady. (n.d.). *Arapaho Ethnobotany.* Retrieved August 5, 2024, from theplantlady.net: http://theplantlady.net/resources/Arapaho%20 Ethnobotany.pdf

The Plant Lady. (n.d.). *Comanche Ethnobotany.* Retrieved August 5, 2023, from theplantlady.net: http://theplantlady.net/resources/Comanche%20 Ethnobotany.pdf

The Red Road. (2023). *Education of the First People*. Retrieved September 16, 2023, from The Red Road: https://theredroad.org/issues/native-american-education/

The SOAP Project. (n.d.). *The SOAP Project*. Retrieved August 9, 2023, from soapproject.org: https://www.soapproject.org/

Tidd, J. (2022). Native American boarding schools in Kansas supported US land grab and forced cultural assimilation. *The Topeka Capital-Journal*. Retrieved June 2, 2023, from https://www.cjonline.com/story/news/state/2022/05/12/report-native-american-boarding-schools-kansas-child-labor/9733760002/

Timbisha Shoshone Tribe. (n.d.). *Timbisha Shoshone Tribe*. Retrieved June 18, 2023, from http://www.timbisha.org/: http://www.timbisha.org/

Tkacik, C. (2018, February 10). *Maryland recognition of Accohannock tribe sparks debate within community of Native Americans*. Retrieved April 22, 2023, from The Baltimore Sun: https://www.baltimoresun.com/maryland/bs-md-accohannock-eastern-shore-indians-20180115-story.html

tmchippewa.com. (n.d.). *Turtle Mountain Band of Chippewa*. Retrieved May 26, 2023, from tmchippewa.com: https://tmchippewa.com/

Tohono O'odham Nation. (2016). *Tohono O'odham Nation*. Retrieved September 4, 2023, from tonation-nsn.gov: http://www.tonation-nsn.gov/

Tolowa Dee-ni' Nation. (n.d.). *Tolowa Dee-ni' Nation*. Retrieved October 30, 2023, from /www.tolowa-nsn.gov: https://www.tolowa-nsn.gov/

Tonkawa Tribe of Oklahoma. (2022). *Tonkawa Tribe of Oklahoma*. Retrieved August 7, 2023, from tonkawatribe.com: https://tonkawatribe.com/

Tooker, E. (1961). *An Ethnography of the Huron Indians, 1615-1649*. Washington: Smithsonian Institution Bureau of American Ethnology Bulletin 190. Retrieved May 30, 2023, from bulletin1901964smit.pdf

Torres Martinez Desert Cahuilla Indians. (n.d.). *Torres Martinez Desert Cahuilla Indians*. Retrieved September 25, 2023, from torresmartinez.org: https://torresmartinez.org/

Toupal, R. (2006). *At Ethnobotany of Indiana Dunes National Lakeshore: A Baseline Study Emphasizing Plant Relationships of the Miami and Potawatomi Tribes*. Bureau of Applied Research in Anthropology University of Arizona. Retrieved June 5, 2023, from

https://www.csu.edu/cerc/researchreports/documents/AnEthnobotanyIndi
anaDunesNationalLakeshoreVolume1.pdf

touringohio.com. (2023). *Wyandot Indians.* Retrieved May 30, 2023, from
touringohio.com: http://touringohio.com/history/wyandot.html

Trahant, M. (2018). The Story of Indian Health is Complicated by History,
Shortages & Bouts of Excellence. *American Academy of Arts & Sciences*, 116-
123. Retrieved November 12, 2023, from https://watermark.silver
chair.com/daed_a_00495.pdf?token=AQECAHi208BE49Ooan9kkhW_Ercy
7Dm3ZL_9Cf3qfKAc485ysgAAAz0wggM5BgkqhkiG9w0BBwagggMqMII
DJgIBADCCAx8GCSqGSIb3DQEHATAeBglghkgBZQMEAS4wEQQMfrk
ZPfg2kUwoRsr8AgEQgIIC8OKAnjMPK-uxSxjYiY8yKbvomIqSZrz-
AVllaasgTT

Train, P., Henrichs, J., & Archer, W. (1941). *Medicinal Uses of Plants by Indian
Tribes of Nevada.* Washington, DC: U.S. Department of Agriculture.
Retrieved June 11, 2023

travelalaska.com. (n.d.). *Alaska Native Culture Fact Sheet.* Retrieved November
15, 2023, from www.travelalaska.com: https://www.travelalaska.com/
sites/default/files/2022-01/Alaska%20Native%20Culture%20
Fact%20Sheet.pdf

tribalnations.mt.gov. (n.d.). *Crow Nation.* Retrieved May 27, 2023, from
Governor's Office of Indian Affairs: https://tribalnations.mt.gov/
Directory/CrowNation

tribalsolar.org. (2020). *Manzanita Band of the Kumeyaay Nation.* Retrieved
September 26, 2023, from tribalsolar.org: https://tribalsolar.org/2020-
grantees/manzanita-band-of-the-kumeyaay-nation/

Tribe Facts. (2018, December 21). *Kiowa Tribe of Oklahoma: Facts, History and
Culture.* Retrieved August 1, 2023, from Only Tribal:
https://www.onlytribal.com/kiowa-tribe.asp#:~:text=Culture%20and%20
Lifestyle%201%20Daily%20life%20and%20food,The%20role%20of%20the
%20horse%20...%20More%20items

Trinidad Rancheria. (2023). *Trinidad Rancheria.* Retrieved September 28, 2023,
from trinidad-rancheria.org: https://trinidad-rancheria.org/

Tulalip Tribes. (2016-2023). *Tulalip Tribes.* Retrieved October 30, 2023, from
www.tulaliptribes-nsn.gov: https://www.tulaliptribes-nsn.gov/

Tule River Tribe. (2023). *Tule River Reservation.* Retrieved October 20, 2023, from tulerivertribe-nsn.gov: https://tulerivertribe-nsn.gov/

Tuolumne Tribal Council. (n.d.). *The Tuolumne Band of Me-Wuk Indians.* Retrieved October 18, 2023, from https://mewuk.com/: https://mewuk.com/

Tuscarora Nation of North Carolina. (2023). *Tuscarora Nation of North Carolina.* Retrieved July 9, 2023, from tuscaroranationnc.com/: https://tuscaroranationnc.com/

Tuscarora Tribe of NC. (2019). *Tuscarora Tribe of NC.* Retrieved July 28, 2023, from tuscarora-tribe-nc.com: http://www.tuscarora-tribe-nc.com/

Two Eagles Smoke Shop. (2023). *About Us.* Retrieved July 28, 2023, from Two Eagles Smoke Shop: https://www.twoeaglessmokeshop.com/about

U.S. Census Bureau. (2021). *Cold Springs Rancheria.* Retrieved October 19, 2023, from censusreporter.org: https://censusreporter.org/profiles/25000US0720-cold-springs-rancheria/

U.S. Department of the Interior. (n.d.). *Office of Subsistence Management.* Retrieved November 21, 2023, from /www.doi.gov: https://www.doi.gov/subsistence

umt.edu. (2004). *Kiowa Ethnobotany.* Retrieved August 6, 2023, from cfcumt.edu: https://files.cfc.umt.edu/cesu/NPS/UMT/2004/Campbell_Etnobotony%20Report/chapterten.pdf

United Auburn Indian Community. (n.d.). *United Auburn Indian Community.* Retrieved October 15, 2023, from www.auburnrancheria.com: https://www.auburnrancheria.com/

United Auburn Indian Community. (n.d.). *United Auburn Indian Community.* Retrieved October 18, 2023, from /www.auburnrancheria.com: https://www.auburnrancheria.com/

United Indian Health Services. (2022). *Big Lagoon Rancheria.* Retrieved September 24, 2023, from /unitedindianhealthservices.org: https://unitedindianhealthservices.org/index.php/consortium-tribes-2/big-lagoon/

United Indian Health Services. (2022). *Elk Valley Rancheria.* Retrieved October 5, 2023, from unitedindianhealthservices.org:

https://unitedindianhealthservices.org/index.php/consortium-tribes-2/elk-valley/

Universary of Colorado. (n.d.). *History of the Northern Arapaho Tribe*. Retrieved July 29, 2023, from The Arapaho Project: https://verbs.colorado.edu/ArapahoLanguageProject/RMNP/history/history.htm

University of Montana. (2023). *Gros Ventre and Assiniboine Tribes (Fort Belknap)*. Retrieved August 5, 2023, from Ethnobotany Gardens: https://www.umt.edu/native-garden/circles/gros-ventre-assiniboine.php

uppersiouxcommunity-nsn.org. (n.d.). *Upper Siuox Community*. Retrieved May 27, 2023, from uppersiouxcommunity-nsn.org: https://www.uppersiouxcommunity-nsn.gov/

US Department of the Interior. (2021, September 29). *Department of the Interior Announces Final Federal Recognition Process to Acknowledge Indian Tribes*. Retrieved August 29, 2023, from US Department of the Interior: https://www.doi.gov/pressreleases/department-interior-announces-final-federal-recognition-process-acknowledge-indian-tribes

U-S-History.com. (2023). *Spokane Indian Tribe*. Retrieved October 26, 2023, from www.u-s-history.com: https://www.u-s-history.com/pages/h1570.html

Utah.gov. (2023). *Skull Valley Band of Goshute & Confederated Tribes of the Goshute*. Retrieved August 14, 2023, from Utah Division of Indian Affairs: https://indian.utah.gov/skull-valley-band-of-goshute/

Ute Indian Tribe. (2023). *Ute Indian Tribe*. Retrieved August 18, 2023, from www.utetribe.com: http://www.utetribe.com/

Ute Mountain Ute Tribe. (2020). *Ute Mountain Ute Tribe*. Retrieved August 18, 2023, from utemountainutetribe.com: https://www.utemountainutetribe.com/

UVE. (2023). *UVE*. Retrieved September 20, 2023, from facebook.com: https://www.facebook.com/UVEhub/

uvm.edu. (2013). *Vermont*. Retrieved April 17, 2023, from Eugenics: Compulsory Sterilization in 50 American States: https://www.uvm.edu/~lkaelber/eugenics/VT/VT.html

Varela, B. (2014, April 21). *The Choctaw tribe and their medicine wheel*. Retrieved July 10, 2023, from Moorpark College Reported:

https://moorparkreporter.com/4001994/news/the-choctaw-tribe-and-their-medicine-wheel/

Viejas Band of Kumeyaay. (2022). *Viejas Band of Kumeyaay Indians.* Retrieved September 26, 2023, from iejasbandofkumeyaay.org: https://viejasbandofkumeyaay.org/

wampanoagtribe-nsn.gov. (n.d.). *Wampanoag Tribe of Gay Head (Aquinnah).* Retrieved April 21, 2023, from wampanoagtribe-nsn.gov: https://wampanoagtribe-nsn.gov/

Warren, B. (2021, September 22). *Native Americans face a deadly drug crisis. How tapping into culture is helping them heal.* Retrieved July 12, 2023, from Louisville Courier Journal: https://www.courier-journal.com/in-depth/news/investigations/2021/09/22/culturally-competent-care-for-addiction-treatment-helps-native-americans-heal/7498590002/

Warren, R. (2004). *Illinois Indians in the Illinois Country.* Retrieved May 31, 2023, from Illinois Periodicals Online: https://www.lib.niu.edu/2004/iht1110419.html

Washoe Tribe of California and Nevada. (2020). *Washoe Tribe of Nevada and California.* Retrieved October 30, 2023, from washoetribe.us: https://washoetribe.us/

Wea Indian Tribe of Indiana. (2005-2020). *The Wea Indian Tribe of Indiana, Inc.* Retrieved June 19, 2023, from https://www.weaindiantribe.com: https://www.weaindiantribe.com

Weiser, K. (2021). *The Conanche-Horsemen of the Plains.* Retrieved July 31, 2023, from Legends of America: https://www.legendsofamerica.com/na-comanche/

Weiser-Alexander, K. (2021). *The Pennacook Tribe of New England.* Retrieved April 18, 2023, from Legends of America: https://www.legends ofamerica.com/pennacook-tribe/

Welch, J. (2013). *Sprouting Valley:Historical Ethnobotany of the Northern Pomo from Potter Valley, California.* Retrieved October 22, 2023, from ethnobiology.org: https://ethnobiology.org/sites/default/files/publications/contributions/Sprouting-Valley-2013-online.pdf

White Mountain Apache Tribe. (2022). *White Mountain Apache Tribe.* Retrieved August 30, 2023, from www.wmat.us: www.wmat.us

Whiting, A. (1978). *Ethnobotany of the Hopi*. New York: AMS Press. Retrieved August 31, 2023, from https://archive.org/details/ethnobotanyofhop 0000whit/mode/2up?view=theater

Wigle, J. (2014, July 23). *Tuscarora Reservation*. Retrieved April 28, 2023, from A Place for Haudenosaunee to meet: http://www.tuscaroras.com/ jtwigle/pages/tuscarora-rez.shtml

Wikipedia. (2023, September 7). *Hupa*. Retrieved October 7, 2023, from en.wikipedia.org: https://en.wikipedia.org/wiki/Hupa

Wikipedia. (2023, August 1). *Mono People*. Retrieved October 19, 2023, from en.wikipedia.org: https://en.wikipedia.org/wiki/Mono_people

Wikipedia. (2023, July 30). *Picayune Rancheria of Chukchansi Indians*. Retrieved October 21, 2023, from en.wikipedia.org: https://en.wikipedia.org/wiki/ Picayune_Rancheria_of_Chukchansi_Indians

Wikipedia. (2023, August 14). *Pomo*. Retrieved October 22, 2023, from en.wikipedia.org: https://en.wikipedia.org/wiki/Pomo# Villages_and_communities

Wikipedia.org. (2023, March 18). *Accomac People*. Retrieved April 22, 2023, from wikipedia.org: https://en.wikipedia.org/wiki/Accomac_people

Wikipedia.org. (2023). *Inaja Band of Diegueno Mission Indians*. Retrieved September 26, 2023, from wikipedia.org: https://en.wikipedia.org/ wiki/Inaja_Band_of_Diegueno_Mission_Indians

Wikipedia.org. (2023, February 16). *Pequots*. Retrieved April 18, 2023, from wikipedia.org: https://en.wikipedia.org/wiki/Pequots

wikipedia.org. (2023, October 12). *Samish People*. Retrieved October 25, 2023, from https://en.wikipedia.org/wiki/Samish_people

Wikipedia.org. (2023). *Shoshone*. Retrieved June 13, 2023, from https://en.wikipedia.org/wiki/Shoshone: https://en.wikipedia.org/wiki/Shoshone

wikipedia.org. (2023, October 12). *Wiyot*. Retrieved October 31, 2023, from en.wikipedia.org/: https://en.wikipedia.org/wiki/ Wiyot#Culture_and_religion

Wikipedia.org. (n.d.). *Tanana Athabaskans*. Retrieved November 15, 2023, from en.wikipedia.org: https://en.wikipedia.org/wiki/Tanana_Athabaskans

Wikiwand. (n.d.). *Missouria*. Retrieved July 23, 2023, from Wikiwand: https://www.wikiwand.com/en/Missouria

Wikiwand.com. (n.d.). *Ewiiaapaayp Band of Kumeyaay Indians*. Retrieved September 26, 2023, from www.wikiwand.com: https://www.wikiwand.com/en/Cuyapaipe_Band_of_Mission_Indians

Wildschut, W., & Ewers, J. (1960). *Crow Indian Medicine Bundles*. Museum of the American Indian, Heye Foundation.

Wilson, C., & Sabo III, G. (2008). *The Quapaw Indiuans*. Retrieved September 10, 2023, from archeology.uark.edu: http://archeology.uark.edu/indiansof arkansas/index.html?pageName=The+Quapaw+Indians

Wilton Rancheria. (2023). *Wilton Rancheria*. Retrieved October 18, 2023, from wiltonrancheria-nsn.gov: https://wiltonrancheria-nsn.gov/

winnebagotribe.com. (2023). *Honor. Tradition. Pride*. Retrieved May 29, 2023, from winnebagotribe.com: https://winnebagotribe.com/

Wintu Tribe of Northern California. (2023). *Wintu Tribe of Northern California*. Retrieved November 1, 2023, from wintutribe.com: https://wintutribe.com/

Wiyot Tribe. (n.d.). *Wiyot Tribe*. Retrieved September 28, 2023, from http://www.wiyot.us/: http://www.wiyot.us/

Wiyot Tribe. (n.d.). *Wiyot Tribe*. Retrieved October 31, 2023, from wiyot.us: http://wiyot.us/

Woodrow, N. (2013). *An Ethnobotanical Research Study on Western Mono and Yokut Traditional Plant Foods and Their Miscellaneous Usage*. Retrieved October 25, 2023, from underc.nd.edu: https://underc.nd.edu/assets/174546/fullsize/woodrow_underc_w_2013.pdf

Woods, A., & Philip, A. (2021, June 9). *The Bureau of Indian Education hasn't told the public how its schools are performing. So we did it instead*. Retrieved September 17, 2023, from azcentral: https://www.azcentral.com/story/news/local/arizona-investigations/2021/06/09/analysis-bie-schools-test-scores-reveals-successes-and-failures/7536092002/

World Atlas. (2017). *The Erie People*. Retrieved April 23, 2023, from World Atlas: https://delawaretribe.org/wp-content/uploads/LENAPE-MEDS.pdf

worldhistory.us. (2018, November 13). *Coeur d'Alene Indians.* Retrieved
August 12, 2023, from worldhistory.us: https://worldhistory.us/american-
history/coeur-dalene-indians.php

Wrangell Cooperative Association. (2023). *Wrangell Cooperative Association.*
Retrieved November 16, 2023, from www.wcatribe.org:
https://www.wcatribe.org/

*Wyandot Nation of Kansas Website.* (2013). Retrieved May 30, 2023, from
wyandot.org: https://www.wyandot.org/

Wyandotte Nation. (2022). *We are Wyandotte.* Retrieved May 30, 2023, from
Wyandotte Nation: https://wyandotte-nation.org/

Wynandotte of Anderdon Nation. (n.d.). *Kwe: Kwe-Welcome.* Retrieved July 28,
2023, from wyandotofanderdon.com:
https://www.wyandotofanderdon.com/wp/

Yale University. (2023, October 16). *Fort Mojave delegation celebrates Indigenous
history during Yale event.* Retrieved October 19, 2023, from news.yale.edu:
https://news.yale.edu/2023/10/16/fort-mojave-delegation-celebrates-
indigenous-history-during-yale-visit?page=8

Yavapai Prescott Indian Tribe. (n.d.). *Yavapai Prescott Indian Tribe.* Retrieved
September 12, 2023, from https://ypit.com: https://ypit.com/

Yavapai-Apache Nation. (2023). *Yavapai-Apache Nation.* Retrieved August 30,
2023, from yavapai-apache.org: https://yavapai-apache.org/

Yocha Dehe Wintun Nation. (2023). *We are the Yocha Dehe Wintun Nation.*
Retrieved November 2, 2023, from yochadehe.gov: https://yochadehe.gov/

Yomba Shoshone Tribe. (2017). *Yomba Shoshone Tribe.* Retrieved June 18, 2023,
from http://www.yombatribe.org/: http://www.yombatribe.org/

Yurok Tribe. (2023). *The Yurok Tribe.* Retrieved September 24, 2023, from
www.yuroktribe.org: https://www.yuroktribe.org/

Milton Keynes UK
Ingram Content Group UK Ltd.
UKHW022323260224
438533UK00002B/42